KU-431-128

Progress in Pathology

Volume 6

Edited by

Nigel Kirkham MD FRCPath
Consultant Histopathologist
Royal Sussex County Hospital
Brighton, UK

Neil A. Shepherd MB BS FRCPath
Consultant Histopathologist &
Visiting Professor of Pathology
Gloucestershire Royal Hospital
Gloucester, UK

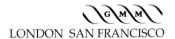
LONDON SAN FRANCISCO

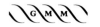

© 2003

Greenwich Medical Media Limited
4th Floor, 137 Euston Road,
London
NW1 2AA

870 Market Street, Ste 720
San Francisco
CA 94109, USA

ISBN 1 8411 01 486

First published 2003

While the advice and information in this book is believed to be true and accurate, neither the authors nor the publisher can accept any legal responsibility or liability for any loss or damage arising from actions or decisions based in this book. The ultimate responsibility for the treatment of patients and the interpretation lies with the medical practitioner. The opinions expressed are those of the authors and the inclusion in this book of information relating to a particular product, method or technique does not amount to an endorsement of its value or quality, or of the claims made by its manufacturer. Every effort has been made to check drug dosages; however, it is still possible that errors have occurred. Furthermore, dosage schedules are constantly being revised and new side-effects recognised. For these reasons, the medical practitioner is strongly urged to consult the drug companies' printed instructions before administering any of the drugs mentioned in this book.

Apart from any fair dealing for the purposes of research or private study, or criticism or review, as permitted under the UK Copyright Designs and Patents Act 1988, this publication may not be reproduced, stored, or transmitted, in any form or by any means, without the prior permission in writing of the publishers, or in the case of reprographic reproduction only in accrodance with the terms of the licences issued by the appropriate Reproduction Rights Organisations outside the UK. Enquiries concerning reproduction outside the terms stated here should be sent to the publishers at the London address printed above.

The rights of Nigel Kirkham and Neil Shepherd to be identified as editors of this work have been asserted by them in accordance with the Copyright Designs and Patents Act 1988.

The publishers makes no representation, express or implied, with regard to the accuracy of the information contained in this book and cannot accept any legal responsibility or liability for any errors or omissions that may be made.

A catalogue record for this book is available from the British Library.

Distributed worldwide by Plymbridge Distributors Ltd
and in the USA by Jamco Distribution

Typeset by Charon Tec Pvt. Ltd, Chennai, India
Printed in China

Visit our website at:
www.greenwich-medical.co.uk

Contents

Contributors

Malcolm R. Alison BSc PhD DSc
FRCPath
Department of Histopathology
Imperial College
London, UK

Kirsten A. Atkins MD
Assistant Professor of Pathology
Virginia Commonwealth University
Richmond, USA

Suhaill I. Baithun MB ChB FRCPath
Senior Lecturer in Pathology &
Honorary Consultant Pathologist
The Royal London Hospital
London, UK

Paul S. Bass BSc FRCPath
Consultant Histopathologist &
Honorary Senior Lecturer
Southampton University Hospital Trust
Southampton, Hampshire, UK

Alan W. Bates PhD
Consultant Histopathologist &
Honorary Clinical Senior Lecturer
in Pathology
The Royal London Hospital
London, UK

Laurence J. R. Brown BSc MB BS
FRCPath
Consultant Histopathologist &
Honorary Senior Lecturer
Leicester Royal Infirmary
Leicester, UK

Natalie C. Direkze MA MB BS MRCP
Clinical Research Fellow
Cancer Research UK and
Department of Histopathology
Imperial College
London, UK

Anthony J. Freemont BSc MD FRCP
FRCPath
Professor of Osteoarticular Pathology
University of Manchester
Manchester, UK

Allan G. Howatson BSc MB ChB
FRCSEd FRCPath
Consultant Paediatric Pathologist
The Royal Hospital for Sick Children
Glasgow, UK

G. Harry Millward-Sadler BSc MB ChB
FRCPath MHSM
Consultant & Honorary Senior Lecturer
Department of Pathology
Southampton University Hospitals
Southampton, UK

Andrew G. Nicholson MB BS MRCPath
DM
Consultant Histopathologist
Royal Brompton Hospital
London, UK

Richard Poulsom BSc PhD MRCPath
Histopathology Unit
Cancer Research UK
London, UK

Sean L. Preston BSc MB BS MRCP
Histopathology Unit
Cancer Research UK and
Department of Histopathology
Barts and the London Queen Mary's
School of Medicine & Dentistry
London, UK

Alexandra J. Rice BA MB BChir
MRCPath
Consultant Histopathologist
St Mary's Hospital
London, UK

Mary E. Rogerson FRCP
Consultant Nephrologist
Southampton University Hospital Trust
Southampton, Hampshire, UK

Mary N. Sheppard FRCPath
Consultant Histopathologist
Royal Brompton & Harefield Trust
London, UK

Kassiani Skordilias MSc MRCPath
Consultant Histopathologist
Central Manchester & Manchester
    Children's University Hospitals
Manchester, UK

Athol U. Wells MB ChB FRACP MD
Interstitial Lung Disease Unit
Royal Brompton Hospital
London, UK

Mark A. Whittaker MRCPath
Consultant Histopathologist
Royal Hospital Haslar
Gosport, Hampshire, UK

Nicholas A. Wright MS DSc MD PhD
    FRCP FRCS FRCPath FMedSci
Histopathology Unit
Cancer Research UK and
Department of Histopathology
Barts and the London Queen Mary's
    School of Medicine and Dentistry
London, UK

Preface

Our aim is to offer reviews of topics on areas of diagnostic difficulty and to balance these with contributions on areas of scientific advance. The first diagnostic challenge in this Volume is that of small round cell tumours in childhood, where we have a comprehensive review of the subject. This is followed by equally thorough reviews of lupus nephritis and the interstitial pneumonias.

Joint diseases do not offer the glamour of the complex diagnostic classifications of, for instance, lymphomas but are important and potentially disabling to the patient. The pathologist has much to offer in the examination of biopsies and joint aspirates. Here we are fortunate to have a full account, with pointers to a possible place for molecular diagnosis in the near future.

Liquid-based cytology has been widely promoted as the future for cervical cytopathology, where screening programmes seem likely to pursue this technology. We have a thorough description of this advancing area backed up by a chapter in which the diagnosis and differential diagnosis of cervical glandular intra-epithelial neoplasia is presented. The Volume continues with a consideration of metastatic tumours in the urinary tract.

The autopsy has been very much in the news recently and mainly for the wrong reasons. To help redress this balance we have two chapters from expert authors, the first describing the autopsy and maternal death, and the second looking at sudden cardiac deaths. The Volume concludes with a review of the rapidly progressing field of stem cell biology of which we will plainly see much more, and probably very soon.

We trust that our readers will find the book both informative and enjoyable to read. We look forward to meeting you again with Volume 7 of *'Progress in Pathology'*.

N.K. and N.A.S.
Brighton and Gloucester July 2003

1

The diagnostic challenge of paediatric small round cell tumours

K. Skordilias A.G. Howatson

On writing about paediatric small round cell tumours (SRCTs) one cannot avoid the obvious question: 'Why another chapter on SRCTs of childhood?' There are three practical answers to this question. First, as diagnostic paediatric pathologists, we experience the challenge of correctly diagnosing these tumours on a daily basis.[1,2] Second, we acknowledge that many general pathologists received their training in rotations with limited exposure to paediatric material. Third, recent studies have drawn major conclusions regarding the diagnosis, prognosis and treatment of these tumours.

In the preparation of this chapter, every effort was made to provide a systematic and ordered approach to the differential diagnosis of paediatric SRCTs on biopsy specimens. We have tried to address problems and questions that commonly arise during the day-to-day practice and summarise information concerning the solid SRCTs published in generally available texts. A large body of information is available on leukaemias and lymphomas of childhood, which will not be considered further here. In fact, the next edition of this title, Progress in Pathology 7, will feature a comprehensive article on lymphoma/leukaemia in childhood.

SPECIMEN HANDLING

In dealing with the specimen, the pathologist should appreciate that taking a biopsy from a paediatric patient is not a trivial procedure. The clinical need is urgent for most of the cases and the sample provided is invariably smaller than

Kassiani Skordilias MSc MRCPath, Consultant Histopathologist, Central Manchester and Manchester Children's University Hospitals, Manchester, UK

Allan G. Howatson BSc MB ChB FRCSEd FRCPath, Consultant Paediatric Pathologist, The Royal Hospital for Sick Children, Glasgow, UK

Table 1.1 Samples required for the application of specialized techniques

Samples required in order of priority
Formalin fixed
Tissue culture for karyotyping
Trial-specific specimens
Frozen tissue for long-term storage (liquid nitrogen)
Glutaraldehyde for electron microscopy
Imprints
±Frozen section

the pathologists would like. The biopsy may have to be divided into even smaller samples to allow the application of specialised techniques. It is clear that if maximum benefit is to be obtained from such small samples, good communication is essential between pathologists, radiologists and surgeons.

Core or wedge biopsies must reach the pathology department fresh in an unfixed state, accompanied by a request form containing relevant information. According to clearly defined protocols,[3–8] the tissue submitted should provide several samples as seen in Table 1.1. These protocols include recommendations on the collection of clinical and pathological data with diagnostic and prognostic significance. The documents are evidence based and define the minimum standards for reporting each tumour group.

When the tissue is insufficient to cover all the options then flexibility and thought are required in deciding what to do rather than following prescribed lists of procedures. Light microscopy and cytogenetics are usually the most important, providing a diagnosis in the majority of the cases. Priority should always be given to the production of paraffin blocks for morphological and immunohistochemical assessment because SRCTs are undifferentiated and crush artefact is often present adding to the diagnostic difficulty. Furthermore, it is important to harvest tissue samples for specific procedures approved by the national bodies co-ordinating clinical trials of treatment. If there is strong clinical suspicion of neuroblastoma for example, then tissue needs to be submitted for N-myc analysis.[7] Little requirement is left for the urgent frozen section diagnosis today. Rapid processing facilities are available in most departments.

THE DIFFERENTIAL DIAGNOSIS

Paediatric SRCTs comprise a group of diverse primitive or undifferentiated neoplasms composed of sheets of small cells with round nuclei and inconspicuous cytoplasm.

The most common neoplasms presenting as SRCTs are lymphoblastic lymphomas/leukaemias, Ewing's sarcoma (ES)/peripheral neuroectodermal tumour (PNET), rhabdomyosarcomas and neuroblastomas. Most rhabdomyosarcomas and neuroblastomas show characteristic patterns of differentiation by light microscopy. However, a number of other paediatric tumours that are not usually problematic can on occasion present as SRCTs and cause diagnostic difficulty, particularly when they present in unusual sites or clinical context. The differential diagnosis, therefore, needs to be expanded beyond the traditional

Table 1.2 The differential diagnosis of SRCTs

Lymphoblastic lymphoma/leukaemia
Rhabdomyosarcoma
Neuroblastoma
ES/PNET
DSRCT
Small cell osteosarcoma
Synovial sarcoma
Wilms' tumour
Renal sarcomas

group to include peculiar variants, such as Wilms' tumour, renal sarcomas, desmoplastic small round cell tumour (DSRCT), small cell osteosarcoma and monophasic synovial sarcoma (Table 1.2).

THE CONTRIBUTION OF CLINICAL INFORMATION

Despite the effort of clinicians not to overload pathologists with clinical information, when one is confronted with an SRCT on an urgent core biopsy the contribution of clinical information cannot be overemphasised.

The minimum dataset required includes age, site, family history, radiological appearances and tumour markers.

Each neoplastic category has a distinct age distribution and this is particularly true for renal neoplasms. Anaplastic Wilms' tumours are virtually non-existent in infancy [9–13] while clear cell sarcoma of the kidney (CCSK) is unheard of in the first 3 months of life.[12–14]

Some anatomical sites are commonly associated with a specific type of tumour. For example, embryonal rhabdomyosarcomas typically arise in sites of embryonic tissue fusion; that is, the head and neck region and the genitourinary tract. A vaginal mass in an infant will most likely be an embryonal rhabdomyosarcoma. Imaging techniques are particularly helpful in establishing the actual site of the tumour and its extent. Information provided regarding the appearances of the tumour together with the differential diagnosis could be of great assistance in difficult cases. Multiple intra-abdominal masses in an adolescent male, for example, are suggestive of a DSRCT.[15]

Tumour markers also contribute to the differential diagnosis. Increased AFP levels in a patient with a hepatic tumour mass are suggestive of a hepatoblastoma while increased blood catecholamines associated with a suprarenal mass in an infant are diagnostic of a neuroblastoma.

Although most of the common childhood cancers occur sporadically, rare cases of host susceptibility are well documented. Familial and hereditary conditions associated with malignancy are important disorders to identify among paediatric patients because careful screening, examination and counselling can detect early signs of cancer and improve the chance of successful treatment. Twenty-five per cent of patients with Beckwith–Wiedemann syndrome (macrosomia, hemihypertrophy, exomphalos, neonatal hypoglycaemia, large tongue and creased ear lobes) develop a tumour (Wilms' tumour, hepatoblastoma and adrenal carcinoma) before the age of 5.[16,17]

MORPHOLOGICAL ASSESSMENT AND DIAGNOSTIC CLUES

The gross appearances are of limited value in facilitating the diagnosis of an SRCT on a small biopsy specimen. Imaging techniques, however, can provide relevant information regarding the macroscopical appearances (such as multi-centricity, organ of origin, texture, calcification, extent of tumour, etc.).

RHABDOMYOSARCOMA

Rhabdomyosarcoma is the most frequent soft tissue tumour of childhood with a peak incidence during the first decade.[18] The tumour is non-familial in most cases. The familial forms are associated with the Li–Fraumeni syndrome and the siblings are at increased risk for the development of various types of neoplasms.[19] Although they occur more commonly in the soft tissues they have been described in virtually every organ.[20] Cutaneous rhabdomyosarcomas have been seen in association with patients having epidermal naevi and those with von Recklinghausen's disease.[18,21]

The histological subtyping in rhabdomyosarcoma began in 1958 with the description of four major groups, namely botryoid, embryonal, alveolar and pleomorphic, known as the conventional scheme.[22] The WHO adapted this classification in 1969[23] but in subsequent decades, schemes based on tumour architecture, histology, clinical behaviour and cellular differentiation had been introduced. It was not until 1994 that a systematic review of all the available schemes was conducted in order to compare their reproducibility and prognostic significance.[24] A modification of the conventional scheme achieved a fair to good observer agreement and demonstrated a highly significant correlation with relation to survival. As a result of this, the International Classification of Rhabdomyosarcoma was introduced (Table 1.3).[25]

The embryonal rhabdomyosarcoma is composed of rhabdomyoblasts at varying stages of muscle development. Usually, they consist of small, round- to spindle-shaped cells with hyperchromatic nuclei and indistinct cytoplasm. Cellularity is variable with alternating densely packed, hypercellular areas and loosely textured myxoid areas.[20] The botryoid rhabdomyosarcoma is a subtype of embryonal rhabdomyosarcoma seen in certain sites, such as vagina and

Table 1.3 International classification of rhabdomyosarcoma[25]

Superior prognosis Botryoid rhabdomyosarcoma Spindle cell rhabdomyosarcoma
Intermediate prognosis Embryonal rhabdomyosarcoma
Poor prognosis Alveolar rhabdomyosarcoma Undifferentiated rhabdomyosarcoma
Subtypes whose prognosis is not presently known Rhabdomyosarcoma with rhabdoid features

urinary bladder. The neoplasm extends to just beneath the overlying mucosa/epithelium where it is separated by a compressed layer of tumour cells called the cambium layer. A spindle cell variant with a better prognosis occurs primarily in the paratesticular region.[26]

The alveolar rhabdomyosarcoma tumour cells are poorly differentiated round to oval, forming aggregates, delimited by dense collagenous septa and showing central loss of cohesion. The solid variant of this tumour lacks an alveolar pattern entirely and it is composed of densely packed groups of neoplastic cells with little or no fibrosis.[27] Pleomorphic rhabdomyosarcoma occurs rarely in infants and children.[28]

The histological subtypes that most commonly cause diagnostic confusion are the solid variant of alveolar rhabdomyosarcoma and the most undifferentiated form of embryonal rhabdomyosarcoma. Cases of the former have been misdiagnosed as embryonal rhabdomyosarcoma before molecular genetics revealed the characteristic translocation. Reticulin is a reliable stain that will display a pericellular distribution in embryonal rhabdomyosarcomas in contrast to outlining cellular aggregates in alveolar rhabdomyosarcoma (Figs 1.1 and 1.2). The importance of this distinction lies with the much more aggressive behaviour and worse prognosis associated with alveolar rhabdomyosarcoma compared to the embryonal subtype.[29–32]

NEUROBLASTOMA

This neoplasm commonly presents as an abdominal mass in a patient with increased urine vanillyl mandelic acid (VMA) and homovanillic acid (HVA) levels. On imaging the tumour may show calcification and necrosis. Rarely it may invade or surround the kidney, mimicking a Wilms' tumour.[33]

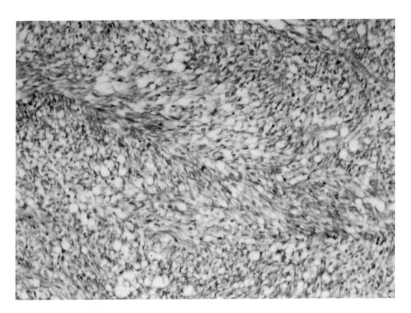

Fig. 1.1 Reticulin staining displaying a pericellular distribution in embryonal rhabdomyosarcoma.

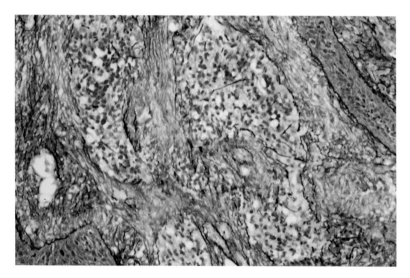

Fig. 1.2 Reticulin stain outlining cellular aggregates in alveolar rhabdomyosarcoma.

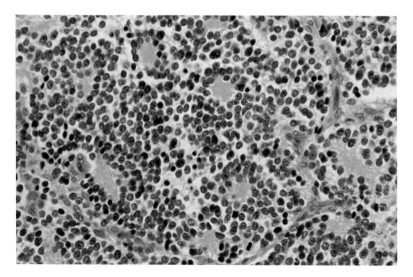

Fig. 1.3 Neuroblasts polarised towards a central point forming a Homer–Wright rosette with a solid fibrillary central core.

The tumour is composed of small primitive neuroblasts, with densely speckled nuclei and little cytoplasm, sometimes admixed with larger cells with features of ganglion cell differentiation. Neuroblasts may be polarised towards a central point forming a Homer–Wright rosette with a solid fibrillary central core (Fig. 1.3). An eosinophilic, acellular fibrillary matrix is often present and fibrovascular septa commonly divide the neoplasm into lobules. Necrosis and calcification are so common as to be helpful in the differential diagnosis of SRCTs.

EWING'S SARCOMA/PRIMITIVE NEUROECTODERMAL TUMOURS

ES/PNET and Askin tumour (thoracopulmonary PNET) represent a group of SRCTs with overlapping clinical and pathological features.

These neoplasms typically arise in the same age group; that is, childhood to young adulthood. ES is classically a primary bone neoplasm where PNET usually arises in soft tissues. ES, however, may present at an extra-osseous site and rare cases of PNET arise in bone.[34,35] These features suggest that the two tumours are related. Indeed the most notable feature shared by ES and PNET is a unique chromosomal translocation. The t(11;22)(q24;12) translocation was identified in ES in 1983[36] and the identical translocation was identified in PNET and Askin tumour in 1984[37] and 1985,[38] respectively. Nevertheless, there is no universal agreement as to whether there is any clinical significance in differentiating between these entities. Some have suggested rosette formation as a diagnostic feature of PNET while others require immunohistochemical evidence of neural differentiation, with or without rosettes.[35] The criteria used, however, appear random and will become irrelevant if future studies fail to reveal prognostic significance. Weiss suggests the classification of these tumours as members of the ES/PNET family, followed by a comment on the presence or absence of morphological, immunohistochemical or ultrastructural features supporting neural differentiation.[39]

ES comprises about 5% of all primary bone tumours but together with osteogenic sarcoma, encompasses the majority of bone tumours in children. The tumour occurs in the medullary cavity of the metaphyseal region of long bones and shows areas of necrosis. Correlation with radiological imaging studies is essential in reaching the diagnosis. The tumour typically presents as a poorly defined laminated lesion with periosteal reaction, sometimes associated with a soft tissue mass. The differential diagnosis includes osteomyelitis and Langerhans cell histiocytosis.[40] Microscopically it is composed of tightly packed round cells with clear or speckled nuclei, without nucleoli. A two-cell population is sometimes present composed of large viable cells and small hyperchromatic necrotic cells (Fig. 1.4). Mitotic count is usually low (<1/10 hpf). Necrosis is often seen, but calcification is not prominent, a feature that may be helpful in the differential diagnosis with neuroblastoma.[39] Cytoplasmic glycogen can be demonstrated on PAS and a lack of background reticulin fibres on reticulin.

PNET is a tumour showing a lobular diffuse and discohesive growth pattern with haemorrhage but no calcification. The tumour lobules are separated by dense fibrovascular septa which may undergo hyalinisation. Both Homer–Wright and perivascular pseudo-rosettes may be seen.[41] The cells are small containing a round to oval nucleus with coarse chromatin and small nucleoli, surrounded by a small rim of eosinophilic cytoplasm. The presence of intercellular fibrillary material is extremely unusual as is the presence of ganglion cells.[42]

DESMOPLASTIC SMALL ROUND CELL TUMOUR

DSRCT is a highly aggressive tumour of uncertain origin. The tumour occurs more commonly in males, presenting with abdominal distension and pain associated with an abdominal mass. At laparotomy, a variably sized mass associated

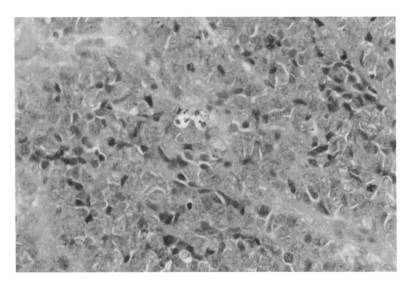

Fig. 1.4 A two-cell population is sometimes present in ES, composed of large viable cells and small hyperchromatic necrotic cells.

with numerous smaller peritoneal implants may involve any portion of the peritoneal cavity.[15]

DSRCT has a distinctive low-power appearance with sharply outlined trabeculae of tumour cells delimited by a desmoplastic stroma (Fig. 1.5). Central necrosis is common and may be associated with calcification in some of the larger trabeculae. The tumour cells are uniform with scanty cytoplasm, hyperchromatic nuclei, indistinct nucleoli and frequent mitoses. Diagnostic confusion tends to arise when the clinical presentation is atypical as in an extra-abdominal location (such as pleura,[43] central nervous system[44] and lymph node[45]).

OSTEOSARCOMA

Osteosarcoma is the commonest malignant bone tumour of childhood, displaying a diversity of histological subtypes, which is beyond the scope of this chapter. The subtype of osteosarcoma that enters the differential diagnosis of SRCTs is the small cell variant. The tumours are usually large (>6 cm) showing a mixed pattern of blastic and sclerotic changes with cortical distortion and often extension through the periosteum. Subperiosteal new bone formation results in either the classical 'Codman's triangle' or bony spiculation. The bone marrow cavity is often involved with transepiphyseal spread. 'Skip lesions', composed of tumour nodules separated by apparently normal marrow, are not uncommon.[40]

The small size and uniformity of the tumour cells as well as their diffuse growth pattern closely simulate the appearance of ES and lymphoma. The histological diagnosis of osteogenic sarcoma is dependent upon the identification of tumour osteoid in the tissue of interest, associated with the appropriate background. In a review of 72 cases of osteosarcoma of bone, in 1997, the investigators suggested making the diagnosis of osteosarcoma only if mineralized

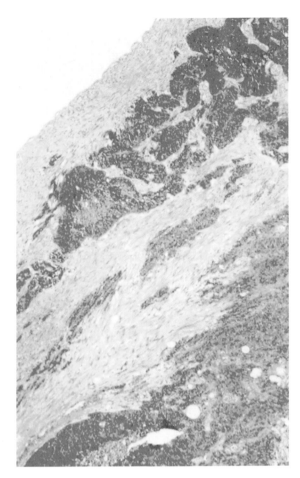

Fig. 1.5 DSRCT has a distinctive low-power appearance with sharply outlined trabecula of tumour cells delimited by a desmoplastic stroma.

matrix is identified.[35,46] Some authors[35] actually suggest that if the diagnosis is doubtful then it is better to err by making the diagnosis of ES. Indeed, we agree that the relationship between ES and the small cell variant of osteosarcoma needs additional study and clarification. Could they represent unusual examples of a bone-forming ES?

SYNOVIAL SARCOMA

Synovial sarcoma is a well-defined entity that has been described extensively in the literature.[47–50] It is seen in adolescents and young adults, presenting as a palpable, deep-seated swelling or mass associated with pain or tenderness, usually arising in the vicinity of large joints, especially the knee. Since it is a slow-growing mass it tends to be sharply circumscribed, round or multilobular.[47]

Unlike most other types of sarcoma, the tumour is composed of two morphologically distinct cell populations: epithelial and spindle cells. Depending on the relative prominence of the two cellular components, synovial sarcomas have been broadly classified into: biphasic, monophasic (fibrous and epithelial) (Fig. 1.6) and poorly differentiated types. The poorly differentiated type is the one that enters the differential diagnosis of SRCTs and is characterised by a

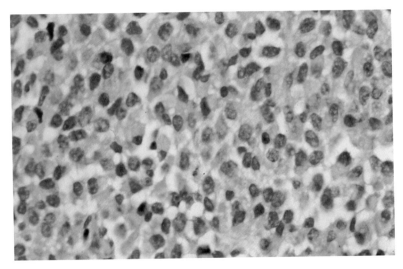

Fig. 1.6 Monophasic synovial sarcoma composed of small cells.

small cell population. The tumours often have a rich vascular background with dilated thin vascular spaces resembling hemangiopericytoma. The diagnosis can be very difficult but the identification of a low-grade component that is typical of monophasic or biphasic synovial sarcoma may be helpful.[47]

WILMS' TUMOUR

Wilms' tumour is one of the commonest malignant, solid, extracranial tumours of childhood, with an incidence of 1 in 10000 children.[12]

The tumour usually displays the classic triphasic appearance including blastema, epithelial and stromal elements but not all Wilms' tumours are triphasic. Biphasic and monophasic cases are by no means rare. The tumours display histological diversity with variable degrees of differentiation (purely blastemal to highly differentiated stromal and epithelial tumours) and patterns of differentiation (diverse spectrum of cell types and organisation patterns). The pattern that is more likely to be included in the differential diagnosis of SRCTs is the diffuse blastematous one.

The blastematous subtype comprises monomorphous sheets of intermediate-sized cells, often with non-cohesive infiltrative margins resembling those of lymphoma. Under such circumstances the identification of any of the three organoid blastemal patterns may provide a clue to the differential diagnosis. The serpentine pattern is most distinctive for Wilms' tumour, characterised by anastomosing cords of blastemal cells separated by myxoid stroma. The nodular pattern is similar to the serpentine but with rounded nests and the basaloid pattern displays an outlining of a layer of cuboidal or columnar cells.[13]

The identification of an epithelial (tubular or glomeruloid) or a stromal (myxoid, fibrous, smooth muscle or adipose cells) component is diagnostic of the triphasic pattern. However, glomeruloid and tubular structures should be differentiated from entrapped renal parenchyma.

CLEAR CELL SARCOMA OF THE KIDNEY (CCSK)

The CCSK is a rare neoplasm with approximately 20 new cases annually in the USA.[13] This means that a pathologist is likely to encounter no more than one or two cases in a lifetime, thus increasing the potential for diagnostic error.[13]

The classic pattern of CCSK is composed of cords and nests of polygonal cells with finely granular chromatin and small or absent nucleoli. The cytoplasm is clear as the name of the tumour implies and the cords are separated by fibro-vascular septa displaying a network of parallel vessels connected at frequent intervals by transverse arcades. However, the name can be misleading because not all tumours are composed of cells with clear or vacuolated cytoplasm. CCSK is a morphological mimic and may present with a number of histological variations[12] that invite confusion with Wilms' tumour or other neoplastic entities entering the differential diagnosis of SRCT. The sclerosing variant of CCSK, for example, may easily be confused with the blastematous component of Wilms' tumour. The sarcoma cells have a tendency to surround and isolate individual nephrons or collecting ducts, a feature that may simulate a triphasic appearance to the inexperienced. To add to the confusion, the entrapped tubules may also show embryonal metaplastic changes. On the other hand, blastemal elements are always more densely cellular than the sarcoma cells, composed of packed cells with overlapping nuclei.[13]

IMMUNOHISTOCHEMISTRY

Usually the pathologist has formulated a differential diagnosis based on the light microscopy and the clinical data, by the time an immunohistochemical request is made. An initial limited panel is often the first step towards refining or confirming the diagnosis. If this results in unexpected findings, a second more comprehensive panel may be used. In any case a multiple antibody panel should be applied, as reliance on one antibody can be misleading.

THE INITIAL PANEL

The initial panel may consist of CD99, cytokeratin, desmin, leucocyte common antigen (LCA), muscle-specific actin (MSA), neurone-specific enolase (NSE), synaptophysin, TdT and vimentin. This panel would help to differentiate between lymphoblastic leukaemia/lymphoma, rhabdomyosarcoma, neuroblastoma, ES/PNET and DSRCT (Table 1.4).

COMMONLY USED ANTIBODIES

CD99
CD99 is a transmembrane glycoprotein product of the MIC2 gene.[51-54] CD99 is a highly sensitive marker, consistently expressed in 85–95% of the ES/PNET family in which it demonstrates a uniform and strong membranous staining.[54,55] Lack of staining with any of the available antibody preparations in the market

Table 1.4 Initial panel of immunohistochemical antibodies for the differential diagnosis of SRCTs

	CD99	CK	DES	LCA	TdT	MSA	NSE	VIM
Lymphoblastic lymphoma	+	–	–	+	+	–	–	–
Neuroblastoma	–	–	–	–	–	–	+	–
ES/PNET	+	±	–	–	–	–	±	+
Rhabdomyosarcoma	±	±	+	–	–	+	±	+
DSRCT	±	+	+	–	–	–	+	+

may be an indication for additional studies to support the diagnosis.[56] Unfortunately, this antibody is not specific for ES/PNET. It has been found to be expressed by virtually all other SRCTs that enter the differential diagnosis, with the exception of neuroblastoma.[57-64] In rhabdomyosarcomas, the expression is cytoplasmic rather than membranous. It has been speculated that CD99 detection is influenced by the more widespread use of antigen-retrieval techniques, such as heat-induced epitope retrieval.[51]

Cytokeratins
Cytokeratins comprise a group of peptides ranging from low to high molecular weight. They are very useful antibodies since different tumours can be distinguished by the various cytokeratins they express. Using a cocktail, cytokeratin is demonstrable in DSRCTs.[15,51] It can also be focally and less consistently present in ES/PNET[4] and rhabdomyosarcomas.[63] Cytokeratin is negative in neuroblastoma and most lymphomas/leukaemias, with the exception of anaplastic large cell lymphoma.[51]

Desmin
Desmin is an intermediate filament and serves as an integral part of the cytoskeleton of cardiac, smooth and skeletal muscle.[51] It is a particularly sensitive marker for rhabdomyosarcoma[51,64] but is not diagnostic of this tumour since it has been shown to be expressed by many other tumours, such as PNET.[51,65] Desmin positivity is a characteristic finding in DSRCT being present in 90% of the cases.[15] It appears that antigen retrieval is an important technique in identifying desmin expression.[51]

Epithelial membrane antigen
Epithelial membrane antigen (EMA) is an antibody to milk fat globule membranes and is characteristically positive in epithelial malignancies.[51] It is also positive in some soft tissue tumours, including synovial sarcoma[51] and DSRCT.[15] Anaplastic large-cell lymphoma expression of EMA is also well documented. ES/PNET, rhabdomyosarcomas and neuroblastomas are typically negative.[51]

CD45 (Leucocyte Common Antigen)
CD45 (LCA) is commonly used to detect leukaemias and lymphomas. Rhabdomyosarcoma, neuroblastoma, ES/PNET and DSRCT are all negative for CD45.[51] LCA-negative lymphoblastic leukaemias and lymphomas, however,

are well described.[66] Misdiagnoses usually arise when the haematological malignancy also lacks expression; therefore, the antibody is best if used in a panel with TdT, B- and T-cell markers.

Muscle-Specific Actin

MSA is an antibody recognizing the alpha and gamma smooth muscle actins.[51] It is a useful marker for rhabdomyosarcoma especially in combination with desmin[63,64] and can help to distinguish rhabdomyosarcoma from DSRCT which is typically negative.[15] Myogenic-regulatory proteins, however, are expressed much earlier than structural proteins such as desmin and actin.[35,51] MyoD1 and myogenin belong to the family of myogenic-regulatory factors that are involved in skeletal muscle differentiation and they are expressed in less-differentiated forms of rhabdomyosarcoma that lack morphologic evidence of rhabdomyogenous differentiation.[51,67]

MyoD1

MyoD1 in particular is expressed in primitive cells and is absent from cells exhibiting morphologic features of differentiation.[51,68] Several studies have demonstrated specificity of MyoD1 as a marker for rhabdomyosarcoma[51,67–69] but strict adherence to nuclear staining is necessary because strong cytoplasmic positivity has been described in non-rhabdomyomatous tumours, such as neuroblastoma.[51] Occasional MyoD1-positive Wilms' tumours have also been described.[51,70]

Myogenin

It is interesting that myogenin may stain alveolar rhabdomyosarcoma more diffusely and strongly than the embryonal type, providing a possible means of immunohistochemically distinguishing the two subtypes.[71]

Neurone-specific enolase

NSE is an antibody which, despite its name, has been shown to be ubiquitously present, being more useful in identifying neuroblastic and neuroendocrine tumours.[51] It is expressed in neuroblastoma, ES/PNET, DSRCT and sporadically in rhabdomyosarcomas (intense cytoplasmic positivity in the alveolar subtype).[4,35,51] It is, therefore, quite obvious that NSE should not be used and interpreted alone.

S100

S100 is a calcium-binding acidic protein that is present in both central and peripheral nervous systems. PNET, neuroblastomas and DSRCT are positive.[51] The presence of S100 reactivity in dendritic cells which surround the tumour cell aggregates in peripheral neuroblastomas is characteristic.[35]

Synaptophysin

Synaptophysin is a transmembrane glycoprotein originally isolated from the presynaptic vesicles of neurones. It is a highly specific marker of neuroendocrine differentiation.[51] Neuroblastomas and DSRCTs express synaptophysin.[72] PNETs are variably positive whereas ES and rhabdomyosarcomas are negative in general.[51,73]

Vimentin

Vimentin is an intermediate filament that is consistently expressed by rhabdomyosarcoma, ES/PNET and DSRCT.[51] The antibody is probably more helpful when not expressed and this is the case for a minority of neoplasms, including neuroblastoma and lymphoblastic leukaemias.[73]

SPECIFIC TUMOURS

RHABDOMYOSARCOMA

Immunohistochemistry is pivotal in making or confirming the diagnosis. It has been recommended that a panel of three antibodies should be applied when the diagnosis is uncertain, including polyclonal desmin, MSA and CD99.[64] Rhabdomyosarcomas express polyclonal desmin in 99% of the cases, MSA in 94% (compared with 4% positivity to a smooth muscle actin) and CD99 in 14% of the tumours.[51] Myoglobulin is positive in 78% of the cases (predominately present in the more-differentiated cases).[51,66] MyoD1 is a good marker for rhabdomyosar-comas as long as one adheres to the requirement of nuclear positivity. It should be remembered that antigen retrieval is essential for the identification of monoclonal desmin and CD99 expression.[51] In the rare cases of CD99 positivity, additional positivity to MSA and desmin is supportive of the diagnosis of rhabdomyosarcoma.[35] Furthermore, CD99-positive rhabdomyosarcomas produce a weak and granular cytoplasmic positivity instead of strong membranous positivity seen in ES/PNET.[51] Finally, although strong expression of myogenic antigens is not diagnostic for rhabdomyosarcomas, the absence of staining by any of the other antibodies in the initial panel, is strongly supportive of that diagnosis.

NEUROBLASTOMA

The tumours are positive for NSE, synaptophysin, Leu 7, chromogranin, Protein Gene Product 9.5 and NB84 and are negative for actin, desmin, vimentin and low-molecular-weight cytokeratin.[51,74,75] Glial fibrillary acid protein (GFAP) highlights the fibrillary background. Rarely neuroblastomas may display rhabdomyomatous differentiation and the use of other antibodies, such as actin and desmin will prevent confusion.[76] Neuroblastomas are negative for vimentin and CD99 distinguishing the tumour from ES.[51] The presence of CD99 positivity virtually excludes the diagnosis of neuroblastoma.[35,77,78]

EWING'S SARCOMA/PERIPHERAL NEUROECTODERMAL TUMOUR

Immunohistochemical confirmation of the diagnosis of ES/PNET is essential, with the use of antibodies including CD99, vimentin, NSE, desmin, MSA and cytokeratin.[51,78–80] Both stain for vimentin and CD99 in 95% of the cases, exhibiting strong membranous staining,[51] a pattern which can be useful in ruling out a blastematous Wilms' tumour[61] (Fig. 1.7). Vimentin positivity is either focally or diffusely positive in a dot-like or perinuclear pattern. Consistent with their presumed neuroectodermal origin, PNETs express NSE, S100 (40%), synaptophysin (40%), chromogranin (20%), neurofilament (40%) and GFAP (<10%).[73,81] Less than 10% demonstrate cytokeratin, EMA and desmin positivity.[51]

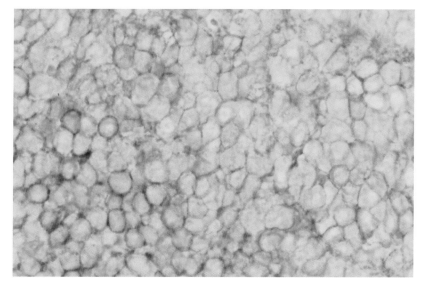

Fig. 1.7 Ewing's sarcoma showing strong membranous positivity to CD99.

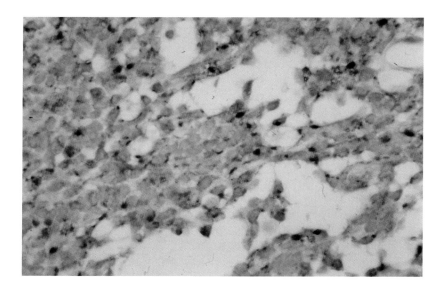

Fig. 1.8 DSRCTs display a dot-like positivity to desmin.

DESMOPLASTIC SMALL ROUND CELL TUMOUR

This tumour demonstrates a distinct immunophenotype, with co-expression of epithelial, neural and muscle markers. The co-expression of desmin, cytokeratin, vimentin and NSE helps to confirm the diagnosis in atypical presentations.[51] Desmin displays a globoid or dot-like positivity (Fig. 1.8), but there is no specific antibody for DSRCT, which may show an immunoprofile similar to that of ES/PNET, Wilms' tumour and synovial sarcoma.[15,51] It is worth

15

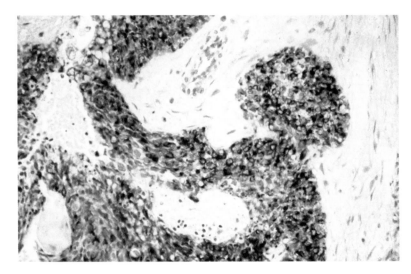

Fig. 1.9 DSRCTs showing strong cytokeratin expression.

noting that DSRCT is not positive for MyoD1, myogenin or myoglobulin, suggesting that the desmin expression is not an indication of true muscle differentiation.[51] MSA is positive in 16% of the cases, which can be useful in distinguishing rhabdomyosarcoma from DSRCT.[82] The tumour expresses a mixture of CAM5.2 and AE1/AE3 cytokeratins (Fig. 1.9) but it does not express CK5/CK6 or CK20. Vimentin and EMA also display cytoplasmic positivity.[51] In 20–35% of the cases, there is expression of CD99 with a cytoplasmic or membranous pattern.[15,82]

SMALL CELL OSTEOSARCOMA

The differential diagnosis of small cell osteosarcoma includes ES and mesenchymal chondrosarcoma.[35] Although foci showing frank spindling of tumour cells and/or the presence of osteoid eliminate the diagnosis of ES, both ES and osteosarcoma tumour cells may contain glycogen, show reactivity to CD99 but exhibit an otherwise non-specific immunoprofile. Only a minority of osteosarcomas show immunoreactivity to osteocalcin, a bone-specific protein produced by osteoblasts that has been shown to be highly specific and sensitive for conventional osteosarcoma.[46,83]

POORLY DIFFERENTIATED SYNOVIAL SARCOMA

The monophasic spindle cell morphological appearance and the poorly differentiated subtype can be confused with other SRCTs. Immunohistochemical expression of cytokeratin (Fig. 1.10) and vimentin in combination with a lack of CD99 and neural markers can help confirm the diagnosis of synovial sarcoma.[51] However, the monophasic pattern can be negative for cytokeratin and as with DSRCT the poorly differentiated subtype can express CD99 (Fig. 1.11).[51,60] The diagnosis of synovial sarcoma can be very difficult in the absence of a biphasic pattern.

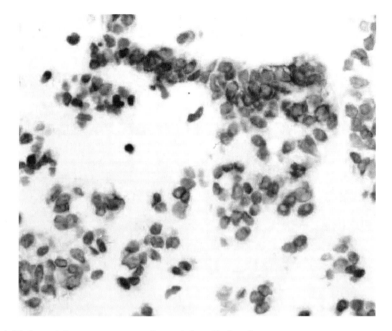

Fig. 1.10 Synovial sarcomas expressing cytokeratin locally.

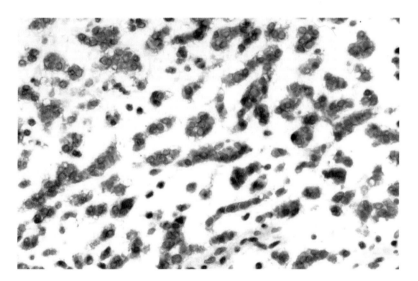

Fig. 1.11 Synovial sarcoma expressing CD99 showing strong cytoplasmic and membranous positivity.

WILMS' TUMOUR

The differential diagnosis includes PNET, neuroblastoma, DSRCT and rhabdomyosarcoma. Wilms' tumours do not exhibit any specific immunophenotype. They are positive for cytokeratin and lack expression of CD99, a feature helpful in the distinction with ES/PNET. The blastemal component may be positive for desmin but is negative for myogenin and myoD1, which are more specific markers of rhabdomyomatous differentiation.[84] In the differential diagnosis with

CCSK, CD34 can be helpful in highlighting the complex capillary network, characteristic of CCSK.

ELECTRON MICROSCOPY

In recent years, electron microscopy (EM) has been used less in many areas of diagnostic pathology but this is not the case for paediatric pathology where it remains an essential tool. EM is central to the diagnosis of metabolic, degenerative, pulmonary, renal, neuromuscular, dermatological and infectious diseases affecting children.[85,86] In paediatric oncology, newer techniques (such as immunohistochemistry and molecular studies) appear to predominate in the diagnosis of SRCTs. They are widely available, less expensive and more extensively investigated than EM. However, recent studies have challenged some assumptions regarding antibody specificities, arguing that the dramatic shift towards immunohistochemistry may not be fully justified.

In difficult cases, EM may provide significant information regarding the nature of a tumour. A particular strength of EM is that it will often provide a correct answer even when a particular diagnosis is not under direct consideration by the pathologist.[87] Immunohistochemistry, on the other hand, depends on the pathologist's opinion regarding the selection of which antibodies are going to be useful in the differential diagnosis.

A recent study measured the level of confidence with which an SRCT diagnosis can be made by comparing the utility of immunohistochemistry and EM.[88] Of 50 poorly differentiated SRCTs, in which the diagnosis was uncertain by routine light microscopy, following the application of immunohistochemistry and EM, only two cases remained without a confident specific diagnosis. The ancillary studies resulted in a revision of the best guess diagnosis in 22% of the cases and this figure would have been higher, had these provisional diagnoses not been made by an experienced paediatric pathologist. More specifically, EM was found to be superior to immunohistochemistry for the diagnosis of ES/PNET, rhabdomyosarcomas and Wilms' tumour and equally as good for the diagnosis of neuroblastoma. The primary weakness of EM was in the diagnosis of lymphomas.[88]

EM can assist in the identification of neural differentiation with the demonstration of distinctive neurosecretory granules and microtubule-bearing neuritic processes. It may even be of practical importance in distinguishing PNET from ES, should this need arise in the future. The identification of early myogenic differentiation in poorly differentiated rhabdomyosarcomas is also possible, by detecting specific myofilament arrays, Z-band material and monoparticulate glycogen (as opposed to rosetted glycogen seen in PNET/ES).[87] Monophasic blastemal Wilms' tumours can be confidently identified with EM by the demonstration of the distinctive flocculent coating of basement membrane-like material surrounding the cells. It was also felt that EM proved more robust in the sense that even when it could not establish the diagnosis, it could at least establish that the tumour was truly undifferentiated.[88]

An assumption often made is that sampling difficulties may influence the performance of EM.[87] Our experience as well as that of other investigators[87] indicates that with reasonable attention to specimen collection and sample sectioning such problems can generally be avoided or easily overcome. Small disrupted specimens, such as those obtained from aspiration biopsies, actually pose little problem for EM because the technique focuses on the study of cells rather than organisational patterns.[87,89] On balance, however, it is fair to record that the results reflect the training and experience of the operators.

CLINICAL USE OF CYTOGENETICS

Only a small percentage of SRCTs will defy precise diagnosis even when immuno-histochemistry and EM are both used.[87] Molecular genetics has an increasing number of applications in tumour analysis and there is no other field where this is more apparent than paediatric oncology. Studies of paediatric tumours have identified novel genes, advanced our understanding of oncogenesis and introduced diagnostic and prognostic markers useful in patient management.[90]

The volume of cytogenetic information in paediatric oncology is overwhelming so we have focused only on the molecular changes relevant to the differential diagnosis of our group of SRCTs.

TECHNIQUES

Genetic changes in paediatric tumours are detected by a variety of techniques.

FLUORESCENCE IN SITU HYBRIDISATION

Fluorescence *in situ* hybridisation (FISH) can be applied to both fresh and archival material. In this technique a probe for a specific gene is labelled and detected using a secondary reagent conjugated to a fluorochrome. The technique allows the examination of individual cells, which is an advantage that permits normal cells to be distinguished from tumour cells, thus detecting heterogeneity within tumour cells.[90]

Reverse transcriptase-polymerase chain reaction (RT-PCR) can detect characterized translocations more readily than FISH, allowing the distinction between the translocated and non-translocated signals often present in the same nucleus. However, because RNA is used as the starting material, the sample needs to be as fresh as possible and great care should be taken to avoid contamination.[90]

KARYOTYPE ANALYSIS

Karyotype analysis has traditionally been used to detect structural and numerical chromosomal abnormalities on a metaphase spread, which requires viable tumour cells set-up in short-term culture. The usefulness of this technique in paediatric oncology is restricted by certain limitations, in that skilled personnel are required for the preparation of metaphase spreads, the identification of chromosome bands and interpretation of abnormalities. The technique is difficult to apply to solid tumours because it relies on actively dividing cells that usually comprise only a small population of the overall tumour and metaphase spreads are frequently of poor quality. This means that milligrams of fresh tumour may be required which may not be available from biopsy specimens.

It is not unusual to find the surrounding connective tissue fibroblasts growing instead of the desired tumour cells and, therefore, the overall success rate of karyotypic analysis of solid tumours can be as low as 20–30%. In addition, the procedure is time consuming, often requiring 2 weeks before a result is available. The information available includes modal chromosome number, abnormalities of individual chromosomes, deletions, translocations, double minutes and homogeneously staining regions.[90]

SPECIFIC TUMOURS

A brief review of the most common SRCTs and their molecular markers is shown in Table 1.5.

RHABDOMYOSARCOMA

The diagnostic difficulty with rhabdomyosarcoma is not limited to making the diagnosis but also includes rendering the correct subtype. In about 70% of

Table 1.5 Molecular genetics in SRCTs

Rhabdomyosarcoma	
Alveolar	t(2;13) (q35;q14) in 70%
	t(1;13)(p36;q14)
Embryonal	cx, +8, +2, +11, rea(12)(q13)
Neuroblastoma	Hyperdiploid, no or few rearrangements, dmins, hsr, with or without deletion of 1(p) or LOH(1p), 17q translocation, N-Myc amplification
ES	t(11;22)(q24;q12) in 90%
	+8, der(16)t(1;16)(q21;q13)
	t(21;22)(q22;q12)
PNET	t(11;22)(q24;q12)
DSRCT	t(11;22)(p13;q21)
Osteosarcoma	Extreme complexity, numerous unidentified markers, i(6p), i(14q), −13, −3, −5 −4, −10, −15, −22
Synovial sarcoma	t(X;18)(p11;q11) in <90%
Wilms' tumour	
Genes associated with WARG phenotype	Locus at (11)(p13), WT1 locus
Genes associated with Beckwith–Wiedemann syndrome	Locus at (11)(p15), WT2 locus
Sporadic Wilms'	Near diploid or pseudo-diploid, +12 (most frequent), +6, +7, +8, +12, +13, +17, +20, rea(11)(p13 or p15) LOH (11)(p) der(16)t(1;16)(q10–21;q10–13) may be the sole change, i(1q)

This table is a modified from Heimand Mitelman (1995) showing abnormalities in order of frequencies of occurrence (*Applied Cytogenetics* – Journal of the Association of Genetic Technologists 1997; 23(6): 167–180).

alveolar rhabdomyosarcomas, a translocation at t(2;13)(q35;q14) is seen.[90,91] In this translocation, the PAX3 gene on chromosome 2 is fused with the FKHR gene on chromosome 13 resulting in a chimeric transcription factor.[90] A less frequently observed translocation is t(1;13)(p36;q14) seen in up to 20% of the cases.[90,92] In this translocation, the PAX3 gene is replaced by the similar PAX7 gene on chromosome 1.[93] Other abnormalities have also been detected including N-myc amplification.[90,94] In contrast to alveolar rhabdomyosarcoma, no consistent genetic changes have been found in embryonal rhabdomyosarcoma.[90] These tumours are usually hyperdiploid with extra copies of chromosomes 2, 8, 9, 11, 12 and 13, 17, 18, 19 and losses of material on chromosomes 10, 14, 15, 16.[90,91,95] A theme pattern emerging is that embryonal rhabdomyosarcoma is character-ized more by whole chromosome gains or losses and the alveolar subtype more by translocations and amplifications. In both subtypes, however, chromosomes 2, 12 and 13 tend to be involved.[90]

NEUROBLASTOMA

There is no specific molecular marker for neuroblastoma. A notable molecular finding, however, is the oncogenic activation of the N-myc gene which when amplified confers a growth advantage to the neoplastic cells *in vitro*, implying a role in the malignant progression of this tumour. N-myc amplification has been found in up to 50% of advanced stage neuroblastomas, with more than 10 copies of the gene correlating with poor prognosis.[90] The converse, that is, lack of amplification does not necessarily indicate good prognosis. Deletions of chro-mosome 1p are the most frequent genetic changes in neuroblastoma and have been identified by cytogenetics and FISH.[90,96,97] The frequency of this change varies between 20% and 90% of cases, depending on the series. The deletions occur more commonly in tumours that are advanced stage, near diploid and are usually associated with poor prognosis and N-myc amplification.[90,97] The puta-tive tumour suppressor gene(s) on chromosome 1p is not as yet identified. Gain of material from chromosome 17 is also an unfavourable prognostic indicator. This abnormality is identified in 90% of high-grade tumours.[90]

FISH shows that chromosomal abnormalities appear to be limited to neuro-blasts and differentiating ganglion cells, but are not found in Schwann cells implying that the latter is a reactive population.[90,98] Tumours with trisomy by FISH show evidence of maturation.[90]

EWING'S SARCOMA/PERIPHERAL NEUROECTODERMAL TUMOUR

In part because of the genetic abnormalities that they have in common, ES and PNET are regarded as related tumours.[39] Both tumours show a reciprocal translocation involving chromosome 22 at q12. The other chromosome most commonly involved is 11 at q24.[90] The t(11;22)(q24;q12) is seen in approximately 90% of cases.[90] The translocation induces fusion of the FLI-1gene on chromo-some 11 with the Ewing's sarcoma gene on chromosome 22, resulting in a chimeric protein, which plays a critical role in oncogenesis.[90,99] The target genes affected are largely unknown apart from the C-myc gene. Five less common translocations have been reported which remarkably maintain a common theme of fusing a portion of the Ewing's sarcoma gene to another gene similar to the FLI-1 gene.[90]

DESMOPLASTIC SMALL ROUND CELL TUMOUR

The DSRCT is also characterized by a t(11;22) translocation but one involving chromosome 11p13 rather than 11q24 as seen in ES. In this case, the EWS gene on chromosome 22 is fused with the Wilms' tumour suppressor gene on chromosome 11, resulting in a chimeric protein. This fusion transcript is unique to DSRCT.[90]

SYNOVIAL SARCOMA

A translocation at t(X;18)(p11;q11) has been found in up to 80% of cases, an abnormality which can be detected by FISH.[47,90] The result is fusion of the SYT gene on chromosome 18 to SSX1 or SSX2 genes on the X chromosome. The reciprocal translocation does not lead to a hybrid transcript. Another variant translocation has also been identified located at t(5;18)(q11;q11).[90]

WILMS' TUMOUR

The genetic events leading to Wilms' tumour are surprisingly complex and involve at least four distinct genetic loci. Wilms' tumour patients with WAGR syndrome (Wilms' tumour, Aniridia, Genitourinary abnormalities, mental Retardation) have a constitutional deletion of 11p13, which suggests that critical genes for the normal development of the kidney, eye and gonads are mapped to this chromosomal location.[90] The WT1 gene has many of the properties expected for a tumour suppressor gene and is also altered in sporadic and hereditary Wilms' tumour, with both large and small deletions and point mutations.[90,100] However, linkage studies have shown no linkage to chromosome 11 in some families with Wilms' tumour suggesting that mutations in other genetic loci may also play a role. In addition, an unidentified gene on short arm of chromosome 11 at band 11p15 has also been associated with the development of sporadic Wilms' tumour. Loss of heterozygosity of the long arm of chromosome 16 has been observed in about 20% of tumours and p53 mutations have been associated with the anaplastic Wilms' variant.[90]

CONCLUSIONS

Rendering a definitive diagnosis may be particularly challenging even for experienced paediatric pathologists because SRCTs may not only show complete absence of differentiation but they may also mimic patterns of differentiation usually associated with other tumours. While light microscopy and morphological features remain at the heart of the diagnostic process, immunohistochemistry, EM and cytogenetics have greatly improved our ability to separate and classify SRCTs. The use of these ancillary tools has become important not only in confirming or diagnosing challenging cases but also in assessing prognosis and suggesting therapy. Histopathology is vital for the clinical management of children with malignant disease and diagnostic accuracy is pivotal.

KEY POINTS

1. Paediatric SRCTs comprise a group of diverse primitive or undifferentiated neoplasms, typically composed of sheets of small cells with round nuclei and inconspicuous cytoplasm.
2. The most common neoplasms presenting as SRCTs are lymphomas/ leukaemias, ES/PNET, rhabdomyosarcomas and neuroblastomas.
3. A number of other paediatric tumours can, on occasion, present as SRCTs and cause diagnostic difficulty, particularly when they present in unusual sites or clinical context.
4. The pathologist formulates a differential diagnosis based on the light microscopy and the clinical data before an immunohistochemical request is made.
5. An initial panel of antibodies might reasonably consist of CD99, cyto-keratin, desmin, LCA, MSA, NSE, synaptophysin, TdT and vimentin. Interpretations of these techniques have pitfalls of their own.
6. Only a small percentage of SRCTs will defy precise diagnosis when immuno-histochemistry and EM are both used.
7. Molecular studies of paediatric tumours have identified novel genes, advancing our understanding of oncogenesis and introducing diagnostic and prognostic markers useful in patient management.

REFERENCES

1. Royal College of Paediatrics and Child Health. The Future of Paediatric Pathology Services. London, 2002
2. Parkes SE, Muir KR, Cameron AH *et al*. The need for specialist review of pathology in paediatric cancer. Br J Cancer 1997; 75: 1156–1159
3. International Society of Paediatric Oncology. Nephroblastoma (Wilms' tumour). Clinical Trial and Study. UKCCSG Protocol 2002; No: WT 2202 02
4. Askin FB, Perlman EJ. Neuroblastoma and peripheral neuroectodermal tumors. Am J Clin Pathol 1998; 109 (4 suppl 1): S23–S30
5. Wold LE. Practical approach to processing osteosarcomas in the surgical pathology laboratory. Pediatr Dev Pathol 1998; 1: 449–454
6. Stocker JT, Mosijczuk AD. Handling the pediatric tumour (editorial). Am J Clin Pathol 1998; 109 (4 suppl 1): S1–S3
7. Joshi VV. Peripheral neuroblastic tumors: pathologic classification based on recommendations of International Neuroblastoma Pathology Committee (modification of Shimada Classification). Pediatr Dev Pathol 2000; 3: 184–199
8. Qualman SJ, Coffin CM, Newton WA *et al*. Intergroup rhabdomyosarcoma study: update for pathologists. Pediatr Dev Pathol 1998; 1: 550–561
9. Murphy WM, Beckwith JB, Farrow GM. Tumors of the kidney. In Tumors of the Kidney, Bladder and Related Urinary Structures. Washington DC: Armed Forces Institute of Pathology, 1994; 1–192
10. Schmidt D, Beckwith JB. Histopathology of childhood renal tumors. Hematol Oncol Clin North Am 1995; 9: 1179–1200
11. Bonadio JF, Storer B, Norkool P, Farwell VT, Beckwith JB, D'Angio GH. Anaplastic Wilms' tumor: clinical and pathologic studies. J Clin Oncol 1985; 3: 513–520
12. Charles AK, Vujavic GM, Berry PJ. Renal tumours of childhood. Histopathology 1998; 32: 293–309
13. Beckwith JB. Renal tumors. In Stocker JT, Askin FB (Eds) Pathology of Solid Tumours in Children. London: Chapman & Hall Medical, 1998; 1–23

14. Newbould MJ, Kelsey AM. Clear cell sarcoma of the kidney in a 4 month-old infant: a case report. Med Pediatr Oncol 1993; 21: 525–528

15. Gerald WL, Ladanyi M, de Alava E *et al*. Clinical, pathologic and molecular spectrum of tumors associated with t(11;22) (p13;q12): desmoplastic small round-cell tumor and its variants. J Clin Oncol 1998; 16: 3028–3036

16. Steenman M, Westerveld A, Mannens M. Genetics of Beckwith–Wiedemann syndrome-associated tumour: common genetic pathways. Gene Chromosom Cancer 2000; 28: 1–13

17. Abelson HT. Oncology. In Berhan RE, Kliegman RM (Eds) Nelson Essentials in Paediatrics. Philadelphia: WB Saunders Company, 1998; 583–608

18. Siegal GP. Primary tumors of muscle. In Stocker JT, Askin FB (Eds) Pathology of Solid Tumours in Children. London: Chapman & Hall Medical, 1998; 161–181

19. Strong LC, Williams WR, Taisky MA. The Li–Fraumeni syndrome: from clinical epidemiology to molecular genetics. Am J Epidemiol 1992; 135: 190–199

20. Rhabdomyosarcoma. In Weiss SW, Goldblum JR (Eds) Enzinger and Weiss's Soft Tissue Tumors. St Louis: Mosby, 2001; 785–835

21. Srouji MN, Donaldson MH, Chatten J *et al*. Perianal rhabdomyosarcoma in childhood. Cancer 1976; 38: 1008–1012

22. Horn RC, Enterline HT. Rhabdomyosarcoma: a clinicopathological study of 39 cases. Cancer 1958; 11: 181–199

23. Enzinger FM, Lattes R, Torloni H. Histological typing of soft tissue tumors. In International Histological Classification of Tumors, No. 3. Geneve: World Health Organisation, 1969

24. Asmar L, Gehan EM, Newton Jr WA *et al*. Agreement among and within groups of pathologists in the classification of rhabdomyosarcoma and related childhood sarcomas; report of an international study of four pathology classifications. Cancer 1994; 74: 2579–2588

25. Newton Jr WA, Gehan EA, Webber BL *et al*. Classification of rhabdomyosarcomas and related sarcomas: pathologic aspects and proposal for a new classification – an Intergroup Rhabdomyosarcoma Study. Cancer 1995; 76: 1073

26. Cavazzana AO, Schmidt D, Ninfo V *et al*. Spindle cell rhabdomyosarcoma: a prognostically favorable variant of rhabdomyosarcoma. Am J Surg Pathol 1992; 16: 229–235

27. Sartelet H, Lantuejoul S, Armari-Alla C *et al*. Solid alveolar rhabdomyosarcoma of the thorax in a child. Histopathology 1998; 32: 165–171

28. Kobet R, Newton Jr WA, Hamoudi AB *et al*. Childhoood rhabdomyosarcoma with anaplastic (pleomorphic) features: a report of the Intergroup Rhabdomyosarcoma Study. Am J Surg Pathol 1993; 17: 443–453

29. Tsokos M. The diagnosis and classification of childhood rhabdomyosarcoma. Semin Diagn Pathol 1994; 11: 26–38

30. Douglass EC, Rowe ST, Valentine M *et al*. Variant translocations of chromosome 13 in alveolar rhabdomyosarcoma. Gene Chromosom Cancer 1991; 3: 480–482

31. Douglass EC, Shapiro DN, Valentino M *et al*. Alveolar rhabdomyosarcoma with the t(2;13): cytogenetic findings and clinicopathologic correlations. Med Pediatr Oncol 1993; 21: 83–87

32. Parham DM, Shapiro DN, Downing JR *et al*. Solid alveolar rhabdomyosarcoma with the t(2;13): report of two cases with diagnostic implications. Am J Surg Pathol 1994; 18: 474–478

33. Panuel M, Bourliere-Najean B, Gentet JC. Aggressive neuroblastoma with initial pulmonary metastases and kidney involvement simulating Wilms' tumor. Eur J Radiol 1992; 14: 201–203

34. Dehner LP. Primitive neuroectodermal tumor and Ewing's sarcoma. Am J Surg Pathol 1993; 17: 1–13

35. Devoe K, Weidner N. Immunohistochemistry of small round-cell tumors. Semin Diagn Pathol 2000; 17: 216–224

36. Aurias A, Rimbaut C, Buffe D *et al*. Chromosomal translocations in Ewing's sarcoma. N Engl J Med 1983; 309: 496–497

37. Whang-Peng J, Triche TJ, Knutsen T *et al*. Chromosome translocation in peripheral neuroepithelioma. N Engl J Med 1984; 311: 584–585

38. Seemayer TA, Vekemans M, de Chadarevian JP. Histological and cytogenetic findings in a malignant tumor of the chest wall and lung (Askin tumour). Virchows Arch 1985; 408: 289–296

39. Primitive neuroectodermal tumors and related lesions. In Weiss SW, Goldblum JR (Eds) Enzinger and Weiss's Soft Tissue Tumors. St Louis: Mosby, 2001; 1265–1321

40. Siegal GP. Primary tumors of bone. In Stocker JT, Askin FB (Eds) Pathology of Solid Tumours in Children. London: Chapman & Hall Medical, 1998; 183–212

41. Schmidt D, Herrmann C, Jurgens H et al. Malignant peripheral neuroectodermal tumor and its necessary distinction from Ewing's sarcoma: a report from the Kiel Pediatric Tumor Registry. Cancer 1991; 68: 2251–2259

42. Askin FB. Neuroblastoma and peripheral neuroectodermal tumors: a clinicopathological review. In Stocker JT, Askin FB (Eds) Pathology of Solid Tumours in Children. London: Chapman & Hall Medical, 1998; 25–50

43. Parkash V, Gerald WL, Parma A et al. Desmoplastic small round cell tumor of the pleura. Am J Surg Pathol 1995; 19: 659–665

44. Tison V, Cerasoli S, Morigi et al. Intracranial desmoplastic small cell tumor: report of a case. Am J Surg Pathol 1996; 20: 112–117

45. Backer A, Mount SL, Zarka MA et al. Desmoplastic small round cell tumour of unknown primary origin with lymph node and lung metastases: histological, cytological, ultrastructural, cytogenetic and molecular findings. Virchows Arch 1998; 432: 135–141

46. Nakajima H, Sim FH, Bond JR et al. Small cell osteosarcoma of bone, review of 72 cases. Cancer 1997; 79: 2095–2106

47. Malignant soft tissue tumors of uncertain type. In Weiss SW, Goldblum JR (Eds) Enzinger and Weiss's Soft Tissue Tumors. St Louis: Mosby, 2001; 1483–1571

48. Cadman NL, Soule EH, Kelly PJ. Synovial sarcoma: an analysis of 134 tumors. Cancer 1965; 18: 613–627

49. Cagle LA, Mirra JM, Storm FK et al. Histologic features relating to prognosis in synovial sarcoma. Cancer 1987; 59: 1810–1814

50. Dardick I, Ramjohn S, Thomas MJ et al. Synovial sarcoma: interrelationship of the biphasic and monophasic subtypes. Pathol Res Pract 1991; 187: 871–885

51. Belchis D. Immunohistochemistry of pediatric small round cell tumors. In Dabbs DJ (Ed.) Diagnostic Immunohistochemistry. Philadelphia: Churchill Livingstone, 2002; 517–535

52. Wick MR. Immunohistology of neuroendocrine and neuroectodermal tumors. Semin Diagn Pathol 2000; 17: 194–203

53. Amann G, Zoubek A, Salzer-Kuntschik M et al. Relation of neurological marker expression and EWS gene fusion in MIC2/CD99-positive tumors of the Ewing family. Hum Pathol 1999; 30: 1058–1064

54. Perlman EJ, Dickman PS, Askin FB et al. Ewing's sarcoma-routine diagnostic utilization of MIC2 analysis: a Pediatric Oncology Group/Children's Cancer Group Inter-group study. Hum Pathol 1994; 25: 304–307

55. Ambros IM, AmbrosPF, Stehl S et al. MIC2 is a specific marker for Ewing's sarcoma and peripheral primitive neuroectodermal tumors: evidence for a common histogenesis of Ewing's sarcoma and peripheral primitive neuroectodermal tumors from MIC2 expression and specific chromosome aberration. Cancer 1991; 67: 1886–1893

56. Dehner LP. On trial: a malignant small cell tumor in a child: four wrongs do not make a right. Am J Clin Pathol 1998; 109: 662–668

57. Soslow RA, Bhargave V, Warnke RA. MIC2, TdT, bcl-2 and CD34 expression in paraffin-embedded high-grade lymphoma/acute lymphoblastic leukemia distinguishes between distinct clinicopathological entities. Hum Pathol 1997; 28: 1158–1165

58. Lumadue JA, Askin FB, Perlman EJ. MIC2 analysis of small cell carcinoma. Am J Clin Pathol 1994; 102: 692–694

59. Nicholson SA, McDermott MB, Swanson PE et al. CD99 and cytokeratin-20 in small cell and basaloid tumors of skin. Appl Immunohistochem Mol Morphol 2000; 8: 37–41

60. Folpe AI, Schmidt RA, Chapman D, Gown AM. Poorly differentiated synovial sarcoma: immunohistochemical distinction from primitive neuroectodermal tumors and high grade malignant peripheral nerve sheath tumors. Am J Surg Pathol 1998; 22: 673–682

61. Ramani P, Rampling D, Link M. Immunohistochemical study of 12E7 in small round-cell tumours of childhood: an assessment of its sensitivity and specificity. Histopathology 1993; 23: 557–561

62. Devaney K, Vinh TN, Sweet DE. Small cell osteosarcoma of bone: an immunohisto-chemical study with differential diagnostic considerations. Hum Pathol 1993; 24: 1211–1225

63. Hibshoosh H, Lattes R. Immunohistochemical and molecular genetic approaches to soft tissue tumor diagnosis: a primer. Semin Oncol 1997; 24: 515–525

64. Qualman SJ, Coffin CM, Newton WA et al. Intergroup rhabdomyosarcoma study: update for pathologists. Pediatr Dev Pathol 1998; 1: 550–561

65. Parham DM, Dia P, Kelly DR et al. Desmin positivity in primitive neuroectodermal tumors of childhood. Am J Surg Pathol 1992; 16: 483–492

66. Ozdemirli M, Farburg-Smith JC et al. Precursor B-lymphoblastic lymphoma presenting as a solitary bone tumor and mimicking Ewing's sarcoma: a report of four cases and review of the literature. Am J Surg Pathol 1998; 22: 795–804

67. Wang NP, Manx J, McNutt MA et al. Expression of myogenic regulatory proteins (myogenin and MyoD1) in small blue round cell tumors of childhood. Am J Pathol 1995; 147: 1799–1810

68. Cui S, Hamo H, Havada T et al. Evaluation of new monoclonal anti-MyoD1 and anti-myogenin antibodies for the diagnosis of rhabdomyosarcoma. Pathol Int 1999; 49: 62–68

69. Dias P, Parham DM, Shapiro DN et al. Myogenic regulatory protein (MyoD1) expression in childhood solid tumors: diagnostic utility in rhabdomyosarcoma. Am J Pathol 1990; 137: 1283–1291

70. Dias P, Parham DM, Shapiro DN et al. Monoclonal antibodies to the myogenic regulatory protein MyoD1: epitope mapping and diagnostic utility. Cancer Res 1992; 52: 6431–6439

71. Dias P, Chen B, Dilday B et al. Strong immunostaining for myogenin in rhabdomyosarcoma is significantly associated with tumors of the alveolar subclass. Am J Pathol 2000; 156: 399–408

72. Miettinen M. Synaptophysin and neurofilament proteins as markers for neuroendocrine tumors. Arch Pathol Lab Med 1987; 111: 813–818

73. Coffin C, Dehner L. Neurogenic tumors of soft tissue. In Coffin C, Dehner L, O'Shea P (Eds) Pediatric Soft Tissue Tumors: A Clinical, Pathological and Therapeutic Approach. Baltimore: Williams & Wilkins, 1997; 80–132

74. Carter RL, al-Sams SZ, Corbett RP, Clinton S. A comparative study of immunohisto-chemical staining for neuron specific enolase, protein gene product 9.5 and S100 protein in neuroblastoma, Ewing's sarcoma and other round cell tumours in children. Histopathology 1990; 19: 461–467

75. Shimada H, Ambros IM, Dehner LP et al. Terminology and morphologic criteria of neuroblastic tumors: recommendations by the International Neuroblastoma Pathology Committee. Cancer 1999; 86: 349–363

76. Layfield LJ, Glasgow BJ. Rhabdomyomatous differentiation in a neuroblastoma: a potential pitfall in the cytologic diagnosis of small round cell tumors of childhood. Diagn Cytopathol 1991; 7: 193–197

77. Weidner N, Tjoe J. Immunohistochemical profile of monoclonal antibody O13: antibody that recognizes glycoprotein p30/32^{MIC2} and is useful in diagnosing Ewing's sarcoma and peripheral neuroepithelioma. Am J Surg Pathol 1994; 18: 486–494

78. Stevenson AJ, Chatten J, Bertoni F et al. CD99 (p30/32^{MIC2}) neuroectodermal/Ewing's sarcoma antigen as an immunohistochemical marker. Review of more than 600 tumors and the literature experience. Appl Immunohistochem 1994; 2: 231–240

79. Halliday BE, Stagel DD, Elsheikh TE, Silverman JF. Diagnostic utility of MIC-2 immunohistochemical staining in the differential diagnosis of small blue cell tumors. Diagn Cytopathol 1998; 19: 410–416

80. Fellinger EJ, Garin-Chesa P, Glasser DB et al. Comparison of cell surface antigen HBA71 (p30/32 MIC2), neuron-specific enolase and vimentin in the immunohistochemical analysis of Ewing's sarcoma of bone. Am J Surg Pathol 1992; 16: 746–755

81. Meis-Kindblom JM, Stenman G, Kindblom LG. Differential diagnosis of small round cell tumors. Semin Diagn Pathol 1996; 13: 213–241

82. Ordonez NG. Desmoplastic small round cell tumor. II: an ultrastructural and immunohistochemical study with emphasis on new immunohistochemical markers. Am J Surg Pathol 1998; 22: 1314–1327

83. Dickersin GR, Rosenberg AE. The ultrastructure of small cell osteosarcoma, with a review of the light microscopy and differential diagnosis. Hum Pathol 1991; 22: 267–275

84. Folpe AL, Patterson K, Gown AM. Antibodies to desmin identify the blastemal component of nephroblastoma. Mod Pathol 1997; 10: 895–900

85. Papadimitriou JM, Henderson DW, Spangolo DV. Diagnostic Ultrastructure of Non-neoplastic Diseases. Edinburgh: Churchill Livingstone, 1992

86. Erlandson RA. Diagnostic Transmission Electron Microscopy of Tumors: With Clinicopathological, Immunohistochemical and Cytogenetic Correlations. New York: Raven Press, 1994

87. Mireau GW, Weeks DA, Hicks MJ. Role of electron microscopy and other special techniques in the diagnosis of childhood round cell tumors. Hum Pathol 1998; 29: 1347–1355

88. Mierau GW, Berry PJ, Malott RL, Weeks DA. Appraisal of the comparative utility of immunohistochemistry and electron microscopy in the diagnosis of childhood round cell tumors. Ultrastruct Pathol 1996; 20: 507–517

89. Yardi HM, Dardick I. Guides to Clinical Aspiration Biopsy. Diagnostic Immunocytochemistry and Electron Microscopy. New York: Igaku-Shoin, 1992

90. Thorner PS, Squire JA. Molecular genetics in the diagnosis and prognosis of solid pediatric tumors. Pediatr Dev Pathol 1998; 1: 337–365

91. Douglass EC, Valentine M, Etcubanas et al. A specific chromosomal abnormality in rhabdomyosarcoma. Cytogenet Cell Genet 1987; 45: 148–156

92. Whang-Peng J, Knutsen T, Theil K, Horowitz ME, Tiche TJ. Cytogenetic studies in subgroups of rhabdomyosarcoma. Gene Chromosom Cancer 1992; 5: 299–310

93. Davis RJ, D'Cruz CM, Lovell MA, Biegel JA, Barr FG. Fusion of PAX7 to FKHR by the variant t(1;13)(p36;q14) translocation in alveolar rhabdomyosarcoma. Cancer Res 1994; 54: 2869–2872

94. Driman D, Thoner PS, Greeenberg ML, Chilton-MacNeill S, Squire J. MYCN gene amplification in rhabdomyosarcoma. Cancer 1994; 73: 2231–2237

95. Weber-Hall S, Anderson J, McManus A et al. Gains, losses and amplications of genomic material in rhabdomyosarcoma analysed by comparative genomic hybridization. Cancer Res 1996; 56: 3220–3224

96. Gehring M, Berthold F, Edler L, Schwab M, Amler LC. The 1p deletion is not a reliable marker for the prognosis of patients with neuroblastoma. Cancer Res 1995; 55: 5366–5369

97. Maris JM, White PS, Beltinger CP et al. Significance of chromosome 1p loss of heterozygosity in neuroblastoma. Cancer Res 1995; 55: 4464–4669

98. Ambros IM, Zellner A, Roald B et al. Role of ploidy, chromosome 1p and Schwann cells in the maturation of neuroblastoma. N Engl J Med 1996; 334: 1505–1511

99. Zucman J, Delattre O, Desmaze C et al. Cloning and characterisation of the Ewing's sarcoma and peripheral neuroepithelioma t(11;22) translocation breakpoints. Gene Chromosom Cancer 1992; 5: 271–277

100. Mrowka C, Schel A. Wilms' tumor suppressor gene WT1: from structure to renal pathophysiologic features. J Am Soc Nephrol 2000; 11: S106–S115

2

Systemic lupus erythematosus and the kidney – lupus nephritis

M.A. Whittaker P.S. Bass M.E. Rogerson

INTRODUCTION

The term 'lupus' is derived from the Latin word for 'wolf' and has been used for centuries to describe a variety of skin conditions characterized by ulceration – literally a wolf's bite! Initially considered a chronic skin condition, lupus erythematosus was noted to exhibit more systemic, visceral involvement in the late 19th century. Iverson and Brun[1] first described percutaneous needle biopsy of the kidney as early as 1951. In 1957, Muehrcke *et al.*[2] published a comprehensive description of the renal biopsy findings characterizing lupus nephritis, which saw the tentative beginnings of a role for renal histopathology in the diagnosis and treatment of lupus nephritis. Today, percutaneous renal biopsy forms an important part of the staging and prognostication for patients suffering with systemic lupus erythematosus (SLE) affecting the kidney.

DEFINITION

SLE is best defined as a remitting and relapsing multisystem inflammatory syndrome with a complex and multifactorial pathogenesis. However, despite considerable work in this field, the precise aetiology still remains obscure. The clinical features of SLE are extremely variable and can closely resemble other connective tissue and non-connective tissue diseases. Consequently, the American College of Rheumatology (ACR) has published a list of criteria that

Mark A. Whittaker MRCPath, Consultant Histopathologist, Royal Hospital Haslar, Gosport, Hampshire, UK

Paul S. Bass BSc FRCPath, Consultant Histopathologist and Honorary Senior Lecturer, Southampton University Hospital Trust, Southampton, Hampshire, UK

Mary E. Rogerson FRCP, Consultant Nephrologist, Southampton University Hospital Trust, Southampton, Hampshire, UK

Table 2.1 ACR criteria for the diagnosis of lupus (revised 1982)

1. Butterfly malar rash
2. Discoid lupus
3. Photosensitivity
4. Oral ulcers
5. Arthritis
6. Serositis (pleuritis or pericarditis)
7. Renal disease (proteinuria and/or cellular casts)
8. Neurologic disorder (seizures or psychosis in absence of other cause)
9. Haemopoietic disorder (anaemia, leucopaenia, lymphopaenia, thrombocytopaenia)
10. Immunologic disorder (LE cell preparation, raised anti-DNA antibody, anti-Smith antibody, false-positive syphilis serology)
11. Positive immunofluoresence for antinuclear antibodies

can be applied to SLE to distinguish it from other closely related conditions. These were updated in 1982 and 1997[3,4] and are shown below (Table 2.1). SLE is characterized by inflammation and involvement of many organs and systems. The skin and musculoskeletal systems are usually involved, but there is often involvement of the heart, lungs, kidneys and central nervous system. The presence of four or more of the ACR criteria is usually taken as establishing the diagnosis with about 95% sensitivity and 96% specificity. The ACR criteria originally evolved to aid in distinguishing SLE from other connective tissue disorders, but over time they have become established as diagnostic criteria for this most protean of conditions.

EPIDEMIOLOGY

SLE is recognized worldwide, although its geographical incidence varies greatly. In the UK, the prevalence is reported as around 12 cases per 100 000 population.[5] However, there are striking sexual and racial differences. The disease is more common in women with the incidence reported as 45.4 cases per 100 000 in woman compared to 3.7 cases per 100 000 in men.[6] Similarly, Afro-Caribbeans living in the UK are far more prone to this illness than Caucasians – 206 and 36.2 cases per 100 000, respectively[7] – although paradoxically the disease appears to be rare in Africa.[8] There is recent evidence that the incidence of SLE has increased approximately three-fold over the last two decades in both Europe and America.[9,10]

Most affected women will develop their illness between the ages of 15 and 40 years suggesting a link to female sex hormones. Genetic factors appear to be important. Monozygotic twins show 25% concordance for the development of SLE and healthy relatives of SLE sufferers often have detectable autoantibodies characteristic of SLE, albeit at low titres. There is a weak association with HLA-DR and some patients have inherited deficiencies of complement components. Infectious agents have been considered, but no convincing evidence has emerged. Drugs may occasionally precipitate a lupus syndrome, but this rarely affects the kidney.[5]

CLINICAL MANIFESTATIONS OF LUPUS

The classical presentation of a young woman with a butterfly rash, non-deforming arthropathy, fever, pericarditis and photosensitivity is rare. More often, the disease presents in a subtle and confusing fashion with apparently non-specific features that make the diagnosis difficult to reach. Patients may present with pyrexia of unknown origin, neuropsychiatric symptoms, abnormal urinary sediment or even pulmonary embolism. In such circumstances, a diagnosis of SLE may not even be considered initially, although nearly all of these patients will have autoantibodies in their serum, which may prove helpful. Although many conditions are characterized by different autoantibodies, some autoantibodies are highly suggestive, if not virtually diagnostic of SLE. The presence of double-stranded DNA (dsDNA) and antibodies to the Smith antigen (anti-Sm) fall into this category.[5]

CLINICAL MANIFESTATIONS OF LUPUS NEPHRITIS

In most cases, a diagnosis of SLE will be reached on the basis of clinical and laboratory indices. Less than half of all SLE patients will have renal abnormalities early in the course of their disease, but with follow-up, as many as 50–80% of adults will develop overt renal features at some time.[11] Nearly, all SLE patients will show abnormalities on renal biopsy, even in the absence of overt renal symptomatology.[12,13] The main presenting feature is that of proteinuria, although any renal 'syndrome' may be seen including microscopic haematuria, nephrotic syndrome and rarely, in more severe forms, acute renal failure. Clearly, in more established and long-standing cases, chronic renal failure may occur. It is perhaps worth noting that, although SLE is rare in children, nearly 80% of those who are diagnosed with this condition will develop lupus nephritis. The prognosis for these patients is closely related to the severity of their renal disease.[5]

PATHOGENESIS OF SYSTEMIC LUPUS ERYTHEMATOSUS

The fundamental underlying defect in SLE appears to be that of an autoimmune disorder and a large number of autoantibodies are seen. While it is important not to overlook the role of other autoantibodies, such as those directed against phospholipids, the cardinal feature of SLE is the production of antibodies directed against nuclear constituents, so-called antinuclear antibodies (ANAs).[14]

Many ANAs are non-specific and may be seen in apparently healthy individuals, particularly with increasing age. Others are seen in a range of connective tissue diseases, such as systemic sclerosis or Sjogren's syndrome, while some are relatively specific or even almost pathognomonic of SLE. Anti-dsDNA, seen in 70% of cases, and anti-Sm, seen in 30% of cases, would fall into this latter category.[15] Although anti-dsDNA titres often rise prior to relapses in SLE,[16] there is a lack of definitive proof for ANAs being directly pathogenic in lupus nephritis.

Infusion of pure ANA immune complexes rarely leads to glomerular localisation or lupus nephritis experimentally.[17] Free DNA is not present in the circulation of patients with SLE and other studies have shown that 'naked' DNA is very poorly immunogenic.[17,18]

Evidence suggests that the autoantigen response in SLE is T-cell dependent.[19] This is based on the observation that anti-DNA-specific CD4 positive T-helper cells are seen and the autoantibodies produced are predominantly of T-cell-dependent IgG isotypes.[20] If DNA is poorly immunogenic, how do anti-DNA-specific T-cells develop? Immunologic tolerance for DNA can be broken if DNA is complexed with DNA-binding proteins, such as histones or nucleosomes.[21] Interestingly, it has been shown that high-affinity anti-DNA antibodies bind even more strongly to nucleosomes than they do to DNA.[22] As many as 80% of SLE patients will express nucleosome-specific antibodies that will not react with nucleosome constituents, that is DNA or histones.[23] The bottom line is that many ANAs are also directed against, and bind to, nucleosomes.

Nucleosomes are formed of a central histone protein octamer around which is wound two superhelical turns of DNA. Adjacent nucleosomes are joined by stretches of linker DNA. The N-terminal regions of the core histones are located on the outside of the histone and create regions of strong positive (cationic) charge.[24] These are involved not only with DNA binding, but appear to be pivotal in the pathogenesis of lupus nephritis. As stated previously, infusion of anti-dsDNA immune complexes does not result in significant glomerular localisation of antibody, or in fact, lead to nephritis experimentally. What has been shown is that ANAs often bind to circulating nucleosome particles, and it is the nucleosomes that actually mediate binding of ANAs to the glomerular basement membrane (GBM).[25] This occurs via the positively charged N-terminal regions of the core histone proteins interacting with anionic (negatively charged) residues of heparan sulphate, and to a lesser extent, collagen IV, within the GBM. Enzymatic removal of heparan sulphate considerably reduces binding of nucleosome-complexed ANAs, indicating the importance of this mechanism in the localisation of ANAs to the GBM.[26] A particularly fascinating development is the demonstration that heparin, which has a similar structure to heparan sulphate, inhibits binding of nucleosome-complexed ANA to the GBM, and reduces the severity of glomerulonephritis (GN) in lupus-prone mice.[27]

Where do nucleosome particles come from? The most likely source would appear to be via apoptosis. Apoptosis is programmed cell death and is an active process requiring enzyme activity. One such enzyme is endonuclease, which causes internucleosomal fragmentation of DNA, therefore, producing nucleosome-sized fragments. These fragments are usually clustered together with other degraded cell constituents into membrane-bound apoptotic bodies that bud from the surface of the dying cell. Adjacent cells prevent the release of this potentially immunogenic material by rapidly phagocytosing the apoptotic bodies. However, if the processes of apoptosis or phagocytosis are disturbed, then the systemic release of nucleosomes could occur. There is evidence that apoptosis is indeed disturbed in SLE patients.[25]

Disturbances in apoptosis could precede the development of SLE in an additional way. The mature population of adult T-lymphocytes is achieved through the process of deletion of autoreactive T-cells in the foetal thymus and the major mechanism for such deletion is apoptosis. A disturbance in apoptosis could result in the persistence of autoreactive T-cells, which survive thymic deletion. These T-cells may persist into adult life in a state of suppression, with the emergence of autoreactive T-cells, and subsequently, the production of autoantibodies if this suppression fails.[5,28]

A different hypothesis to explain the production of autoantigens is that of antigenic mimicry. If viral or bacterial peptides contain sequences that are similar or identical to native antigens, there may be activation of T-cells and inadvertent production of autoantibodies. Similarly, there is a possibility that the autoantibodies arise as a result of direct polyclonal B-cell activation, perhaps as a result of exposure to superantigens.[5]

The currently favoured hypotheses regarding the aetiology of SLE include those of disturbed apoptosis leading to nucleosome fragment release with subsequent activation of T-cells. It may be that apoptotic cleavage of DNA into nucleosome-sized fragments, and its subsequent processing into small peptide fragments for display in MHC Class II molecules by antigen presenting cells, exposes novel antigenic sites to the immune system that favour a strong T-cell response.[29]

One should not forget the potential effects of autoantigens directed against non-nuclear antigens. Antiphospholipid antibodies (APA) are seen in 25–50% of SLE patients and are mainly directed against β2-globulin phospholipid-carrier protein. These APAs prolong clotting times *in vitro* (activated partial thromboplastin time (APTT)), but are associated with increased risk of thrombosis *in vivo*.[15] Consequently, these patients are at increased risk of such events as renovascular thrombosis, stroke, foetal loss and non-bacterial thrombotic endocarditis (Libman–Sacks endocarditis). Antibodies directed against red blood cells, leucocytes, lymphocytes or platelets can result in various cytopaenias.

MEDIATION OF GLOMERULAR INJURY IN LUPUS NEPHRITIS

There is no reason to suppose that the mechanism of injury in lupus induced GN is any different to that of many other forms of immune complex-mediated GN. There is a Type III hypersensitivity reaction with subsequent activation of complement, release of cytokines and recruitment of inflammatory cells, which results in tissue damage. It is important to remember that the mesangial matrix is essentially basement membrane material and contains heparan sulphate that may interact with histone proteins within nucleosomes in much the same manner as occurs at the GBM.

LABORATORY INVESTIGATIONS IN SYSTEMIC LUPUS ERYTHEMATOSUS

The cardinal feature of SLE is the presence of ANA. However, while most patients with SLE will have ANAs, it is not true to say that most patients with ANAs will have SLE.[15] Up to one-third of healthy patients will have low titres of ANA detectable on screening. The method for detecting ANA is not specified in the ACR criteria and several techniques exist that may give differing results.

The Farr assay will detect high-affinity ANA, immunofluoresence (IF) will detect moderate and high-affinity ANA and enzyme-linked immunosorbent assay (ELISA) will detect low- and high-affinity ANA. The most common screening test performed in the UK is IF with test serum applied to rodent liver or human epithelial (HEp2) tissue. Those samples found to be ANA positive on this initial screening test will then be subjected to more specific assays, such as ELISA or Farr assay, which are commonly used for this purpose.[15]

INDICATIONS FOR RENAL BIOPSY

The diagnosis of SLE is usually, but not always, already established in patients presenting with renal signs and symptoms. Some authors question the need for renal biopsy in such patients, arguing that the disease can be diagnosed and managed on the basis of its clinical presentation alone.[30] The majority of clinicians, however, feel that renal biopsy is extremely valuable in the assessment and management of lupus nephritis.[5,13,31–33] Generally, patients who have an abnormal urine sediment, significant proteinuria (with or without haematuria) or a raised creatinine will undergo renal biopsy. Histology enables characterisation of the severity, distribution and type of renal lesion, which provides prognostic information and informs the choice of initial treatment protocols. With newer and more effective treatment regimes available to clinicians, the clinical course of these patients has changed significantly and is now more difficult to evaluate using clinical parameters alone.[34] For this reason, renal biopsy appears even more important today in providing relevant prognostic information and the majority of clinicians will continue to advocate the use of this diagnostic/ prognostic tool.

PATHOLOGICAL CHANGES OF LUPUS NEPHRITIS

GLOMERULAR CHANGES IN LUPUS NEPHRITIS

The plethora of clinical symptoms and the diversity of autoantibodies seen in SLE patients are recapitulated in the renal biopsy appearances. The World Health Organization (WHO) classification of renal lupus is based purely on glomerular findings and divides lupus nephritis into five categories on the basis of light microscopic (LM), immunohistochemical (IP or IF) and electron microscopic (EM) findings (Table 2.2).[35] This has been modified into a more detailed and expanded WHO classification, but the original classification is more widely used, although more limited in value.[5] In order to classify lupus nephritis accurately, it is mandatory to perform all three investigations (LM, IP/IF and EM) on patients known or suspected to have SLE.

WHO CLASS I (NORMAL)

This is a very rare finding on renal biopsy as patients with normal urine and renal function are unlikely to be biopsied in normal clinical practice and even

Table 2.2 WHO classification of lupus nephritis[34]

Class	Light microscopy	Immunohistology	Electron microscopy
I	No lesion	No lesion	No lesion
II	Purely mesangial disease IIa Normocellular IIb Hypercellular	Mesangial IgG, C3	Mesangial deposits
III	Focal segmental necrosis and proliferation	Granular capillary and mesangial Ig, C3	Mesangial and subendothelial deposits
IV	Mesangial proliferation; membranoproliferative and/or crescentic pattern	Same as Class III 'full-house' pattern	Mesangial and sub-endothelial proliferation; subepithelial deposits
V	Diffuse membranous thickening	Membranous granular IgG, C3	Subepithelial deposits; often mesangial deposits

patients without evidence of renal disease will usually show minor histological changes. There are no glomerular abnormalities by light microscopy, immuno-histology or electron microscopy.

WHO CLASS II (MESANGIAL DISEASE)

This category is subdivided into Class IIa and b according to the absence or presence of mesangial hypercellularity, respectively. Mesangial immune deposits can be detected by immunohistology and electron microscopy, but no significant subendothelial deposits are present. Mesangial hypercellularity is defined as more than three or four mesangial cell nuclei in a mesangial tuft, away from the vascular pole, in a 3 μm section. The changes can range from focal to diffuse (affecting few or many glomeruli) and segmental to global (affecting part or all of a glomerulus). This pattern usually forms a background pattern in other, higher WHO classes but, in itself, rarely transforms to a higher class.[36] Clinically, many of these patients will be asymptomatic, but around 30% will show mild proteinuria or haematuria, although the vast majority will have normal renal function. The prognosis for this WHO class is, therefore, excellent.

WHO CLASS III (FOCAL PROLIFERATIVE GLOMERULONEPHRITIS)

Most authorities consider Classes III and IV lesions to be qualitatively similar processes.[5,36] Class III lupus nephritis is characterized by segmental hypercellularity, often associated with necrosis, in up to 50% of the glomeruli sampled. The hypercellularity is composed of endothelial and mesangial cells as well as infiltrating neutrophils and mononuclear inflammatory cells – so-called endocapillary proliferation. Mesangial deposits can be identified with immunohistology, but in addition deposits are also located on the GBM, seen in a subendothelial location with electron microscopy. At times, the subendothelial deposits can be so large as to be visible by light microscopy. If the deposits encircle a capillary wall, this can appear as a 'wire-loop' lesion, a glassy, eosinophilic thickened capillary wall. These are seen as large or confluent subendothelial electron dense deposits. Another pattern seen may be that of a so-called 'hyaline thrombus', where a subendothelial deposit of immunoglobulin may become so massive as to protrude into the capillary lumen and occlude it with a glassy eosinophilic mass. Clinically, these patients usually present with mild to moderate proteinuria and/or haematuria, although some will present with nephrotic syndrome. A degree of renal impairment is seen in approximately 25% of patients. However, the prognosis is good, unless there is transformation to the more aggressive Class IV disease, which seems to occur in approximately 30% of cases.

WHO CLASS IV (DIFFUSE PROLIFERATIVE GLOMERULONEPHRITIS)

As previously noted, Class IV lupus nephritis is similar to Class III, but varies in severity and degree. Arbitrarily, over 50% of glomeruli must be affected by this endocapillary proliferation to fall into this group (compared to less than 50% in Class III), so clearly these two classes form a spectrum of disease, albeit with different natural histories if left untreated. The capillary wall changes tend to be more pronounced in Class IV lesions with more frequent wire loops and hyaline thrombi. Necrosis is also more widespread and crescent formation (proliferation of tuft parietal epithelial cells and inflammatory cells within Bowman's capsule) more likely (Fig. 2.1). By immunohistology, the presence of more diffuse capillary wall deposits is seen, again demonstrated in a subendothelial location by electron microscopy. Mesangial deposits, as expected, are also present. In a similar fashion to Class III lupus nephritis, the presence of prominent mesangial and subendothelial deposits in Class IV lesions can lead to an appearance closely mimicking membranoproliferative GN with an expanded, hypercellular mesangium and double contoured GBM seen on PAS/Silver staining. The presence of large numbers of crescents is a poor prognostic sign. Tubulointerstitial inflammation is most pronounced in Class IV lesions compared to other classes and there may also be immune deposits within vessel walls and tubular basement membranes

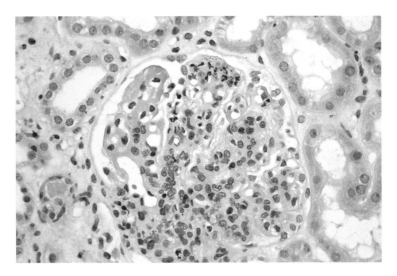

Fig. 2.1 WHO Class IV lupus nephritis. Note the wire loops and necrosis in the capillary tuft. H&E ×400.

(Fig. 2.2). Clinically, this class is the most severe form of lupus nephritis with most patients presenting with proteinuria and haematuria, and 50% with the nephrotic syndrome.[33] Three quarters will have impaired renal function and renal failure is a common outcome, if these patients remain untreated.

WHO CLASS V (MEMBRANOUS GLOMERULONEPHRITIS)

By light microscopy, the Class V lesion is almost indistinguishable from idiopathic membranous GN (Fig. 2.3). In well-established lesions, there is diffuse capillary wall thickening with spike formation seen on PAS/Silver staining. At later stages, intramembranous immune complex deposits may impart a chain/loop-like appearance with these stains as the deposits become surrounded by GBM

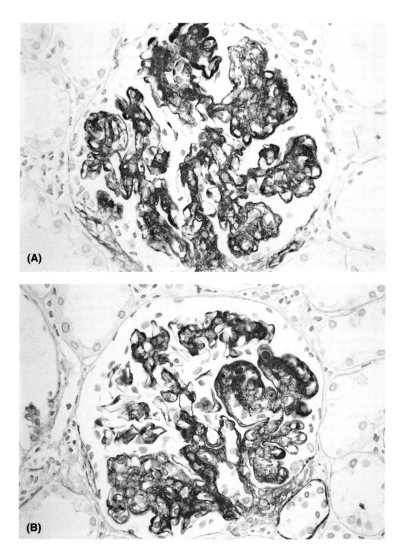

(A)

(B)

Fig. 2.2 WHO Class IV lupus nephritis. Immunoperoxidase staining showing strong granular deposits of (A) C3 and (B) IgM. Immunoperoxidase ×400.

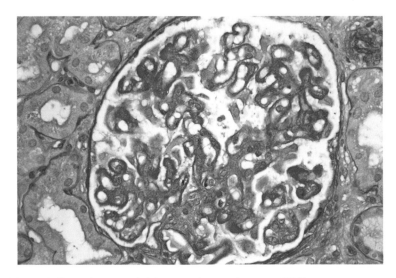

Fig. 2.3 WHO Class V lupus nephritis. Note the membranous GN-like appearance. PAS ×400.

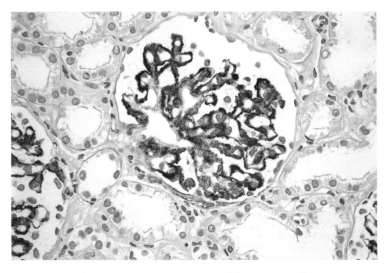

Fig. 2.4 WHO Class V lupus nephritis. Immunoperoxidase staining showing strong granular deposits of IgG. Immunoperoxidase ×400.

material. However, unlike primary membranous disease, Class V lupus nephritis is nearly always associated with at least mild mesangial hypercellularity and matrix expansion. Immunohistology will demonstrate capillary wall immune complex deposition but, in this instance, unlike Class IV lupus nephritis, the deposits will be seen in a subepithelial location (Fig. 2.4). Immune complexes will also be found in the mesangium. Clinically, as in primary membranous GN, Class V lupus nephritis presents with proteinuria, mainly within the nephrotic range and generally progresses slowly. Transformation to a more aggressive, proliferative Class III or IV nephritis is uncommon. Renal insufficiency is also uncommon, as is significant tubulointerstitial damage with which it correlates. One relatively common complication that supervenes on Class V lupus nephritis (and in other causes of the nephrotic syndrome) is that of renal vein thrombosis. This is reported to occur in between 10% and 50% of cases.[5] This possibility should always be considered in cases of membranous-type lupus nephritis.

WHO CLASS VI (ADVANCED SCLEROSING GLOMERULOPATHY)

This class was introduced into the modified WHO classification and is worth mentioning if only for completeness sake. This represents the end stage of lupus nephritis and is characterized by glomerulosclerosis, tubular atrophy and interstitial fibrosis. The kidney may be so scarred that the underlying aetiology is difficult to ascertain, but immunohistochemistry may demonstrate the presence of immune complexes within glomeruli to hint at the diagnosis. Clinically, this class of lupus nephritis usually presents with proteinuria and hypertension and progresses remorselessly to chronic renal failure.

MIXED FORMS

As previously stated, a continuum exists between Classes III and IV lupus nephritis, and unsurprisingly other mixed forms of lupus nephritis occur. Most commonly, these are mixtures of Class V and Classes III and IV. In this instance, the prognosis of the glomerular lesion is that of the disease with the worse prognosis.

TUBULOINTERSTITIAL CHANGES IN LUPUS NEPHRITIS

One drawback with the WHO classification of lupus nephritis is that it concentrates on glomerular changes and largely ignores important changes within the tubulointerstitium. About 50% of patients with nephritis, more in Class IV, will have immune deposits within the tubular basement membrane and a chronic inflammatory cell infiltrate within the interstitium.[5] As the disease progresses, more chronic changes ensue and the interstitium becomes expanded with fibrous tissue and tubules become atrophic. It has been shown that damage to the tubulointerstitial compartment of the kidney correlates much more closely with impaired renal function than does glomerular damage. The mechanism appears to be that interstitial events may lead to destruction of peritubular capillaries, which are derived from the efferent glomerular arteriole. Loss of these capillaries leads firstly to tubular ischaemia and atrophy, and secondly to a rise in glomerular capillary pressure, which may damage the glomerulus. Glomerulosclerosis may follow, leading to a reduction in numbers of glomeruli, and ultimately, causing impairment of glomerular filtration rate/renal function.[37] Clearly, avoiding chronic damage to this compartment is crucial to maintain satisfactory renal function.

VASCULAR CHANGES IN LUPUS NEPHRITIS

The most common abnormality seen in renal vessels is immune complex deposition within the intima and media of arterioles, arteries and veins. This is demonstrated by immunohistology in Classes III and IV disease, but appears to have no clinical significance.[36] Much more uncommonly, in severe Class IV nephritis, arterioles may show immune complex deposition associated with fibrinoid degeneration, although lacking the inflammatory infiltrate seen in true vasculitis. This is an extremely poor prognostic feature.[36]

IMMUNOHISTOLOGY AND ELECTRON MICROSCOPY IN LUPUS NEPHRITIS

Classically, immune complexes in lupus nephritis are granular and are present not only within the mesangium, but also capillary walls depending on WHO class. IgG is usually the dominant immunoglobulin, but one would expect to also see IgM and IgA deposition. Early complement components C1q and C4 are also strongly expressed and C3 would be expected to be present. When all of the immunoglobulins and complement components are positive, a 'full house' deposit is said to be present – a classical feature of lupus nephritis that would not normally be expected in any other type of glomerulopathy.

Electron microscopy is the third modality for examination of renal biopsies (the first two being light microscopy/histochemistry and immunohistology). Not all centres perform electron microscopy routinely as it is time consuming and expensive. Also, many types of GN can be adequately diagnosed without using it. However, some renal pathologists will routinely perform all three modalities before making a diagnosis. In the case of lupus nephritis, it is essentially mandatory to enable accurate WHO classification. A recent paper suggested that electron microscopy provides clinically meaningful information in 45% of renal biopsies in general.[38] In lupus nephritis, the important diagnoses to make are those of Class III and, especially, Class IV nephritis with its more aggressive clinical course (Fig. 2.5). The subendothelial location of the immune complex deposits can only really be confirmed with the use of electron microscopy and is a marker of disease activity. Similarly, biopsies classified as Class II (mesangial) or Class V (membranous) nephritis may show the presence of large subendothelial deposits by electron microscopy. In this instance, such a finding may denote the imminent transformation to a more aggressive proliferative lesion, indicating the need for early treatment.[31] Another area in which electron microscopy can be of crucial importance is in the assessment of post-transplant kidneys to distinguish between recurrence of lupus and graft rejection. The histological changes of transplant rejection can closely mimic lupus nephritis and immunohistology may be unsatisfactory due to immunosuppression. The presence of electron dense deposits within glomeruli can, therefore, provide strong evidence of recurrence of an immune complex-mediated disease.[39]

PROGNOSIS OF LUPUS NEPHRITIS

The prognosis of lupus nephritis has altered drastically over the last 30 years. In the 1950s and 1960s, the 5-year survival for all patients with lupus nephritis was only 44%. For those with the most severe form of diffuse proliferative lupus

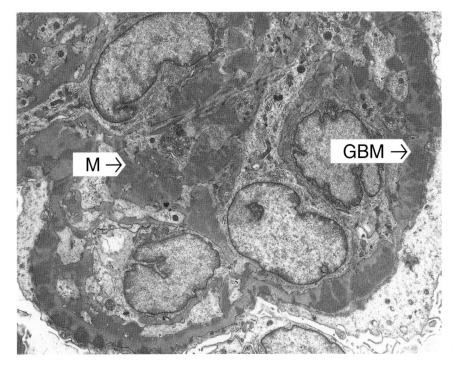

Fig. 2.5 WHO Class IV lupus nephritis. Electron photomicrograph showing both mesangial (M) and GBM electron dense deposits. EM ×4000.

nephritis (WHO Class IV), this figure fell to 17%.[40] However, the advent of new therapeutic regimes, particularly steroids, has altered this outlook, such that in the early 1990s, the figures were 92% and 82%, respectively.[40] Consequently, the clinical course of lupus nephritis has now changed as a result of better management, such that the outcome for patients with Class IV nephritis now differs very little from lupus nephritis as a whole.[5,40] Today, almost all patients with renal involvement will receive treatment including those with mild Class II nephritis. What has been shown is that early treatment results in better preservation of renal function compared to late treatment.[32]

NATURAL HISTORY OF LUPUS NEPHRITIS

Although the short- and medium-term outcome has been studied extensively, the long-term outlook for patients with lupus nephritis has not. In one of the few papers to examine this, Bono *et al.* studied 110 patients over a median period of 15.5 years, and found that in more recent years, the survival of patients had improved significantly.[41] The principal causes of death were sepsis, myocardial infarction and cerebrovascular accidents.[42] However, the risks for these outcomes were no different for patients with end-stage renal disease (ESRD) caused by lupus nephritis than for ESRD due to other causes.[42] Among the long-term surviving patients, 38% had normal urine and renal function, 62%

had persistent proteinuria and 18% had impaired but stable renal function.[41] If ESRD does develop, it occurs during the first decade of the disease, with very few, if any, patients developing renal failure after more than 10 years.[41] Such findings suggest that in the long term, this disease fizzles out, with or without permanent renal damage. It is interesting to note that between 1982 and 1995, the incidence of ESRD due to lupus nephritis increased steadily, almost doubling, despite the introduction of new, more effective treatment regimes during this period.[43] This increase is directly comparable to the increase in ESRD due to other forms of renal disease, probably a reflection of improved patient survival.[41]

ACTIVITY AND CHRONICITY INDICES

The WHO classification is a useful prognostic tool. A more controversial tool is the activity and chronicity index scoring suggested by the American National Institute of Health (NIH) (Table 2.3).[5] Some feel that this may be a more accurate indicator of long-term prognosis than the WHO classification,[44] although this is not universally accepted.[45] Activity indices, of which there are six (see Table 2.3), reflect acute, potentially reversible renal damage and are scored out of 24. The four indices of chronicity reflect permanent damage that cannot be reversed and are scored out of 12. Each feature is graded from 0 (absent), 1 (mild), 2 (moderate) or 3 (severe) and the scores added together in each index to give a semi-quantitative outcome. Some studies have suggested that a high-chronicity index (>3) predicts a poor outcome, especially when combined with a high-activity index (>10).[46,47] Although there is disagreement about the validity of the NIH indices, most clinicians would accept that these indices do provide at least a rough estimate of the potential reversibility of a given lupus nephritis. In the practical environment of everyday practice, such quantitative methods may not be used. In these circumstances, the renal biopsy report would mention the presence or absence of these features, providing useful information as to which patients should perhaps receive aggressive chemotherapy and which should not. New attempts at fine-tuning these indices have been published, but are extremely complex and are as yet clinically unproven.[48]

Table 2.3 National Institute of Health scoring indices in lupus nephritis

Index of activity (0–24)	
Endocapillary hypercellularity	(0–3)
Leucocyte infiltration	(0–3)
Subendothelial hyaline deposits	(0–3)
Fibrinoid necrosis/karyorrhexis	(0–3) × 2
Cellular crescents	(0–3) × 2
Interstitial inflammation	(0–3)
Index of chronicity (0–12)	
Sclerotic glomeruli	(0–3)
Fibrous crescents	(0–3)
Tubular atrophy	(0–3)
Interstitial fibrosis	(0–3)

HISTOLOGICAL DIFFERENTIAL DIAGNOSIS OF LUPUS NEPHRITIS

As might be expected from the description of the various WHO classes of lupus nephritis, the disease is a great mimic of many types of glomerulopathy (Table 2.4). As such, the diagnosis of lupus always needs to be borne in mind, when examining a renal biopsy, especially if the patient is a young female. A particular pointer towards a diagnosis of lupus nephritis is the pattern of immunohistology seen; a 'full house' deposit of immunoglobulin and complement components is highly suggestive. While a diagnosis of lupus nephritis can be suggested on such a basis, a firm diagnosis is the realm of the clinician based on laboratory and ACR clinical criteria.

CURRENT TREATMENT OPTIONS

There is currently no specific cure for SLE or lupus nephritis.[5,49] However, there are two distinct phases in the treatment of lupus nephritis. The first is the induction of remission in the acute phase of disease. The second is the maintenance phase, where there is a requirement for long-term management of chronic, usually low-grade, disease.[5] The drugs currently used in treating lupus nephritis are generally similar for each of these two phases of treatment, but the aim of treatment and drug protocols differ.[5,50] In the induction phase, the patient is at acute risk and control of the disease process is most important, with less regard to side effects of treatment. During the maintenance phase, the reverse is the case, with limitation of side effects being of most importance.[5,49]

CORTICOSTEROIDS

Induction therapy, currently, usually comprises high doses of corticosteroids. Prolonged high-dose oral prednisolone has significant side effects and most clinicians compromise by using pulsed intravenous methylprednisolone with a reducing course of oral prednisolone. This has the benefit of less side effects

Table 2.4 Differential diagnosis of lupus GN

Mesangial disease (WHO Class II)	IgA nephropathy (Berger's disease) Henoch–Schonlein purpura
Focal proliferative GN (WHO Class III)	IgA nephropathy (Berger's disease) Henoch–Schonlein purpura Bacterial endocarditis Vasculitis (i.e. ANCA-related diseases)
Diffuse proliferative GN (WHO Class IV)	Post-infectious GN Membranoproliferative GN Crescentic GN (and its causes)
Membranous GN (WHO Class V)	Idiopathic membranous GN 2° membranous GN (drugs, neoplasia) Membranoproliferative GN

and rapid onset of action in reducing acute lesions. In maintenance therapy, corticosteroids remain the mainstay of therapy, used at a low dose and often on an alternate day regime to minimise side effects.[5,30,50]

CYTOTOXIC AGENTS

For induction purposes, cyclophosphamide appears to be the cytotoxic agent of choice. This is a powerful inhibitor of B-cells, resulting in rapid reduction in autoantibody levels and can be given orally or intravenously. It is usually combined with corticosteroids and helps to prevent progression of chronic lesions.[5,30,50] However, this drug has serious side effects including a 50–70% risk of amenorrhoea/early menopause in women after long-term use.[5,49,51] This risk increases with age. Its use in pregnancy is absolutely contraindicated due to a powerful teratogenic effect, and it is associated with urothelial damage ranging from haemorrhagic cystitis to invasive cancer.[5] Other malignancies are also seen, such as lymphoma and skin cancers.[51] Clearly, its use as a maintenance drug is problematic.

Azathioprine is a much safer drug with no significant risk of sterility and is safe to use in pregnancy.[5] Several studies have examined the efficacy of azathioprine compared to cyclophosphamide in lupus nephritis and no significant difference between the two has emerged. As a result of the more powerful B-cell inhibition shown by cyclophosphamide, this drug tends to be used in the induction phase with a switch to azathioprine in the maintenance phase. It has been shown that the use of corticosteroids with cytotoxic agents improves renal outcome considerably compared to steroids alone.[52,53]

RENAL-REPLACEMENT THERAPY

DIALYSIS

Since the advent of corticosteroids and cytotoxic agents in the treatment of patients with SLE and lupus nephritis, survival figures have improved radically. Consequently, more patients are surviving long enough to develop ESRD, although the actual incidence appears to have been relatively stable for the last 30 years[5,54] at between 10% and 20% of patients. Although not initially considered appropriate for SLE patients because of the systemic nature of their illness, it is now clear that dialysis, both haemodialysis and continuous ambulatory peritoneal dialysis (CAPD), are as effective in these patients as in non-SLE patients. The five-year survival of SLE patients treated with dialysis is at least as good as that for non-SLE patients, and ranges between 80% and 90%.[55,56] The only significant problem appears to be susceptibility to thrombosis in some patients, mainly related to APA, which could be problematic in the arteriovenous shunt required for haemodialysis.[5] In view of this excellent prognosis, it is no longer of paramount importance to prevent ESRD at all costs in patients with already tenuous renal function. Patient survival is no different if ESRD is avoided or not. One benefit of dialysis is the ability to reduce or even stop immunosuppressive drugs, where there is insignificant extra-renal disease, reducing the risk of serious infection.

Recent data for renal transplants suggest that graft and patient survival in SLE is not significantly different to those patients with non-SLE glomerular diseases.[57] Only a few extra precautions need to be considered in SLE patients. Firstly, there may be difficulties in cross matching due to autoantibodies, although in reality, this does not affect graft outcome.[5] Secondly, as in dialysis, there may be APA causing increased susceptibility to renal vessel thrombosis, necessitating the use of anticoagulants. These problems aside renal transplantation is remarkably successful.[5,49]

An intriguing by-product of transplantation in SLE appears to be a very low level of recurrence of lupus nephritis in the transplanted kidney, even where the disease was active at the time of transplantation.[54,58] It has been estimated at around 1%, and even in this circumstance, it very rarely causes graft failure. Why disease activity should be so diminished in transplant patients is unclear; certainly, the post-transplant drug regimes are little different to those used in pre-transplantation, which failed to control the disease progression to ESRD.

EMERGING TREATMENT OPTIONS

There are several, widely diverging, new therapeutic options being actively investigated. Some show considerable promise.

CHEMOTHERAPY/IMMUNOSUPPRESSION

Mycophenolate mofetil is an inhibitor of purine synthesis that has been shown to be more effective than azathioprine in preventing acute rejection of transplanted organs. In murine SLE studies, it is also more effective at preventing progressive lupus nephritis.[59] Human trials are being initiated and appear encouraging.[60,61] Fludarabine is an adenosine analogue, the activity of which depends on kinase enzymes, which are most prevalent in lymphoid cells. It is used in lymphoid malignancies at present, but is being evaluated in several autoimmune diseases, including SLE.[50]

In patients with severe disease that is refractory to treatment, there is considerable interest in bone marrow ablation and restitution.[50] Two methods are being investigated. The first is bone marrow ablation with chemotherapy followed by either allogenic bone marrow transplantation or stem cell reconstitution. The second is high-dose ablative chemotherapy followed by intensive medical support and granulocyte colony stimulating factor (G-CSF) treatment.[62] This technique appears to show only a modest delay in reconstituting peripheral granulocytes and platelets over stem cell re-infusion, and has the advantage of being considerably less expensive than stem cell harvesting and avoids the graft versus host disease of allogenic bone marrow transplantation. Although the results have been promising in terms of sustained remission,[63] there are problems with substantial morbidity and mortality.[64]

LYMPHOCYTE INHIBITORS

A two-stage signalling process is necessary to develop and sustain most antigen-specific humoral and cellular immune responses. After an antigen has been processed and displayed in MHC Class II molecules on the surface of an antigen presenting cell, it interacts with the T-cell receptor (on a T-cell), thus forming the first signal to that T-cell. This first signal causes it to express an activation receptor molecule, CD156 (also called CD40L), on its surface. This receptor forms the basis of the second, co-stimulatory signal, when it interacts with its activating ligand, CD40, present on the surface of the B-cells. This second, co-stimulatory signal leads to full activation of that T-cell and clonal expansion of T-helper cells for development of a highly specific humoral and cellular immune response against the original antigen. At the same time as expressing the activation receptor CD156, the T-cell also expresses an inhibition receptor called CTLA4, which antagonizes T-cell activation, thereby modulating T-helper cell function. The importance of this two-stage activation process became clear, when it was realized that a T-cell that receives the first signal but not the second, co-stimulatory signal, will undergo apoptosis resulting in inhibition of development of antigen-specific T-cells, and consequently, inhibition of a specific humoral and cellular response to a given antigen. Experimentally, antibodies directed against CD156 and also CTLA4 analogue (i.e. a synthetic CTLA4) have profound effects on immune responses without producing generalized immunosuppression.[65] Clearly, these agents are very exciting therapeutic prospects.

COMPLEMENT INHIBITORS

Complement activation by immunoglobulin within immune complexes is integral to the immune-mediated damage seen in lupus nephritis (and other forms of GN). Experimental studies in mice have shown monoclonal antibody directed against C5b, part of the membrane attack complex of complement reduces the severity of lupus nephritis.[66]

IMMUNOMODULANT THERAPY

Reducing ANA titres without the use of general immunosuppressants is desirable but, currently, not achievable. One possible therapy is LJP-394, which can specifically reduce anti-dsDNA titres by targeting anti-dsDNA-specific B-cells.[50,67] LJP-394 binds to B-cell receptors in the absence of a co-stimulatory signal from a T-cell or APC, thus, inducing apoptosis in the anti-dsDNA-specific B-cell population. In mice with overt nephritis, LJP-394 increased animal survival by 300%.[68] In humans, significant falls in anti-dsDNA antibody titres have been observed.

GENE THERAPY

In some animal models, successful gene therapy has already been achieved[69] with Fas-ligand gene transfer in lupus-prone mice. While treatment in humans must wait for adequate delineation of disease promoting genes, the prospects are certainly exciting.

PLASMAPHERESIS

While an obvious rationale for plasma exchange can be seen for lupus, with vast arrays of circulating autoantibodies present in the plasma of sufferers, several controlled trials have failed to demonstrate any benefit from the addition of plasmapheresis to current treatment protocols. As such, there does not appear to be a role for plasma exchange in the treatment of SLE.[5,49,50]

CONCLUSIONS

Most patients with SLE will eventually develop lupus nephritis with overt renal features. These could include proteinuria, nephrotic syndrome, haematuria and even renal failure. Renal biopsy in such patients is useful in providing valuable information about prognosis to clinicians and helps to guide treatment regimes. The histological findings can be interpreted according to the WHO classification and the prognosis for these patients correlates well with the WHO class. It is important to examine these biopsies with light microscopy, immunohistology and electron microscopy. Current treatment protocols make use of cortico-steroids and immunosuppressant drugs, such as azathioprine and cyclophos-phamide, but new therapeutic options are being actively investigated with some showing considerable promise.

KEY POINTS

- SLE is a multisystem autoimmune disorder defined according to criteria set out by the ACR.
- Most patients with SLE will eventually develop features of lupus nephritis.
- SLE is characterized by ANAs directed against anti-dsDNA and the anti-Sm.
- Nucleosomes and disordered apoptosis appear to be pivotal in the patho-genesis of SLE and the localisation of ANA to the GBM in lupus nephritis.
- Renal biopsy can provide useful information about prognosis and can guide treatment regimes.
- Lupus nephritis is classified according to the WHO classification.
- Disease activity can be estimated by American National Institute of Health Activity and Chronicity Index scoring, although this is controversial
- The histopathological differential diagnosis of lupus nephritis includes all types of primary GN, vasculitis and Goodpasture's syndrome.
- Treatment includes corticosteroids and immunosuppressive drugs, such as cyclophosphamide and azathioprine.

REFERENCES

1. Iverson P, Brun C. Aspiration biopsy of the kidney. Am J Med 1951; 11: 324–330
2. Muehrcke RC, Kark RM, Pirani CL, Pollack VE. Lupus nephritis: a clinical and pathological study based on renal biopsies. Medicine 1957; 36: 1–146
3. Tan EM, Cohen AS, Fries JF *et al.* The 1982 revised criteria for the classification of systemic lupus erythematosus. Arthritis Rheum 1982; 25: 1271–1277

4. Hochberg MC. Updating the American College of Rheumatology revised criteria for the classification of systemic lupus erythematosus. Arthritis Rheum 1997; 40: 1725

5. Cameron JS. Glomerular disease: lupus nephritis. In Johnson RJ, Feehally J (Eds) Comprehensive Clinical Nephrology. London: Mosby, 2000

6. Hopkinson ND, Doherty M, Powell RJ. The prevalence and incidence of systemic lupus erythematosus in Nottingham, UK, 1989–1990. Br J Rheumatol 1993; 32: 110–115

7. Johnson AE, Gordon C, Palmer RG, Bacon PA. The prevalence and incidence of systemic lupus erythematosus in Birmingham, England. Relationship to ethnicity and country of birth. Arthritis Rheum 1995; 38: 551–558

8. Fessel WJ. Epidemiology of systemic lupus erythematosus. Rheum Dis Clin North Am 1988; 14: 15–23

9. Uramoto KM, Michet Jr CJ, Thumboo et al. Trends in the incidence and mortality of systemic lupus erythematosus, 1950–1992. Arthritis Rheum 1999; 42: 46–50

10. Voss A, Green A, Junker P. Systemic lupus erythematosus in Denmark: clinical and epidemiological characterization of a county-based cohort. Scand J Rheumatol 1998; 27: 98–105

11. Pollack V, Pirani C. Renal histologic findings in systemic lupus erythematosus. Mayo Clin Proc 1969; 44: 630–644

12. Mahajan SK, Ordenez NG, Feitelson PJ, Lim VS, Spargo BH, Katz AI. Lupus nephropathy without renal involvement. Medicine 1977; 56: 493–501

13. Eiser AR, Katz SM, Swartz C. Clinically occult diffuse proliferative lupus nephritis. An age-related phenomenon. Arch Intern Med 1979; 139: 1022–1025

14. Foster MH. Relevance of systemic lupus erythematosus nephritis animal models to human disease. Semin Nephrol 1999; 19: 12–24

15. Egner W. The use of laboratory tests in the diagnosis of SLE. J Clin Pathol 2000; 53: 424–432

16. Ter Borg EJ, Horst G, Hummel EJ, Limburg PC, Kallenberg CGM. Predictive value of rises in anti-double-stranded DNA antibody levels for disease exacerbations in systemic lupus erythematosus: a long term prospective study. Arthritis Rheum 1989; 33: 634–643

17. Eilat D. Cross reactions of anti-DNA antibodies and the central dogma of lupus nephritis. Immunol Today 1985; 6: 123–127

18. Dziarski R. Autoimmunity: polyclonal activation or antigen induction? Immunol Today 1988; 9: 340–342

19. Carson DA. The specificity of anti-DNA antibodies in systemic lupus erythematosus. J Immunol 1991; 146: 1–2

20. Berden JHM. Nucleosomes and lupus nephritis. In Lewis EJ (Ed.) Lupus Nephritis. Oxford: Oxford University Press, 1999

21. Reeves WH, Satoh M, Wang J, Chou CH, Ajmani AK. Systemic lupus erythematosus. Antibodies to DNA, DNA-binding proteins, and histones. Rheum Dis Clin North Am 1994; 20: 1–28

22. Stemmer C, Richalet-Secordel P, Van-Bruggen MCJ et al. Dual reactivity of several monoclonal anti-nucleosome autoantibodies for double stranded DNA and a short segment of histone H3. J Biol Chem 1996; 271: 21257–21261

23. Chabre H, Amoura Z, Piette JC et al. Presence of nucleosome-restricted antibodies in patients with systemic lupus erythematosus. Arthritis Rheum 1995; 38: 1485–1491

24. Amoura Z, Chabre H, Bach JF, Koutouzov S. Antinucleosome antibodies and systemic lupus erythematosus. Adv Nephrol 1997; 26: 303–316

25. Berden JH, Licht R, Van Bruggen MC, Tax WJ. Role of nucleosomes for induction and glomerular binding of autoantibodies in lupus nephritis. Curr Opin Nephrol Hypertens 1999; 8: 299–306

26. Tumlin JA. Lupus nephritis: novel immunosuppressive modalities and future directions. Sem Nephrol 1999; 19: 67–76

27. Van Bruggen MC, Walgreen B, Rijke TP et al. Heparin and heparinoids prevent the binding of immune complexes containing nucleosomes to the GBM and delay nephritis in MRL/lpr mice. Kidney Int 1996; 50: 1555–1564

28. Marrack P, Hugo P, McCormack J, Kappler J. Death and T cells. Immunol Rev 1993; 133: 119–129

29. Mamula MJ. Lupus autoimmunity: from peptides to particles. Immunol Rev 1995; 144: 301–314

30. Salach RH, Cash JM. Managing lupus nephritis: algorithms for conservative use of renal biopsy. Cleve Clin J Med 1996; 63: 106–115

31. Herrera GA. The value of electron microscopy in the diagnosis and clinical management of lupus nephritis. Ultrastruct Pathol 1999; 23: 63–77

32. Esdaile JM, Joseph L, MacKenzie T, Kashgarian M, Hayslett JP. The benefit of early treatment with immunosuppressive agents in lupus nephritis. J Rheumatol 1994; 21: 2046–2051

33. Stamenkovic I, Favre H, Donath A, Assimacopoulos A, Chatelanat F. Renal biopsy in SLE irrespective of clinical findings: long-term follow up. Clin Nephrol 1986; 26: 109–115

34. Austin HA, Boumpas DT, Vaughan EM, Balow JE. Predicting renal outcomes in severe lupus nephritis: contributions of clinical and histologic data. Kidney Int 1994; 45: 544–550

35. Churg J, Sobin LH. Renal disease: classification and atlas of glomerular diseases. World Health Organisation, Tokyo, Igaku-Shoin, 1982

36. Dische FE. Renal disease in systemic lupus erythematosus. In Dische FE (Ed.) Renal Pathology. Oxford: Oxford University Press, 1995

37. Fine LG, Ong AC, Norman JT. Mechanisms of tubulointerstitial injury in progressive renal diseases. Eur J Clin Invest 1993; 23: 259–265

38. Haas M. A re-evaluation of routine electron microscopy in the examination of native renal biopsies. J Am Soc Nephrol 1997; 8: 70–76

39. Herrera GA, Isaac J, Turbat-Herrera EA. Role of electron microscopy in transplant renal pathology. Ultrastruct Pathol 1997; 21: 481–498

40. Cameron JS. Lupus nephritis: an historical perspective 1968–1998. J Nephrol 1999; 12 (suppl 2): S29–S41

41. Bono L, Cameron JS, Hicks JA. The very long-term prognosis and complications of lupus nephritis and its treatment. QJM 1999; 92: 211–218

42. Ward MM. Cardiovascular and cerebrovascular morbidity and mortality among women with end-stage renal disease attributable to lupus nephritis. Am J Kidney Dis 2000; 36: 516–525

43. Ward MM. Changes in the incidence of end-stage renal disease due to lupus nephritis. Arch Intern Med 2000; 160: 3136–3140

44. Austin HA, Muenz LR, Joyce KM, Antonovych TT, Balow JE. Diffuse proliferative lupus nephritis: identification of specific pathologic features affecting renal outcome. Kidney Int 1984; 25: 689–695

45. Schwartz MM, Lan SP, Bernstein J, Hill GS, Holley K, Lewis EJ. Role of pathology indices in the management of severe lupus glomerulonephritis. Kidney Int 1992; 42: 743–748

46. Austin HA, Muenz LR, Joyce KM, Antonovych TA et al. Prognostic factors in lupus nephritis: contribution of renal histologic data. Am J Med 1983; 75: 382–391

47. Nossent HC, Henzen-Logmans SC, Vroom TM, Berden JH, Swaak TJ. Contribution of renal biopsy data in predicting outcome in lupus nephritis: analysis of 116 patients. Arthritis Rheum 1990; 33: 970–977

48. Hill GS, Delahousse M, Nochy D et al. A new morphologic index for the evaluation of renal biopsies in lupus nephritis. Kidney Int 2000; 58: 1160–1173

49. Berden JH. Nephrology forum: lupus nephritis. Kidney Int 1997; 52: 538–558

50. Balow JE, Boumpas DT, Austin HA. New prospects for treatment of lupus nephritis. Semin Nephrol 2000; 1: 32–39

51. Boumpas DT, Austin HA, Vaughan EM et al. Risk for sustained amenorrhea in patients with systemic lupus erythematosus receiving intermittent pulse cyclophosphamide therapy. Ann Intern Med 1993; 119: 366–369

52. Felson DT, Anderson J. Evidence for the superiority of immunosuppressive drugs and prednisone over prednisone alone in lupus nephritis. Results of a pooled analysis. N Engl J Med 1984; 311: 1528–1533

53. Balow JE, Austin HA, Muenz LR et al. Effect of treatment on the evolution of renal abnormalities in lupus nephritis. N Engl J Med 1984; 311: 491–495

54. Nossent JC. End stage renal disease in patients with systemic lupus erythematosus. In Lewis EJ (Ed.) Lupus Nephritis. Oxford: Oxford University Press, 1999

55. Tax WJ, Kramers C, Van Bruggen MC, Berden JH. Apoptosis, nucleosomes, and nephritis in systemic lupus erythematosus. Kidney Int 1995; 48: 666–673

56. Rumore PM, Steinman CR. Endogenous circulating DNA in systemic lupus erythematosus. Occurrence as multimeric complexes bound to histone. J Clin Invest 1990; 86: 69–74

57. Krishnan G, Thacker L, Angstad JD, Capelli JP. Multicenter analysis of renal allograft survival in lupus patients. Transplant Proc 1991; 23: 1755–1756

58. Ward LA, Jelveh Z, Feinfeld DA. Recurrent membranous lupus nephritis after renal transplantation: a case report and review of the literature. Am J Kidney Dis 1994; 23: 326–329

59. Van Bruggen MC, Walgreen B, Rijke TP, Berden JH. Attenuation of murine lupus nephritis by mycophenolate mofetil. J Am Soc Nephrol 1998; 9: 1407–1415

60. Briggs WA, Choi MJ, Scheel Jr PJ. Successful mycophenolate mofetil treatment of glomerular disease. Am J Kidney Dis 1998; 31: 213–217

61. Chan TM, Li FK, Tang CSD et al. Efficacy of mycophenolate mofetil in patients with diffuse proliferative lupus nephritis. N Engl J Med 2000; 343: 1156–1162

62. Brodsky RA, Petri M, Smith BD et al. Immunoablative high-dose cyclophosphamide with stem-cell rescue for refractory, severe autoimmune disease. Ann Intern Med 1998; 129: 1031–1035

63. Burt RK, Traynor AE, Pope R et al. Treatment of autoimmune disease by intense immunosuppressive conditioning and autologous hematopoietic stem cell transplantation. Blood 1998; 92: 3505–3514

64. Euler HH, Marmont AM, Bacigalupo A et al. Early recurrence or persistence of autoimmune diseases after unmanipulated autologous stem cell transplantation. Blood 1996; 88: 3621–3625

65. Kalled SL, Cutler AH, Datta SK, Thomas DW. Anti-CD40 ligand antibody treatment of SNF1 mice with established nephritis: preservation of kidney function. J Immunol 1998; 160: 2158–2165

66. Wang Y, Hu Q, Madri JA et al. Amelioration of lupus-like autoimmune disease in NZB/WF1 mice after treatment with a blocking antibody specific for complement component C5. Proc Natl Acad Sci USA 1996; 93: 8563–8568

67. Tumlin JA. Lupus nephritis. Novel immunosuppressive modalities and future directions. Sem Nephrol 1999; 19: 67–76

68. Weisman MH, Bluestein HG, Berner CM, de Haan HA. Reduction in circulating dsDNA antibody titre after administration of LJP-394. J Rheumatol 1997; 24: 314–318

69. Hong NM, Masuko-Hongo K, Sasakawa H et al. Amelioration of lymphoid hyperplasia and hypergammaglobulinemia in lupus-prone mice (gld) by Fas-ligand gene transfer. J Autoimmun 1998; 11: 301–307

3

The classification of interstitial pneumonias

A.J. Rice A.U. Wells A.G. Nicholson

INTRODUCTION

Classification of diffuse parenchymal lung diseases has remained both complex and controversial for many decades, with systems differing between countries and also evolving over time as aetiologies became apparent and new entities were recognised. There are, therefore, over 100 entities that could be grouped as diffuse parenchymal lung diseases,[1] within which the histological patterns of interstitial pneumonias are an integral part.

Interstitial pneumonias in an idiopathic setting were subdivided over 30 years ago by Liebow and Carrington into usual interstitial pneumonia (UIP), desquamative interstitial pneumonia (DIP), bronchiolitis obliterans with interstitial pneumonia (BIP), giant cell interstitial pneumonia (GIP) and lymphocytic interstitial pneumonia (LIP).[2] Since this initial classification, BIP is now more commonly termed as organizing pneumonia (OP) and GIP is regarded as a pneumoconiosis associated with hard metal exposure.[3] More recently, papers describing further histological subsets of interstitial pneumonia such as non-specific interstitial pneumonia (NSIP),[4] respiratory bronchiolitis-associated interstitial lung disease (RBILD)[5,6] and acute interstitial pneumonia (AIP)[7] have been recognised, leading to revision of Liebow's classification.[8] Therefore, certain terms have been dropped (e.g. GIP) and new patterns (e.g. NSIP) have been added to subsequent classifications. The situation is further complicated by the fact that terms used more in the clinical setting, such as idiopathic pulmonary fibrosis (IPF) and cryptogenic fibrosing alveolitis (CFA), relate to the same well-defined clinical entity, yet the histological patterns that they encompass

Alexandra J. Rice BA MB BChir MRCPath, Consultant Histopathologist, St Mary's Hospital, London, UK

Athol U. Wells MB ChB FRACP MD, Interstitial Lung Disease Unit, Royal Brompton Hospital, London, UK

Andrew G. Nicholson MB BS MRCPath DM, Consultant Histopathologist, Royal Brompton Hospital, London, UK

Table 3.1 Histological patterns of interstitial pneumonias and clinicopathological counterparts in an idiopathic setting (from Ref. [23])

Histological pattern	Clinicopathological diagnosis
Usual interstitial pneumonia	Cryptogenic fibrosing alveolitis/idiopathic pulmonary fibrosis
Non-specific interstitial pneumonia	Non-specific interstitial pneumonia*
Organizing pneumonia	Cryptogenic organising pneumonia
Diffuse alveolar damage	Acute interstitial pneumonia
Desquamative interstitial pneumonia	Desquamative interstitial pneumonia
Respiratory bronchiolitis	Respiratory bronchiolitis-associated interstitial lung disease
Lymphocytic interstitial pneumonia	Lymphocytic interstitial pneumonia

*Provisional term.

differ. Up until recently, IPF has been said to show only a pattern of UIP,[9] while CFA has encompassed a wider range of patterns, including UIP and DIP.[10] How these clinicopathological entities relate to more recently described patterns, such as NSIP, is also controversial.

There is, therefore, a wealth of published terminology that is not always histogenetically correct (e.g. DIP is neither desquamative nor predominantly interstitial), which is interpreted in different ways by both clinicians and pathologists; yet despite these shortcomings, there is unequivocal evidence that recognition of these patterns provides significant prognostic data.[10–16] Added to this the need for inclusion of recently described entities, such as RBILD[5,6,17,18] and NSIP,[4,10,12–15] plus the impact of high-resolution computerised tomography (HRCT)[19–21] and there was clearly a need for a consensus classification system that was acceptable to clinicians, radiologists and pathologists alike. This has recently been addressed by an ATS/ERS sponsored committee comprising clinicians, radiologists and pathologists who have recently published a consensus document relating to idiopathic interstitial pneumonias, which is summarised in Table 3.1.[22] This chapter first discusses these histological patterns and their relationship to idiopathic disease, then reviews their relationship to connective tissue disorders (CTDs) and interstitial pneumonias in children.

PATTERNS OF INTERSTITIAL PNEUMONIAS IN AN IDIOPATHIC SETTING

USUAL INTERSTITIAL PNEUMONIA

UIP is the most common histological pattern seen in cases of idiopathic interstitial pneumonia, and it is associated with the classic clinical presentation and course of a patient with IPF/CFA.[11,23–26] Fibrosing alveolitis was originally defined by Scadding as a diffuse lung disease characterised by inflammation and fibrosis in the interstitium and alveolar spaces.[27] The prefix 'cryptogenic' was added for those cases where there was no known cause and, despite numerous proposals for a causative agent, no single cause has yet been proven.[28,29] The incidence and

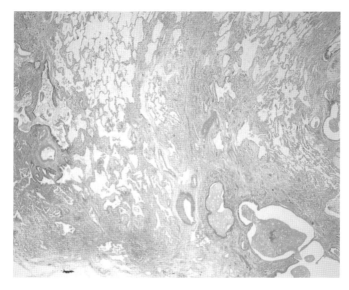

Fig. 3.1 A case of UIP shows patchy inflammation and fibrosis with a subpleural distribution showing areas of honeycombing.

clinical presentation of CFA is well defined and the disease is typically characterised by chronic progression to death with an average survival of 2–3 years from the onset of exertional breathlessness.[9–11,14,16,22] An objective response to treatment is seen in only 20% of patients. Historically, there has been semantic inconsistency in relating histological patterns to clinical disease spectra, IPF equating strictly to the pattern of UIP,[9] but CFA incorporating both DIP and UIP. For patients with CFA, these patterns were thought to represent early (cellular/ desquamative) and late (fibrotic) phases of the disease[25,30–33] rather than distinct conditions.[23] However, it is now generally accepted that UIP and DIP are distinct (although abundant macrophages may occasionally be seen superimposed on a pattern of UIP), supported by recent data on prognosis[10,11,14] and progression of disease on sequential CT scans: cases of DIP, which have a patchy distribution on CT, do not invariably progress to the characteristic subpleural distribution of UIP.[34,35] Therefore, the pattern of DIP should no longer be regarded as a CFA sub-group and its clinicopathological counterpart is described below. UIP should be considered as the predominant histological pattern that equates with CFA/IPF, although it is now clear that some patients with a clinical presentation typical of CFA/IPF have a pattern of NSIP at biopsy.[10,15]

Histologically, UIP is typically within the lower lobes and peripheral, with microscopy showing a subpleural or paraseptal distribution of patchy and heterogenous inflammation and fibrosis, alternating with areas of normal alveolar lung (Fig. 3.1). The essential feature for a diagnosis of UIP is a variation in the age of the fibrosis (sometimes termed *temporal heterogeneity*), with areas of localised fibroblastic proliferation, so-called 'fibroblastic foci', comprising an abundance of plump spindle cells and little intervening collagen, lying immediately adjacent to areas of established fibrosis that are characterised by poorly cellular-hyalinised collagen (Fig. 3.2). Interest has recently focused on these fibroblastic foci as they are thought to represent the sites of repeated and continued lung

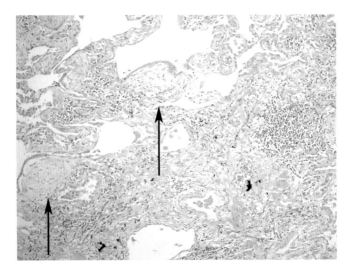

Fig. 3.2 A case of UIP shows fibroblastic foci (arrows) lying immediately adjacent to areas of established fibrosis. This variation in the age of fibrosis is termed 'temporal heterogeneity'.

damage [23,26,36] and there is evidence to suggest that the extent of these foci is associated with mortality and increased rate of disease progression.[37,38] A chronic inflammatory cell infiltrate is also present, mainly comprising small lymphocytes with occasional plasma cells, although this tends to be less than that seen in the other histological patterns of interstitial pneumonia. Although the small lymphocytes in the interstitium are mainly T-cells, aggregates of B-lymphocytes may also be present, although these are not usually prominent in idiopathic disease. As the disease becomes more advanced, there is increased loss of alveolar architecture with the eventual formation of cysts separated by bands of fibrosis, so-called 'honeycombing'. These dilated air-spaces show varying degrees of bronchiolisation and, less commonly, goblet cell hyperplasia. Historically, such cases have always been stated as consistent with CFA and it is true that most cases of end-stage lung are the result of UIP. However, studies looking at the ability to differentiate end-stage UIP from end-stage NSIP have shown poor reproducibility[10] and it is preferable to classify these changes as end-stage lung rather than assign a histological pattern.[8,10,39] Such areas can be avoided by discussion at the time of biopsy in order to select the ideal site (see Practical aspects).[22] Other features seen in UIP are smooth muscle hypertrophy, endarteritis obliterans and type 2 cell hyperplasia, although these are considered secondary phenomena and are not specific to this pattern.

Distinguishing UIP from other patterns is valuable in terms of both prognosis and response to treatment, which are significantly worse in UIP than in other subsets.[10–15] The pattern is quite distinctive but occasionally alveolar macrophages may be numerous, mimicking the pattern of DIP. However, temporal heterogeneity of the underlying fibrosis is not present in DIP. A histological pattern of diffuse alveolar damage (DAD) may be superimposed on a pattern of UIP in patients with acute exacerbations of IPF/CFA,[40–42] but the underlying patchy established fibrosis should still be identifiable, both on biopsy and HRCT. There are also a few occasions when UIP is seen in other disorders, namely drug reactions to cytotoxic drugs and chronic extrinsic allergic alveolitis (EAA). Therefore, correlation with clinical and imaging data is essential before a clinicopathological diagnosis of CFA/IPF is reached.[22] Occasionally, eosinophilic pneumonia-like areas may be seen in UIP.[43]

NON-SPECIFIC INTERSTITIAL PNEUMONIA

Although NSIP had previously been used in relation to HIV infection in the lung,[44] Katzenstein and Fiorelli used the term to describe a group of cases of interstitial pneumonia, which could not be classified according to the recognised subsets at that time. The authors were particular in stating that this was not a specific disease entity, in that some cases were associated with collagen vascular diseases, some with exposure to environmental allergens and some had a history of acute lung injury, with the biopsy perhaps reflecting incomplete resolution of DAD. Despite this, the pattern that they described showed greater response to treatment and a more favourable prognosis than patients with a histological pattern of UIP[4] and the term has subsequently evolved into a recognised pattern of idiopathic interstitial pneumonia.[10–15] However, its clinicopathological counterpart is less well defined and the term NSIP is regarded as provisional in the consensus classification system (Table 3.1).[22]

Histologically, NSIP has a temporally uniform pattern, characterised by expansion of the interstitium by variable amounts of chronic inflammation and fibrosis. The inflammatory cell infiltrate comprises mainly small lymphocytes with occasional plasma cells, while the fibrosis can be predominantly collagenous or fibroblastic in nature. Cases of NSIP with interstitial fibrosis have a worse prognosis than those which are purely inflammatory.[4] The process may be either patchy or diffuse within the pulmonary acinus but is generally more diffuse than UIP, and a key feature in distinguishing NSIP from UIP is the relative absence of temporal heterogeneity, in particular fibroblastic foci, in NSIP. Alveolar macrophages may be present but NSIP lacks the numbers seen in DIP, and no more than 10% of the biopsy shows intra-alveolar organisation, in contradistinction to OP. No hyaline membranes are seen in contrast to AIP, and the density of the interstitial lymphocytic infiltrate is insufficient for a diagnosis of LIP.[22] Although initially subdivided into Grades 1–3 by Katzenstein and Fiorelli,[4] subsequent studies have shown that the survival for the mixed and fibrotic patterns are similar.[10,14] Current practice is to subdivide into two groups, namely cellular NSIP (Fig. 3.3) and fibrotic NSIP (Fig. 3.4).[22]

Clinically, it remains uncertain exactly what the histological pattern NSIP represents, although there is likely to be more than one aetiology. There is already evidence that some cases represent IPF/CFA, although whether these cases are early or inactive phases of IPF remains unclear.[10,15,45,46] Others are likely to be derived from occult hypersensitivity or collagen vascular diseases.[47] Studies are ongoing to determine the nature and frequency of these clinical associations, and a spectrum of CT appearances are now recognised.[46] In the interim, a histological pattern of NSIP should be viewed as a 'holding pattern' from which the clinician can return to the patient to look for such associations, rather than a 'wastebasket' diagnosis alluded to by some.[45]

DIFFUSE ALVEOLAR DAMAGE

The term AIP was introduced to recognise those cases of idiopathic interstitial pneumonia with an acute presentation and rapid clinical progression.[7] The

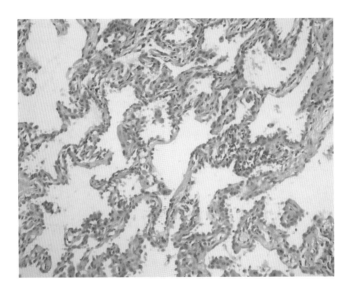

Fig. 3.3 A case of cellular NSIP where there is a diffuse interstitial infiltrate of chronic inflammatory cells and scattered fibroblasts, with minimal deposition of collagen.

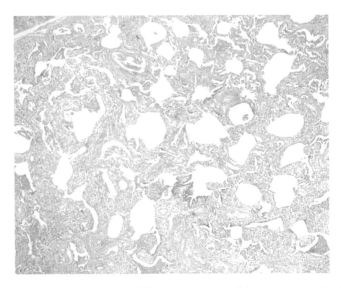

Fig. 3.4 A case of fibrotic NSIP with diffuse involvement of the interstitium by chronic inflammation and fibrosis. The fibrosis is more diffuse in affected areas than those of UIP (Fig. 3.1) and there is no variation in the age of fibrosis.

histological features are identical to those of DAD, the pattern of acute lung injury seen in the acute respiratory distress syndrome (ARDS), but are distinct from other forms of interstitial pneumonia, with which it can enter the clinical differential diagnosis. AIP is now considered to be synonymous with the historical cases of Hamman–Rich disease.[48,49] AIP starts with a flu-like episode, which is succeeded by rapidly progressive severe dyspnoea often leading to death from respiratory failure. The age range is wide and, by definition, patients are previously healthy with no underlying pulmonary disease.[7,49] Thus, AIP differs from

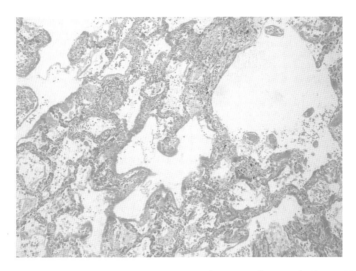

Fig. 3.5 A case of AIP shows the histopathological features of DAD. The interstitium is expanded by plump fibroblasts and a mixed inflammatory cell infiltrate, with abundant hyaline membranes lining alveoli.

the previously described forms of interstitial pneumonia in that it describes the clinicopathological syndrome rather than the histological pattern: it is classified on histology alone as DAD (Table 3.1). HRCT typically shows bilateral infiltrates with ground glass opacification, bronchial dilation and alveolar consolidation.

Histologically, DAD is characterised by marked expansion of the interstitium by a predominantly fibroblastic proliferation with an accompanying inflammatory cell infiltrate of variable intensity. There is hyperplasia of type 2 pneumocytes that can show sufficient cytological atypia, such that they may enter the differential diagnosis of malignancy in cytological specimens. The bronchiolar epithelium may also show squamous metaplasia. Residual foci of hyaline membranes may also be present, though this is probably dependent on the phase of the disease at the time of biopsy (Fig. 3.5). Thrombi are not infrequent within small pulmonary arteries.[7]

In terms of differential diagnosis, UIP should be distinguishable through an absence of temporal heterogeneity and the presence of hyaline membranes, although rare acute exacerbations of UIP may occur as terminal events.[40–42] If patients have long-term survival, the histological pattern may be indistinguishable from NSIP in the residual lung[4] and in such cases, the clinical presentation may be essential in making the diagnosis.[7,49] Likewise, the organising phase of DAD may be indistinguishable from OP due to other chronic causes and again review of clinical and imaging data are essential.[50] However, in cryptogenic organizing pneumonia (COP), the disease has a more patchy and peribronchial distribution and interstitial changes are less prominent.[51]

The long-term sequelae of AIP are varied. Most patients die of their disease, with recent mortality about 70%,[7,49] but a minority recover completely or survive with residual fibrosis. Some may have repeated episodes of AIP and develop chronic progressive fibrosis.[52] Treatment principally involves respiratory support in the acute phase, sometimes with additional immunosuppressive therapy.

Table 3.2 Causes of organizing pneumonia

Primary or idiopathic
Cryptogenic organising pneumonia (idiopathic bronchiolitis obliterans-organising pneumonia)
Secondary
Organising diffuse alveolar damage
Organising infections
Organisation distal to obstruction
Organising aspiration pneumonia
Organising drug reactions, fume and toxic exposures
Connective tissue disease
Extrinsic allergic alveolitis/hypersensitivity pneumonitis
Eosinophilic lung disease
Transplantation
Inflammatory bowel disease
As a secondary reaction in chronic bronchiolitis
As a reparative reaction around other processes (including abscesses, Wegener's granulomatosis, neoplasms and others)

ORGANISING PNEUMONIA

OP is a non-specific pattern of repair seen in response to injury, which may be classified as primary (or idiopathic) or secondary (with recognised cause/association) disease (Table 3.2). OP in an idiopathic setting has been regarded as a distinct clinicopathological entity since Davison *et al.* classified such cases as COP,[53–55] while others have preferred the term idiopathic bronchiolitis obliterans-organising pneumonia (BOOP).[56] However, the term COP is preferred in the consensus classification as it facilitates its distinction from constrictive obliterative bronchiolitis.[22] As the disease is predominantly intra-alveolar and not primarily interstitial, it can be argued that OP should not be included among the histological patterns of interstitial pneumonia, especially as classic clinical cases are unlikely to be clinically mistaken for patients with UIP.[8] Indeed, COP may be equally viewed as a small airways disease.[57] However, some cases mimic UIP clinically and radiologically,[24] and pathologists have sometimes mistaken OP for UIP.[26] Furthermore, some clinical series of IPF/CFA have included cases that, in retrospect, are recognisable as idiopathic BOOP/COP.[11] Therefore, as OP should be considered in the differential diagnosis of a patient with suspected interstitial pneumonia,[58] it is included in the classification system.

COP affects males and females equally and is most common in the fifth and sixth decades. There are no known risk factors and it is not related to smoking. Patients present with an illness of relatively short onset characterised by cough and dyspnoea, sometimes following a viral-like syndrome. There may be a clinical suspicion of infection, but no agent is identified. A number of patterns can be seen on HRCT, but typically there is focal consolidation, variably admixed with patchy or diffuse alveolar ground glass opacification, which can be migratory. Occasionally, COP may present as a solitary focal lesion. Bronchoalveolar lavage (BAL) typically shows a mixed pattern with increased numbers of lymphocytes in almost all cases with variable increases in neutrophils, eosinophils and foamy macrophages[59,60] and, therefore, may be useful in excluding other causes of OP. For example, a strikingly high lymphocyte count is more suggestive of EAA and a marked eosinophilia would favour an eosinophilic pneumonia.

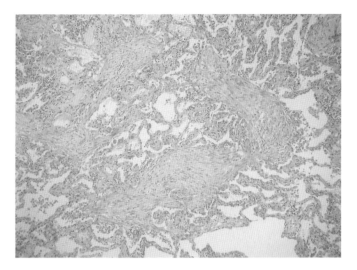

Fig. 3.6 A case of OP shows patchy filling of alveoli by buds of fibroblastic tissue, together with a mild non-specific chronic inflammatory cell infiltrate.

Histologically, the involved bronchioles and alveoli are filled and obstructed by intraluminal polyps of fibroblastic tissue (Masson bodies). These have a loose myxoid quality and contain little collagen. A small amount of fibrin may also be present in some alveoli. There is a mild interstitial inflammatory infiltrate, type 2 cell hyperplasia, and a variable increase in alveolar macrophages (Fig. 3.6). The macrophages often have foamy cytoplasm, representing endogenous lipid pneumonia secondary to bronchiolar obstruction. The alveolar architecture usually remains relatively normal, but there may sometimes be scarring and remodelling, which is associated with a poorer prognosis.[61] In some of these patients, the fibrosis is stable, and possibly represents the effects of prolonged inflammation. In others, it is progressive with development of honeycombing, and is associated with a poor outcome.[62] Features that are not typically seen in OP in an idiopathic setting are granulomas, vasculitis, hyaline membranes and increased numbers of neutrophils or eosinophils.

OP can be differentiated from the exudative phase of DAD as hyaline membranes are not a feature of OP. However, the organising phase of DAD and OP due to other causes are very similar. Features that favour OP in this context include a peribronchiolar patchy distribution, intrabronchiolar buds of fibroblastic tissue and relatively little expansion of the interstitium by oedematous fibroinflammatory tissue. NSIP is more interstitial and there is relatively little (<10%) intra-alveolar organisation. In UIP, the fibroblastic foci may resemble OP, but they are relatively inconspicuous compared to the more mature fibrosis.[22]

As COP is a clinicopathological diagnosis, secondary causes of OP including infection and drugs must be excluded. Some causes, like drug reactions, require clinical input but the histopathologist can help to exclude diseases that show an OP-like histological pattern, including Wegener's granulomatosis, Langerhans cell histiocytosis and lymphoma by careful screening for underlying vasculitis, Langerhans cells and atypical lymphocytes, respectively. Furthermore, large numbers of neutrophils, granulomas or necrosis suggest infection, small poorly formed peribronchial granulomas raise the possibility of EAA and increased eosinophils with eosinophilic abscesses suggest an eosinophilic pneumonia. All these should be carefully looked for in a biopsy where the predominant feature is OP. The prognosis of COP following steroid treatment is very good, although recurrence of disease is not infrequent.[54,55] Cases of secondary OP show a more variable prognosis.[63]

DESQUAMATIVE INTERSTITIAL PNEUMONIA

The term DIP arose as the cells filling alveolar spaces, the predominant feature in DIP, were initially thought to be desquamated pneumocytes. These are now known to be macrophages[64,65] but, despite this misnomer, DIP remains the preferred term.[22] Patients usually present in the fourth or fifth decade, complaining of increasing shortness of breath in association with a dry cough. Clubbing, fever, fatigue and loss of weight may occur.[23] The chest radiograph is sometimes insensitive for the detection of DIP, with appearances ranging from normal to a slight triangular haziness radiating from the hilus along the heart borders to both bases, sparing the costophrenic angles.[23] Widespread ground glass opacification is probably equally as frequent, sometimes having a granular or nodular texture. The HRCT findings of DIP are documented in several studies,[34-66] with ground glass opacification, the cardinal feature. Occasionally, small cysts may be apparent.[35] Pulmonary function tests show a restrictive pattern with a reduction in diffusing capacity and hypoxaemia on blood gas analysis. Published data on BAL findings are sparse and vary in the few published studies, although there is a striking increase in macrophage numbers, compared to healthy cigarette smokers.[65]

Histologically, the major histological feature is the presence of large numbers of macrophages within alveoli (Fig. 3.7), with a diffuse distribution throughout pulmonary acini. These macrophages characteristically have abundant eosinophilic cytoplasm, which may have a glassy appearance and often contains a finely granular light brown pigment that stains for haemosiderin (Fig. 3.7). The alveolar architecture is generally well maintained, although there is usually a mild chronic inflammatory cell infiltrate within the interstitium. The inflammatory cell infiltrate may include a small number of eosinophils and can be accompanied by interstitial fibroblastic proliferation and/or a mild degree of established fibrosis although temporal heterogeneity is not seen. Severe fibrosis and honeycombing are exceptional features and UIP should be thoroughly excluded in these instances. Also, UIP does not typically have an abundance of macrophages. In cases where there is doubt over the histological pattern, correlation with clinical and imaging data is of often value in distinguishing IPF/CFA from DIP. With regard to other histological patterns, DIP should be easily distinguishable from OP, LIP and DAD as a dominant accumulation of macrophages is not seen and other diagnostic histological features (intra-alveolar organisation, dense lymphoid interstitial infiltrate and hyaline membranes) are absent. In relation to NSIP, there may occasionally be an overlap between these patterns as the volume of macrophages is not consistently present throughout all lung fields. However, correlation with the clinical and imaging data in these situations usually leads to successful differentiation.

In addition to the other patterns of interstitial pneumonia, there are several disorders that result in a 'DIP-like reaction' (an accumulation of alveolar macrophages secondary to co-existent disease or a pulmonary insult). These

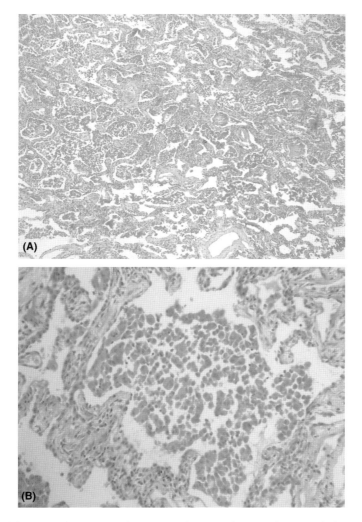

Fig. 3.7 (A) A case of DIP seen at low power shows uniformity of histopathological changes in areas of involved pulmonary acini. (B) Intra-alveolar accumulation of macrophages is the major histological feature.

include Langerhans cell histiocytosis, where nodular aggregates of Langerhans cells may be masked by the accumulation of macrophages,[67] dust inhalation[68] and drug reactions.[69] DIP should, therefore, not be thought of as a specific entity, but as a histological pattern with a variety of clinical associations that need to be considered separately and treated accordingly.

RESPIRATORY BRONCHIOLITIS-ASSOCIATED INTERSTITIAL LUNG DISEASE (RBILD)

Respiratory bronchiolitis (RB) is a common incidental histological finding in heavy smokers and a strong relationship between peribronchiolar fibrosis/inflammation and smoking was reported as early as 1974.[70] However, in 1986 Myers and colleagues described six patients,[5] all heavy smokers, who had clinical, radiological and physiological evidence of chronic interstitial lung disease (ILD) but only RB on open lung biopsy. The term RBILD was later coined in a further series that clarified the histological differences between the incidental changes of smoking, RBILD and DIP.[6] Almost all patients with RBILD are current cigarette smokers aged between 22 and 53 years, with equal sex distribution. The commonest presenting features are a gradual onset of shortness of breath and a prominent cough. Other symptoms include chest pain, weight loss and rarely fever and haemoptysis. Pneumothorax occasionally occurs. Clubbing is extremely rare. Some patients are asymptomatic at presentation and are referred with incidental findings of an abnormal chest radiograph. Routine laboratory studies are non-specific and in general are not helpful. A normal chest radiograph is found in approximately 20% of patients with RBILD. In over half, a diffuse bilateral reticulo-nodular pattern with basal ground glass opacity is found.[18,71,72] HRCT changes in RBILD are sometimes subtle and easily overlooked, and therefore, lung biopsy is occasionally appropriate despite apparently normal HRCT appearances. Varying degrees of patchy ground glass opacity and centrilobular nodules are the most common findings. Several series have noted considerable overlap in the HRCT appearances of RBILD and DIP, which may indicate that the two disorders represent a continuum, with variably severe small airway and parenchymal reaction to cigarette smoke. Similar but less extensive findings are also present in asymptomatic smokers.[5,6,18,72,73] Pulmonary function tests generally show either restriction or a mixed restrictive–obstructive pattern, and reduced gas transfer levels. Mild hypoxaemia may be present at rest or with exercise. BAL may help to distinguish patients with RBILD from healthy smokers or smokers with IPF, especially when macrophage numbers are strikingly increased in isolation.

Histologically, RB is characterised by an accumulation of alveolar macrophages within respiratory bronchioles spilling into neighbouring alveoli (Fig. 3.8). These

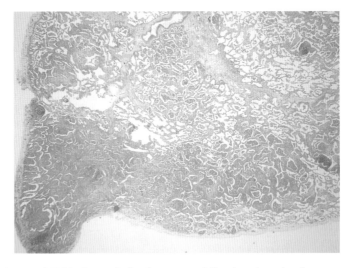

Fig. 3.8 A case of RBILD shows similar features to DIP, other than the changes are patchy and have a centrilobular distribution. Macrophages are identical to those seen in Fig. 3.7(B).

macrophages are pigmented in a similar fashion to those seen in DIP, but the distribution is centriacinar as opposed to the diffuse abnormalities seen in DIP. Their accumulation may be associated with peribronchiolar alveolar septal thickening by fibroblasts and collagen deposition, characteristically radiating from the involved bronchiole (Fig. 3.8). There is usually an accompanying chronic inflammatory cell infiltrate in the wall of the bronchiole and the surrounding alveolar walls. The surrounding pulmonary parenchyma is usually normal but may show mild emphysema.[18] No honeycomb changes have been described and, if present, should raise the possibility of the RB being incidental to a second pathology. In terms of differential diagnosis, there is a strong histological overlap with DIP, the only difference being the patchy peribronchiolar distribution in RBILD. Indeed, cases of RBILD often have areas indistinguishable from DIP. Therefore, although there is no definitive evidence that RBILD progresses to DIP, it seems likely that these two entities overlap, with cigarette smoking being the likely cause in the majority of cases. Nevertheless, it is currently recommended that these patterns should be distinguished as there are differences in the spectrum of associated clinical disorders.[22]

LYMPHOCYTIC INTERSTITIAL PNEUMONIA

LIP is a clinicopathological term initially introduced by Liebow and Carrington in 1969 to describe a dense and diffuse lymphocytic interstitial infiltrate,[2] and, as such, was part of their proposed classification of patterns of interstitial pneumonias. However, because it more frequently enters the differential diagnosis of non-Hodgkin's lymphomas in the lung and historically was thought to be a pre-neoplastic condition that often progressed to lymphoma, it was dropped from ensuing classifications of interstitial pneumonias,[8] and was preferably classified as a lymphoproliferative disease. Subsequent data on the nature of LIP using immunohistochemical and molecular analysis have suggested that cases said to have 'progressed' to lymphoma probably had lymphoma from the outset. While malignant transformation can occur, it is an extremely rare phenomenon,[74,75] and LIP is, therefore, currently recognised as representing diffuse involvement of the lung parenchyma by reactive pulmonary lymphoid hyperplasia, leading to re-inclusion into the consensus classification system. A specific cause for LIP is not known, and its aetiology is most likely multifactorial, although viruses are implicated[76–80] as well as autoimmunity.[81–83] To this end, idiopathic LIP is exceptionally rare, although the pulmonary disease may precede systemic manifestation of the connective tissue disease (CTD). Nevertheless, it remains within the consensus classification system.[22]

Patients with LIP are usually female, with an average age at presentation of about 50 years. Presenting symptoms tend to be dyspnoea, cough and chest pain, with haemoptysis occasionally being described. Many patients with LIP show abnormalities of immunoglobulin production, typically hypergammaglobulinaemia but occasionally hypogammaglobulinaemia, or a monoclonal gammopathy.[84–86] There is usually a restrictive ventilatory defect. Chest X-ray abnormalities are characteristically reticular, coarse reticulo-nodular or fine reticulo-nodular shadowing.[81–84,87,88] The HRCT findings in LIP consist of areas of ground-glass attenuation, poorly defined centrilobular nodules and subpleural small nodules. In addition to surgical lung biopsy, BAL may also be of value as

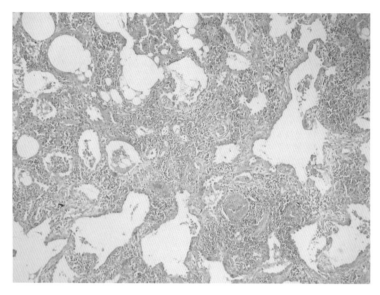

Fig. 3.9 A case of LIP with diffuse expansion of the interstitium by a dense infiltrate of small lymphocytes, plasma cells and histiocytes.

an increase in the total cell count of CD3-positive T-cells and of polyclonal CD20-positive B-cells suggests the diagnosis.[89]

Histologically, LIP is characterised by a dense interstitial lymphoid infiltrate with variable, usually minor, peribronchial involvement. There is no particular accentuation of severity (i.e. peripheral or centriacinar) within the acinus. Granuloma formation is occasionally noted.[81–83] Immunohistochemistry using CD20 shows that B-cells are mainly limited to the germinal centres, often highlighting more follicles than are seen on routine sections. The interstitial lymphocytes are predominantly T-cells mixed with scattered B-cells, plasma cells and histiocytes (Fig. 3.9). Although significant interstitial fibrosis is rarely seen in biopsies, progressive changes have been reported.[82] Amplification of the immunoglobulin heavy chain gene using the polymerase chain reaction generally shows a polyclonal pattern, although occasional oligoclonal patterns are seen[83] and one paper has described minor clones in the infiltrate.[90]

INTERSTITIAL PNEUMONIAS IN ASSOCIATION WITH CONNECTIVE TISSUE DISORDERS

The CTDs comprise a heterogeneous group of diseases, which includes rheumatoid arthritis, systemic sclerosis, polymyositis/dermatomyositis (PM/DM), systemic lupus erythematosus (SLE), Sjogren's syndrome and mixed CTDs (MCTDs). It is well established that some patients with these CTDs will suffer from pulmonary disease at some stage in their disease progression, although both the incidence of pulmonary disease overall and the variety of histopathological entities vary in relation to the different disease types (Table 3.3).[91–96] Furthermore, in some patients, pulmonary manifestations will even precede the CTD.[97–99]

Table 3.3 The prevalence of pulmonary complications in connective tissue diseases

	RA	SLE	SSc	PM/DM	SS
Usual interstitial pneumonia	++	±	+	+	±
Non-specific interstitial pneumonia	+?	+?	++	+?	+?
Lymphocytic interstitial pneumonia/FB	+	±	−	−	++
Organising pneumonia	++	±	±	++	±
Diffuse alveolar damage	+	+	±	±	−
Desquamative interstitial pneumonia/RB-ILD	+*	−	+*	−	−

RA: Rheumatoid arthritis (Refs [4,87,88,95,107,124]); SLE: Systemic lupus erythematosus (Refs [104,109−111,119,125]); SSc: Systemic sclerosis (Refs [18,99,104,154]); PM/DM: Polymyositis/Dermatomyositis (Refs [96,97,105,106]); SS: Sjogren's syndrome [Refs [118,127,153]]; FB: Follicular bronchiolitis, RB-ILD: Respiratory bronchiolitis−associated interstitial lung disease; ++: frequent, +: not infrequent, ±: rare; ?: prevalence currently uncertain; *: Probable incidental to pulmonary symptoms. Updated from Refs [94,100].

Conversely, it should also be recognised that there is a high prevalence of subclinical involvement, which is being increasingly identified with more sensitive diagnostic methods. Therefore, prognostic data from previously published cohorts should not necessarily be applied to more subtle disease and certain histological features, for example, respiratory bronchiolitis in the context of a smoking history may sometimes be incidental to symptomatic respiratory disease.[94,100]

As with idiopathic disease, the term 'fibrosing alveolitis' has been used to describe the histological features when patients present with diffuse fibrotic lung disease,[92,101,102] and terms such as *'fibrosing alveolitis associated with systemic sclerosis'* (FASSc) have been used to distinguish those cases with, in the cited example, systemic sclerosis from those with idiopathic disease (sometimes termed *'lone CFA'* when discussed in this context). Even in studies where cases are subdivided into patterns of interstitial pneumonia, they generally predate recognition of NSIP as histological pattern, a pattern that is likely to have a higher frequency in this group of patients.

USUAL INTERSTITIAL PNEUMONIA IN CONNECTIVE TISSUE DISORDERS

UIP is most frequently seen in patients with lone CFA/IPF,[10,11,13,14] but its incidence in patients with CTDs is less well characterised. For example, a recent study has shown that nearly 80% of cases with FASSc have a pattern of NSIP rather than UIP.[103] UIP was considered the most frequently seen pattern in PM/DM, before NSIP was recognised as a discrete entity,[96,104,105] but a recent study has shown that the majority have an NSIP pattern.[106] In contrast, 1–4% of patients with rheumatoid arthritis appear to develop ILD,[95,107] and patients with UIP have a worse prognosis than those with histological patterns of OP and LIP.[95,96,107] One recent study describes histological variation between UIP in CTDs other than scleroderma when compared to both UIP seen in scleroderma and UIP in IPF.[104] Therefore, although a pattern of UIP is known to occur on a background of CTDs, its prognostic significance is as yet uncertain for most disorders. The histological features of UIP are described earlier and typically there are no clear-cut discriminating features between patients with idiopathic disease and those seen in association with CTDs. However, an increase in the intensity of interstitial chronic inflammation, plus increased numbers of germinal centres, have been described as features linked to background CTDs, particularly it could rheumatoid arthritis. Equally it could be argued that this represents follicular bronchiolitis (FB) superimposed on UIP.

NON-SPECIFIC INTERSTITIAL PNEUMONIA IN CONNECTIVE TISSUE DISORDERS

Even in Katzentstein and Fiorelli's paper on NSIP, a significant number of cases was noted to have CTDs,[4] and NSIP in association with CTDs is increasingly reported in scleroderma,[103] rheumatoid arthritis,[4,108] polymyositis,[96,106] Sjogren's syndrome and SLE.[4,109–111] However, this may not simply be due to increasing recognition, but also because treatment of pulmonary complications is more effective than in idiopathic disease,[112] preventing progression to the generally more fibrotic pattern of UIP. Furthermore, the prognostic significance of NSIP in CTDs and even within the NSIP group between cellular and fibrotic patterns remains uncertain. In patients with FASSc and an NSIP pattern, there are not the significant differences in prognosis between fibrotic NSIP and UIP seen in idiopathic disease, and neither are there prognostic differences between cellular and fibrotic subtypes of NSIP.[103] Again, histological features seen in patients with CTDs cannot be distinguished from idiopathic disease on the basis of the interstitial pneumonia, although the presence of increased numbers of germinal centres again may suggest a background CTD.

DIFFUSE ALVEOLAR DAMAGE IN CONNECTIVE TISSUE DISORDERS

In relation to CTDs, patients with no history of pulmonary involvement may develop acute respiratory failure independent of other recognised causes, with biopsy features showing the histological pattern of DAD. This is best characterised in relation to SLE, where it is termed acute lupus pneumonitis,[109,110,113,114] although other causes of acute respiratory failure are more frequent[115] and some pulmonary manifestations in SLE may be related to non-pulmonary disease.[116] A pattern of DAD is also described in association with PM/DM[96,117] and rheumatoid arthritis.

DIFFUSE PULMONARY LYMPHOID HYPERPLASIA (LYMPHOCYTIC INTERSTITIAL PNEUMONIA AND FOLLICULAR BRONCHIOLITIS) IN CONNECTIVE TISSUE DISORDERS

This term comprises overlapping histological patterns of pulmonary lymphoid hyperplasia that show interstitial (LIP) and peribronchiolar (FB) predominance, respectively. As discussed earlier, recognition of these patterns in a patient with no recognised clinical association should precipitate investigations along these lines, as idiopathic LIP/FB is exceptionally rare. It is most often seen in association with rheumatoid arthritis[87,88] and Sjogren's syndrome,[84,118] but is also rarely described in other CTDs.[119] The histological features of LIP are described earlier, while FB shows a mainly bronchocentric distribution of follicular hyperplasia in bronchial mucosa-associated lymphoid tissue (MALT). LIP also needs to be distinguished from diffuse pulmonary lymphomas manifesting as interstitial lung disease,[83,120] although awareness that the latter may arise in patients with fibrosing alveolitis, both isolated and associated with CTDs,[121–123] should alert the pathologist to undertake the necessary investigations.

ORGANISING PNEUMONIA IN CONNECTIVE TISSUE DISORDERS

OP is not uncommonly seen in association with polymyositis[96,97] and rheumatoid arthritis,[124] but only rarely in association with SLE,[125] systemic sclerosis[126] and Sjogren's syndrome.[127] The clinical outcome in patients with CTDs is similar to that in COP apart from some patients, typically with PM/DM or rheumatoid arthritis, who have associated interstitial fibrosis, denoting a poorer prognosis. This is more likely to represent progression of a single disease process than two distinct patterns.[94] Apart from those with associated interstitial fibrosis, the histological features are generally similar to those seen in patients with idiopathic disease.

DESQUAMATIVE INTERSTITIAL PNEUMONIA AND RESPIRATORY BRONCHIOLITIS IN CONNECTIVE TISSUE DISORDERS

Small numbers of patients with histological patterns of both DIP and RBILD are reported in CTDs, although, where documented, all were smokers.[6,18,23,107,128] Therefore, while bronchiolitic disorders are well described in CTDs,[129] the fact that most cases of DIP and RBILD are caused by smoking implies a lack of true association with the CTD,[17] with no relationship to the patient's symptoms in many cases.[18,128]

OTHER FEATURES IN CONNECTIVE TISSUE DISORDERS

Some patients will show more than one pattern of disease (e.g. pulmonary hypertension superimposed upon a pattern of UIP/NSIP in scleroderma)[128] and these may be central to characterising the key pulmonary complications of an individual connective tissue disease. In terms of combinations of patterns of interstitial pneumonia, a superimposition of two patterns may also sometimes be recognised (e.g. an OP with prominent interstitial fibrosis would favour PM/DM).[62] However, how these multiple patterns relate to pathogenesis in a single CTD is unknown.

INTERSTITIAL PNEUMONIAS IN CHILDREN

Most authors have classified paediatric interstitial lung disease according to systems devised for diseases in adults,[130,131] although additional terms, such as 'chronic pneumonitis of infancy'[132] and 'cellular pneumonitis in infants'[133] have also been proposed. In contrast to adults, there is a comparative lack of data on such investigations as CT scanning in children[134] and tissue sampling is often required in order to reach a diagnosis.[135] As in adults, this usually requires an open or thoracoscopic lung biopsy for cases with an interstitial pneumonia.[134,136]

CRYPTOGENIC FIBROSING ALVEOLITIS AND ITS RELATIONSHIP TO USUAL INTERSTITIAL PNEUMONIA AND NON-SPECIFIC INTERSTITIAL PNEUMONIA IN CHILDREN

Several series of interstitial lung disease in children describe cases of CFA but, as for those in associational with CTDs, most predate recognition of NSIP. Indeed, when strict histological criteria are applied, UIP is exceptionally rare in children. Today, most reported cases of CFA in children would probably be otherwise classified,[137,138] in contrast to UIP being the most frequent pattern of interstitial pneumonia in adults. This may explain why what has been termed CFA in children has a much better prognosis than CFA in adults. Most cases are more appropriately classified as NSIP in terms of histological pattern, although the clinical relevance of NSIP is even less well characterised in children than adults.

DESQUAMATIVE INTERSTITIAL PNEUMONIA AND RESPIRATORY BRONCHIOLITIS-ASSOCIATED INTERSTITIAL LUNG DISEASE IN CHILDREN

RBILD appears to be limited to adults but DIP is well described in children.[139] The histological features are similar to those in adults but the outcome is worse in children, especially in infancy[140] and those with familial disease.[141] Therefore, the aetiology is probably different in children and most likely multifactorial. Some children with a DIP-like pattern have been shown to have surfactant B deficiency. Others have had lipid storage diseases, such as Gaucher's disease,[142] and it has been suggested that hitherto unrecognised defects in metabolism may be responsible for other cases.[138]

LYMPHOCYTIC INTERSTITIAL PNEUMONIA IN CHILDREN

This is the most commonly described pattern of interstitial pneumonia in childhood,[137,138] with similar histological features to those described for adults. The paediatric disease is also nearly always associated with either CTDs or immunodeficiency states, both congenital and acquired. It is a well-described complication of paediatric AIDS and occurs in over 30% of children perinatally affected by HIV. In congenital immunodeficiency, it is likely that lymphocyte dysregulation is involved in its development.[137,143] Familial cases are also described.[144] Again, the histological pattern is similar to that seen in adults.

ORGANISING PNEUMONIA IN CHILDREN

Rare cases have been reported in children and occasional cases of idiopathic acute neutrophilic pneumonia have also been identified in children (AGN, personal observations).

DIFFUSE ALVEOLAR DAMAGE IN CHILDREN

DAD is not infrequently seen in infancy, being the histopathological pattern seen in respiratory distress syndromes, but the majority of these patients do not come to biopsy. However, occasional cases of acute respiratory failure develop in older

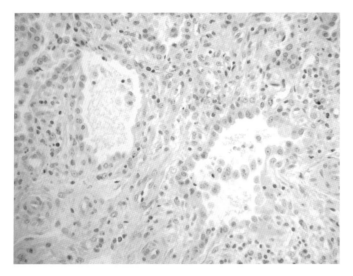

Fig. 3.10 A case of chronic pneumonitis of infancy shows diffuse expansion of the interstitium by plump fibroblasts with little accompanying inflammation. Type 2 cell hyperplasia is marked, and focal proteinosis-like material fills some of the residual air-spaces.

children who are previously well and these patients have shown a pattern of DAD on biopsy. In these instances, when no underlying causes identified, a clinical diagnosis of AIP is appropriate.[7]

CHRONIC PNEUMONITIS OF INFANCY[132] AND CELLULAR INTERSTITIAL PNEUMONITIS IN INFANTS[133]

These appear to differ histologically from interstitial pneumonias in adults but overlap each other. From their original descriptions, it appears that chronic pneumonitis of infancy has a distinct histological pattern, while that of cellular intersititial pneumonitis of infants is more akin to NSIP. Katzenstein *et al.* suggested that some cases of cellular interstitial pneumonitis represent chronic pneumonitis of infancy and also that some previously published reports on paediatric cases of CFA, UIP and DIP represent this condition.[132] Histologically, cases of chronic pneumonitis of infancy show extremely florid type 2 cell hyperplasia and diffuse expansion of the interstitium by fibroblastic tissue with comparatively little interstitial chronic inflammation. Acellular intra-alveolar material resembling that seen in alveolar proteinosis is a frequent finding (Fig. 3.10).[132,137]

PRACTICAL ASPECTS

INTEROBSERVER VARIATION

From the pathologist's perspective, it is important to recognise the various histopathological features in a reproducible fashion. While surprisingly few interobserver variation studies have been performed, agreement between observers, as quantified by kappa coefficients of agreement, is sufficient for diagnostic usage and not dissimilar to agreement reported in studies of HRCT scoring of patterns of interstitial pneumonia.[10,103,145]

INTER-RELATIONSHIP WITH HIGH-RESOLUTION COMPUTERISED TOMOGRAPHY DATA

With advances in imaging, in particular those in HRCT, radiologists have become particularly adept at diagnosing interstitial lung diseases, to such an extent that the diagnosis of typical IPF/CFA and assessment of potential disease reversibility can be made without recourse to biopsy.[21,146,147] It is possible that the recognition of new, clinically distinct histological subsets of interstitial pneumonias may slightly increase the frequency of lung biopsies, but the rapid characterisation of the CT appearances of these entities[22,46,72,148,149] makes this uncertain. Regardless of the frequency of recourse to biopsy, the pathologist must ensure close correlation with both radiologist and clinician when assessing an open or thoracoscopic lung biopsy.[150] Even in cases where there is a reasonable degree of confidence in the histological pattern, it is worth confirming that this is compatible with clinical and radiological data. Furthermore, while there is considerable evidence that histological classification into subsets of interstitial pneumonia is worthwhile, there is overlap between most, if not all, groups, a problem that is compounded by the limitations of sampling at lung biopsy. HRCT may often be of value in narrowing down this differential diagnosis. This is especially true in advanced cases of interstitial lung disease, when the sampled tissue may only reveal honeycombing. In this instance, radiological data is sometimes of more value than the pathology in making the diagnosis,[151] although biopsy of areas showing end-stage lung should ideally be pre-empted by selecting the site of biopsy prior to operation, primarily based upon CT appearances.

WHEN TO BIOPSY

Surgical lung biopsies only occur in a minority of patients in the UK,[22] with criteria for the diagnosis of IPF/CFA met without a tissue diagnosis in many cases.[9] As stated above, the increasing ability of HRCT to provide a secure diagnosis is likely to obviate surgical lung biopsy in an increasing proportion of cases. Indeed, given the high pre-test probability for certain patterns of interstitial pneumonia in particular CTDs, the cardinal indication for surgical lung biopsy is difficulty in reconciling clinical and imaging data, most often in relation to histological patterns other than UIP.[152] However, biopsies may also be warranted to exclude superimposed malignancy, opportunistic infections or drug reactions[92] and surgical lung biopsies will undoubtedly continue in a minority of patients for the foreseeable future.

TYPE OF BIOPSY

Both transbronchial and surgical lung biopsies are sometimes performed in the assessment of parenchymal disease. Transbronchial biopsies are most useful in the diagnosis of Langerhans cell histiocytosis, alveolar proteinosis, malignancy, infections, organising pneumonia and, particularly, granulomatous diseases, especially sarcoidosis and EAA. However, the changes seen in the interstitial pneumonias are often patchy and transbronchial biopsies may not be representative. Therefore, it is best not to assign histological patterns of interstitial pneumonia based upon a transbronchial biopsy. Neither should tissue obtained by transbronchial biopsy be used to assess the degree of fibrosis or inflammation.[22] The open and thoracoscopic surgical techniques allow the surgeon to visualise and sample abnormal areas of lung and the larger size of the biopsy permits a more accurate assessment of the spatial pattern of interstitial disease, although it is important that the surgeon does not biopsy areas of lung that show non-specific end-stage features or honeycombing. Ideally, biopsies should be taken from at least two sites, in order to minimise the risk of sampling error.[15]

GLOSSARY

AIP	Acute interstitial pneumonia
BAL	Bronchoalveolar lavage
BOOP	Bronchiolitis obliterans-organising pneumonia
CFA	Cryptogenic fibrosing alveolitis
COP	Cryptogenic organising pneumonia
CTD	Connective tissue disorder
DAD	Diffuse alveolar damage
DIP	Desquamative interstitial pneumonia
EAA	Extrinsic allergic alveolitis
GIP	Giant cell interstitial pneumonia
IPF	Idiopathic pulmonary fibrosis
LIP	Lymphocytic interstitial pneumonia
NSIP	Non-specific interstitial pneumonia
OP	Organising pneumonia
RB	Respiratory bronchiolitis
RBILD	Respiratory bronchiolitis-associated interstitial lung disease
UIP	Usual interstitial pneumonia

*Liebow and Carrington's classification of interstitial pneumonias used the term BIP (bronchiolitis obliterans-interstitial pneumonia).

REFERENCES

1. Turner-Warwick M. Interstitial lung disease. Sem Respir Med 1984; 6: 1–102
2. Liebow AA, Carrington CB. The interstitial pneumonias. In Simon M, Potchen EJ, Lemay E (Eds.) Frontiers in Pulmonary Radiology. New York: Grune and Stratton, 1969; 102–141
3. Anttila S, Sutinen S, Paananen M, Kreus KE, Sivonen SJ, Grekula A et al. Hard metal lung disease: a clinical, histological, ultrastructural and X-ray microanalytical study. Eur J Respir Dis 1986; 69: 83–94
4. Katzenstein AL, Fiorelli RF. Nonspecific interstitial pneumonia/fibrosis. Histologic features and clinical significance. Am J Surg Pathol 1994; 18: 136–147
5. Myers JL, Veal Jr CF, Shin MS, Katzenstein AL. Respiratory bronchiolitis causing interstitial lung disease. A clinicopathologic study of six cases. Am Rev Respir Dis 1987; 135: 880–884
6. Yousem SA, Colby TV, Gaensler EA. Respiratory bronchiolitis-associated interstitial lung disease and its relationship to desquamative interstitial pneumonia. Mayo Clin Proc 1989; 64: 1373–1380
7. Katzenstein AL, Myers JL, Mazur MT. Acute interstitial pneumonia: a clinicopathologic, ultrastructural, and cell kinetic study. Am J Surg Pathol 1986; 10: 256–267

8. Katzenstein AL, Myers JL. Idiopathic pulmonary fibrosis: clinical relevance of pathologic classification. Am J Respir Crit Care Med 1998; 157: 1301–1315

9. American Thoracic Society. Idiopathic pulmonary fibrosis: diagnosis and treatment. International Consensus Statement. American Thoracic Society (ATS) and the European Respiratory Society (ERS). Am J Respir Crit Care Med 2000; 161: 646–664

10. Nicholson AG, Colby TV, duBois RM, Hansell DM, Wells AU. The prognostic significance of the histologic pattern of interstitial pneumonia in patients presenting with the clinical entity of cryptogenic fibrosing alveolitis. Am J Respir Crit Care Med 2000; 162: 2213–2217

11. Bjoracker JA, Ryu JH, Edwin MK, Myers JL, Tazelaar HD, Schroeder DA *et al.* Prognostic significance of histopathological subsets in idiopathic pulmonary fibrosis. Am J Respir Crit Care Med 1998; 157: 199–203

12. Daniil ZD, Gilchrist FC, Nicholson AG, Hansell DM, Harris J, Colby TV *et al.* A histologic pattern of nonspecific interstitial pneumonia is associated with a better prognosis than usual interstitial pneumonia in patients with cryptogenic fibrosing alveolitis. Am J Respir Crit Care Med 1999; 160: 899–905

13. Nagai S, Kitaichi M, Itoh H, Nishimura K, Izumi T, Colby TV. Idiopathic nonspecific interstitial pneumonia/fibrosis: comparison with idiopathic pulmonary fibrosis and BOOP. Eur Resp J 1998; 12: 1010–1019

14. Travis WD, Matsui K, Moss J, Ferrans VJ. Idiopathic nonspecific interstitial pneumonia: prognostic significance of cellular and fibrosing patterns – survival comparison with usual interstitial pneumonia and desquamative interstitial pneumonia. Am J Surg Pathol 2000; 24: 19–33

15. Flaherty KR, Travis WD, Colby TV, Toews GB, Kazerooni EA, Gross BH *et al.* Histopathologic variability in usual and nonspecific interstitial pneumonias. Am J Respir Crit Care Med 2001; 164: 1722–1727

16. Flaherty KR, Toews GB, Travis WD, Colby TV, Kazerooni EA, Gross BH *et al.* Clinical significance of histological classification of idiopathic interstitial pneumonia. Eur Respir J 2002; 19: 275–283

17. Ryu JH, Colby TV, Hartman TE, Vassallo R. Smoking-related interstitial lung diseases: a concise review. Eur Respir J 2001; 17: 122–132

18. Moon J, duBois RM, Colby TV, Hansell DM, Nicholson AG. Clinical significance of respiratory bronchiolitis on open lung biopsy and its relationship to smoking related interstitial lung disease. Thorax 1999; 54: 1009–1014

19. Johkoh T, Muller NL, Cartier Y, Kavanagh PV, Hartman TE, Akira M *et al.* Idiopathic interstitial pneumonias: diagnostic accuracy of thin-section CT in 129 patients. Radiology 1999; 211: 555–560

20. Wells AU, Rubens MB, du Bois RM, Hansell DM. Serial CT in fibrosing alveolitis: prognostic significance of the initial pattern. Am J Roentgenol 1993; 161: 1159–1165

21. Hansell DM, Wells AU. CT evaluation of fibrosing alveolitis – applications and insights. J Thor Imag 1996; 11: 231–249

22. Travis WD, King TE, Bateman ED, Lynch DA, Capron F, Colby TV *et al.* Consensus classification of idiopathic interstitial pneumonias. Am J Respir Crit Care Med 2002; 165: 277–304

23. Carrington CB, Gaensler EA, Coutu RE, Fitzgerald MX, Gupta RG. Natural history and treated course of usual and desquamative interstitial pneumonia. N Engl J Med 1978; 298: 801–809

24. Muller NL, Guerry-Force ML, Staples CA, Wright JL, Wiggs B, Coppin C *et al.* Differential diagnosis of bronchiolitis obliterans with organizing pneumonia and usual interstitial pneumonia: clinical, functional, and radiologic findings. Radiology 1987; 162: 151–156

25. Crystal RG, Gadek JE, Ferrans VJ, Fulmer JD, Line BR, Hunninghake GW. Interstitial lung disease: current concepts of pathogenesis, staging and therapy. Am J Med 1981; 70: 542–568

26. Katzenstein AL, Myers JL, Prophet WD, Corley LS, Shin MS. Bronchiolitis obliterans and usual interstitial pneumonia. A comparative clinicopathologic study. Am J Surg Pathol 1986; 10: 373–381

27. Scadding JG. Fibrosing alveolitis. Br Med J 1964; 2: 686

28. Turner-Warwick M. In search of a cause of cryptogenic fibrosing alveolitis (CFA): one initiating factor or many? Thorax 1998; 53: S3–S9

29. Britton J, Hubbard R. Recent advances in the aetiology of cryptogenic fibrosing alveolitis. Histopathology 2000; 37: 387–392

30. Scadding JG, Hinson KFW. Diffuse fibrosing alveolitis (diffuse interstitial fibrosis of the lungs): correlation of histology at biopsy with prognosis. Thorax 1967; 22: 291–304

31. Dunnill MS. Pulmonary fibrosis. Histopathology 1990; 16: 321–329

32. Turner-Warwick M, Burrows B, Johnson A. Cryptogenic fibrosing alveolitis: clinical features and their influence on survival. Thorax 1980; 35: 171–180

33. Fishman AP. UIP, DIP and all that. N Engl J Med 1978; 298: 843–845

34. Hartman TE, Primack SL, Kang EY, Swensen SJ, Hansell DM, McGuinness G et al. Disease progression in usual interstitial pneumonia compared with desquamative interstitial pneumonia. Assessment with serial CT. Chest 1996; 110: 378–382

35. Akira M, Yamamoto S, Hara H, Sakatani M, Ueda E. Serial computed tomographic evaluation in desquamative interstitial pneumonia. Thorax 1997; 52: 333–337.

36. Katzenstein AL, Askin FB. Idiopathic Interstitial Pneumonia. In Katzenstein AL, Askin FB (Eds.) Surgical Pathology of Non-neoplastic Lung Disease. Philadelphia: W.B. Saunders, 1997; 49–80

37. King Jr TE, Schwarz MI, Brown K, Tooze JA, Colby TV, Waldron Jr JA et al. Idiopathic pulmonary fibrosis: relationship between histopathologic features and mortality. Am J Respir Crit Care Med 2001; 164: 1025–1032

38. Nicholson AG, Fulford LG, Colby TV, du Bois RM, Hansell DM, Wells AU. The frequency of fibroblastic foci in usual interstitial pneumonia and their relationship to disease progression. Am J Respir Crit Care Med 2002; 166: 173–177.

39. Myers JL. NSIP, UIP, and the ABCs of idiopathic interstitial pneumonias. Eur Resp J 1998; 12: 1003–1004

40. Kondoh Y, Taniguchi H, Kawabata Y, Yokoi T, Suzuki K, Takagi K. Acute exacerbation in idiopathic pulmonary fibrosis. Analysis of clinical and pathologic findings in three cases. Chest 1993; 103: 1808–1812

41. Akira M. Computed tomography and pathologic findings in fulminant forms of idiopathic interstitial pneumonia. J Thorac Imag 1999; 14: 76–84

42. Akira M, Hamada H, Sakatani M, Kobayashi C, Nishioka M, Yamamoto S. CT findings during phase of accelerated deterioration in patients with idiopathic pulmonary fibrosis. Am J Roentgenol 1997; 168: 79–83

43. Yousem SA. Eosinophilic pneumonia-like areas in idiopathic usual interstitial pneumonia. Mod Pathol 2000; 13: 1280–1284

44. Ognibene FP, Masur H, Rogers P, Travis WD, Suffredini, AF et al. Nonspecific interstitial pneumonitis without evidence of *Pneumocystis carinii* in asymptomatic patients infected with human immunodeficiency virus (HIV). Ann Int Med 1988; 109: 874–879

45. Nicholson AG, Wells AU. Nonspecific interstitial pneumonia – nobody said it's perfect. Am J Respir Crit Care Med 2001; 164: 1553–1554

46. MacDonald SL, Rubens MB, Hansell DM, Copley SJ, Desai SR, du Bois RM et al. Nonspecific interstitial pneumonia and usual interstitial pneumonia: comparative appearances at and diagnostic accuracy of thin-section CT. Radiology 2001; 221: 600–605

47. Hartman TE, Swensen SJ, Hansell DM, Colby TV, Myers JL, Tazelaar HD et al. Nonspecific interstitial pneumonia: variable appearance at high-resolution chest CT. Radiology 2000; 217; 701–705

48. Hamman L, Rich A. Acute diffuse interstitial fibrosis of the lung. Bull Johns Hopkins Hosp 1944; 74: 177

49. Olson J, Colby TV, Elliott CG. Hamman–Rich syndrome revisited. Mayo Clin Proc 1990; 65: 1538–1548

50. Myers JL, Colby TV. Pathologic manifestations of bronchiolitis, constrictive bronchiolitis, cryptogenic organizing pneumonia, and diffuse panbronchiolitis. Clin Chest Med 1993; 14: 611–622

51. Colby TV. Pathologic aspects of bronchiolitis obliterans organizing pneumonia. Chest 1992; 102: 38S–43S

52. Vourlekis JS, Brown KK, Cool CD, Young DA, Cherniack RM, King TE et al. Acute interstitial pneumonitis – case series and review of the literature. Medicine 2000; 79: 369–378

53. Davison AG, Heard BE, McCallister WAC, Turner-Warwick MEH. Cryptogenic organising pneumonitis. Quart J Med 1983; 52: 383–394

54. King TEJ, Mortenson RL. Cryptogenic organizing pneumonitis. The North American experience. Chest 1992; 102: 8S–13S
55. Cordier JF. Organising pneumonia. Thorax 2000; 55: 318–328
56. Epler GR, Colby TV, McCloud TC, Carrington CB, Gaensler EA. Bronchiolitis obliterans organising pneumonia. N Engl J Med 1985; 312: 152–158
57. Wright JL, Cagle P, Churg A, Colby TV, Myers J. Diseases of the small airways. Am Rev Respir Dis 1992; 146: 240–262
58. Kitaichi M. Pathologic features and the classification of interstitial pneumonia of unknown etiology. Bull Chest Dis Res Inst, Kyoto Univ 1990; 23: 1–18
59. Costabel U, Teschler H, Guzman J. Bronchiolitis obliterans organizing pneumonia (BOOP): the cytological and immunocytological profile of bronchoalveolar lavage. Eur Respir J 1992; 5: 791–797
60. Nagai S, Aung H, Tanaka S, Satake N, Mio T, Kawatani A et al. Bronchoalveolar lavage cell findings in patients with BOOP and related diseases. Chest 1992; 102: 32S–37S
61. Yousem SA, Lohr RH, Colby TV. Idiopathic bronchiolitis obliterans organizing pneumonia/cryptogenic organizing pneumonia with unfavorable outcome: pathologic predictors. Mod Pathol 1997; 10: 864–871
62. Cohen AJ, King TE, Downey GP. Rapidly progressive bronchiolitis obliterans with organizing pneumonia. Am J Respir Crit Care Med 1994; 149: 1670–1675
63. Lohr RH, Boland BJ, Douglas WW, Dockrell DH, Colby TV, Swensen SJ et al. Organizing pneumonia. Features and prognosis of cryptogenic, secondary, and focal variants. Arch Int Med 1997; 157: 1323–1329
64. Corrin B, Dewar A, Rodriguez-Roisin R, Turner-Warwick M. Fine structural changes in cryptogenic fibrosing alveolitis and asbestosis. J Pathol 1985; 147: 107–119
65. Fromm GB, Dunn LJ, Harris JO. Desquamative interstitial pneumonitis. Characterization of free intraalveolar cells. Chest 1980; 77: 552–554
66. Hartman TE, Primack SL, Swensen SJ, Hansell D, McGuinness G, Muller NL. Desquamative interstitial pneumonia: thin-section CT findings in 22 patients. Radiology 1993; 187: 787–790
67. Bedrossian CW, Kuhn C, Luna MA, Conklin RH, Byrd RB, Kaplan PD. Desquamative interstitial pneumonia-like reaction accompanying pulmonary lesions. Chest 1977; 72: 166–169
68. Herbert A, Sterling G, Abraham J, Corrin B. Desquamative interstitial pneumonia in an aluminum welder. Hum Pathol 1982; 13: 694–699
69. Hamadeh MA, Atkinson J, Smith LJ. Sulfasalazine-induced pulmonary disease. Chest 1992; 101: 1033–1037
70. Niewoehner DE, Kleinerman J, Rice DB. Pathologic changes in the peripheral airways of young cigarette smokers. N Engl J Med 1974; 291: 755–758
71. Holt RM, Schmidt RA, Godwin JD, Raghu G. High resolution CT in respiratory bronchiolitis-associated interstitial lung disease. J Comput Assist Tomo 1993; 17: 46–50
72. Heyneman LE, Ward S, Lynch DA, Remy-Jardin M, Johkoh T, Muller NL. Respiratory bronchiolitis, respiratory bronchiolitis-associated interstitial lung disease, and desquamative interstitial pneumonia: different entities or part of the spectrum of the same disease process? Am J Roentgenol 1999; 173: 1617–1622
73. King TE. Respiratory bronchiolitis-associated interstitial lung disease. Clin Chest Med 1993; 14: 693–698
74. Kradin RL, Young RH, Kradin LA, Mark EJ. Immunoblastic lymphoma arising in chronic lymphoid hyperplasia of the pulmonary interstitium. Cancer 1982; 50: 1339–1343
75. Teruya-Feldstein J, Temeck BK, Sloas MM, Kingma DW, Raffeld M, Pass HI et al. Pulmonary malignant lymphoma of mucosa-associated lymphoid tissue (MALT) arising in a pediatric HIV-positive patient. Am J Surg Pathol 1995; 19: 357–363
76. Kramer MR, Saldana MJ, Ramos M, Pitchenik AE. High titres of Epstein–Barr virus antibodies in adult patients with lymphocytic interstitial pneumonitis associated with AIDS. Respir Med 1992; 86: 49–52
77. Barbera JA, Hayashi S, Hegele RG, Hogg JC. Detection of Epstein–Barr virus in lymphocytic interstitial pneumonia by in situ hybridisation. Am Rev Respir Dis 1992; 145: 940–946
78. Kaan PM, Hegele RG, Hayashi S, Hogg JC. Expression of bcl-2 and Epstein–Barr virus LMP1 in lymphocytic interstitial pneumonia. Thorax 1997; 52: 12–16

79. Andiman WA, Eastman R, Martin K, Katz BZ, Rubinstein A, Pitt J *et al*. Opportunistic lymphoproliferations associated with Epstein–Barr viral DNA in infants and children with AIDS. Lancet 1985; 2: 1390–1393

80. Trovato R, Luppi M, Barozzi P, Da Prato L, Maiorana A, Lico S *et al*. Cellular localization of human herpesvirus 8 in nonneoplastic lymphadenopathies and chronic interstitial pneumonitis by *in situ* polymerase chain reaction studies. J Hum Virol 1999; 2: 38–44

81. Koss MN, Hochholzer L, Langloss JM, Wehunt WD, Lazarus AA. Lymphoid interstitial pneumonia: clinicopathological and immunopathological findings in 18 cases. Pathology 1987; 19: 178–185

82. Strimlan CV, Rosenow EC, Weiland LH, Brown LR. Lymphocytic interstitial pneumonitis. Review of 13 cases. Ann Int Med 1978; 88: 616–621

83. Nicholson AG, Wotherspoon AC, Diss TC, Hansell DM, DuBois R, Sheppard MN *et al*. Reactive pulmonary lymphoid disorders. Histopathology 1995; 26: 405–412

84. Liebow AA, Carrington CB. Diffuse pulmonary lymphoreticular infiltrations associated with dysproteinaemia. Med Clin North Am 1973; 57: 809–843

85. Church JA, Isaacs H, Saxon A, Keens TG, Richards W. Lymphoid interstitial pneumonitis and hypogammoglobulinaemia in children. Am Rev Respir Dis 1981; 124: 491–496

86. Montes M, Tomasi Jr TB, Noehreun TH, Culver GJ. Lymphoid interstitial pneumonia with monoclonal gammopathy. Am Rev Respir Dis 1968; 98: 277–280

87. Yousem SA, Colby TV, Carrington CB. Follicular bronchitis/bronchiolitis. Hum Pathol 1985; 16: 700–706

88. Fortoul TI, Cano-Valle F, Oliva E, Barrios R. Follicular bronchiolitis in association with connective tissue diseases. Lung 1985; 163: 305–314

89. Poletti V, Kitaichi M. Facts and controversies in the classification of idiopathic interstitial pneumonias. Sarcoidosis Vasc Diff Lung Dis 2000; 17: 229–238

90. Kurosu K, Yumoto N, Furukawa M, Kuriyama T, Mikata A. Third complementarity-determining-region sequence analysis of lymphocytic interstitial pneumonia: most cases demonstrate a minor monoclonal population hidden among normal lymphocyte clones. Am J Respir Crit Care Med 1997; 155: 1453–1460

91. Wiedemann HP, Matthay RA. Pulmonary manifestations of the collagen vascular diseases. Clin Chest Med 1989; 10: 677–722

92. Askin FB. Pulmonary disorders in the collagen vascular diseases. Hum Pathol 1990; 21: 465–466

93. Katzenstein AL, Askin FB. Systemic diseases involving the lung. In Katzenstein M, Askin FB (Eds) Surgical Pathology of Non-neoplastic Lung Disease. Philadelphia, PA: Saunders, 1997; 168–192

94. Wells AU. Lung disease in association with connective tissue disorders. In Olivieri D, du Bois RM (Eds) Interstitial Lung Diseases. Sheffield: ERS Journals Ltd, 2001: 137–164

95. Yousem SA, Colby TV, Carrington CB. Lung biopsy in rheumatoid arthritis. Am Rev Respir Dis 1985; 131: 770–777

96. Tazelaar HD, Viggiano RW, Pickersgill J, Colby TV. Interstitial lung disease in polymyositis and dermatomyositis. Clinical features and prognosis as correlated with histologic findings. Am Rev Respir Dis 1990; 141: 727–733

97. Schwarz MI, Matthay RA, Sahn SA, Stanford RE, Marmorstein BL, Scheinhorn DJ. Interstitial lung disease in polymyositis and dermatomyositis: analysis of six cases and review of the literature. Medicine (Baltimore) 1976; 55: 89–104

98. King TE. Connective tissue disease. In Schwarz MI, King TE (Eds) Interstitial Lung Disease. Hamilton, Ontario, BC: Decker Inc, 1998; 645–684

99. Imokawa S, Sato A, Sato J, Tsukamoto K, Todate A, Toyoshima M *et al*. Interstitial pneumonia preceding systemic sclerosis. Nihon Kokyuki Gakkai Zasshi 1998; 36: 969–972

100. Nicholson AG, Colby TV, Wells AU. Histopathological approach to patterns of interstitial pneumonia in patients with connective tissue disorders. Sarcoidosis Vasc Diff Lung Dis 2002; 19: 10–17

101. Fairfax AJ, Haslam PL, Pavia D, Sheahan NF, Bateman JR, Agnew JE *et al*. Pulmonary disorders associated with Sjogren's syndrome. Quart J Med 1981; 50: 279–295

102. Turner-Warwick M. Some connective tissue disorders of the lung. Postgrad Med J 1988; 64: 497–504

103. Bouros D, Nicholson AG, Colby TV, Polychronopoulos V, Pantelidis P, Wells AU et al. Histopathologic subsets of fibrosing alveolitis in patients with scleroderma and their relationship to natural history and treated course. Am J Respir Crit Care Med 2002

104. Nagao T, Nagai S, Kitaichi M, Hayashi M, Shigematsu M, Tsutsumi T et al. Usual interstitial pneumonia: idiopathic pulmonary fibrosis versus collagen vascular diseases. Respiration 2001; 68: 151–159

105. Takizawa H, Shiga J, Moroi Y, Miyachi S, Nishiwaki M, Miyamoto T. Interstitial lung disease in dermatomyositis: clinicopathological study. J Rheumatol 1987; 14: 102–107

106. Douglas WW, Tazelaar HD, Hartman TE, Hartman RP, Decker PA, Schroeder DR et al. Polymyositis–dermatomyositis-associated interstitial lung disease. Am J Respir Crit Care Med 2001; 164: 1182–1185

107. Hakala M, Paakko P, Huhti E, Tarkka M, Sutinen S. Open lung biopsy of patients with rheumatoid arthritis. Clin Rheumatol 1990; 9: 452–460

108. Fujita J, Yamadori I, Suemitsu I, Yoshinouchi T, Ohtsuki Y, Yamaji Y et al. Clinical features of non-specific interstitial pneumonia. Respir Med 1999; 93: 113–118

109. Kim JS, Lee KS, Koh EM, Kim SY, Chung MP, Han J. Thoracic involvement of systemic lupus erythematosus: clinical, pathologic, and radiologic findings. J Comput Assist Tomogr 2000; 24: 9–18

110. Orens JB, Martinez FJ, Lynch JP. Pleuropulmonary manifestations of systemic lupus erythematosus. Rheum Dis Clin North Am 1994; 20: 159–193

111. Murin S, Wiedemann HP, Matthay RA. Pulmonary manifestations of systemic lupus erythematosus. Clin Chest Med 1998; 19: 641–165

112. White B, Moore WC, Wigley FM, Xiao HQ, Wise RA. Cyclophosphamide is associated with pulmonary function and survival benefit in patients with scleroderma and alveolitis. Ann Int Med 2000; 132: 947–954

113. Cheema GS, Quismorio FP. Interstitial lung disease in systemic lupus erythematosus. Curr Opin Pulm Med 2000; 6: 424–429

114. Nadorra RL, Landing BH. Pulmonary lesions in childhood onset systemic lupus erythematosus: analysis of 26 cases, and summary of literature. Pediatr Pathol 1987; 7: 1–18

115. Kim WU, Kim SI, Yoo WH, Park JH, Min JK, Kim SC et al. Adult respiratory distress syndrome in systemic lupus erythematosus: causes and prognostic factors: a single center, retrospective study. Lupus 1999; 8: 552–557

116. Haupt HM, Moore GW, Hutchins GM. The lung in systemic lupus erythematosus. Analysis of the pathologic changes in 120 patients. Am J Med 1981; 71: 791–798

117. Lakhanpal S, Lie JT, Conn DL, Martin WJ. Pulmonary disease in polymyositis/dermatomyositis: a clinicopathological analysis of 65 autopsy cases. Ann Rheum Dis 1987; 46: 23–29

118. Strimlan CV, Rosenov EC, Divertie MB, Harrison Jr EG. Pulmonary manifestations of Sjogren's syndrome. Chest 1976; 70: 354–361

119. Yood RA, Steigman DM, Gill LR. Lymphocytic interstitial pneumonitis in a patient with systemic lupus erythematosus. Lupus 1995; 4: 161–163

120. Nicholson AG, Wotherspoon AC, Diss TC, Butcher DN, Sheppard MN, Isaacson PG et al. Pulmonary B-cell non-Hodgkin's lymphomas. The value of immunohistochemistry and gene analysis in diagnosis. Histopathology 1995; 26: 395–404

121. Nicholson AG, Wotherspoon AC, Jones AL, Sheppard MN, Isaacson PG, Corrin B. Pulmonary B-cell non-Hodgkin's lymphoma associated with autoimmune disorders: a clinicopathological review of six cases. Eur Respir J 1996; 9: 2022–2025

122. Frizzera G. Immunosuppression, autoimmunity and lymphoproliferative disorders. Hum Pathol 1994; 25: 627–629.

123. Orchard TR, Eraut CD, Davison AG. Non-Hodgkin's lymphoma arising in cryptogenic fibrosing alveolitis. Thorax 1998; 53: 228–229

124. Rees JH, Woodhead MA, Sheppard MN, du Bois RM. Rheumatoid arthritis and cryptogenic organising pneumonitis. Respir Med 1991; 85: 243–246

125. Min JK, Hong YS, Park SH, Park JH, Lee SH, Lee YS et al. Bronchiolitis obliterans organizing pneumonia as an initial manifestation in patients with systemic lupus erythematosus. J Rheumatol 1997; 24: 2254–2257

126. Bridges AJ, Hsu KC, Dias-Arias AA, Chechani V. Bronchiolitis obliterans organizing pneumonia and scleroderma. J Rheumatol 1992; 19: 1136–1140

127. Hayashi R, Yamashita N, Sugiyama E, Maruyama M, Matsui S, Yoshida Y *et al*. A case of primary Sjogren's syndrome with interstitial pneumonia showing bronchiolitis obliterans organizing pneumonia pattern and lymphofollicular formation. Nihon Kokyuki Gakkai Zasshi 2000; 38: 880–884

128. Yousem SA. The pulmonary pathologic manifestations of the CREST syndrome. Hum Pathol 1990; 21: 467–474

129. Wells AU, du Bois RM. Bronchiolitis in association with connective tissue disorders. Clin Chest Med 1993; 14: 655–666

130. Bokulic RE, Hilman BC. Interstitial lung disease in children. Pedr Clin N Am 1994; 41: 543–567

131. Fan LL, Langston C. Chronic interstitial lung disease in children. Pediatr Pulmonol 1993; 16: 184–196

132. Katzenstein AL, Gordon LP, Oliphant M, Swender PT. Chronic pneumonitis of infancy. A unique form of interstitial lung disease occurring in early childhood. Am J Surg Pathol 1995; 19: 439–447

133. Schroeder SA, Shannon DC, Mark EJ. Cellular interstitial pneumonitis in infants: a clinicopathologic study. Chest 1992; 101: 1065–1069

134. Bush A, du Bois RM. Congenital and pediatric interstitial disease. Curr Op Pulmonol Med 1996; 2: 347–356

135. Bush A. Diagnosis of interstitial lung disease. Pediatr Pulmonol 1996; 22: 81–82

136. Fan LL. Evaluation and therapy of chronic interstitial pneumonitis in children. Curr Op Pediatr 1994; 6: 248–254

137. Nicholson AG, Kim H, Corrin B, Bush A, duBois RM, Rosenthal M *et al*. The value of classifying interstitial pneumonitis in childhood according to defined histological patterns. Histopathology 1998; 33: 203–211

138. Fan LL. Pediatric interstitial lung disease. In Schwartz MI, King TE Jr. Interstitial Lung Disease 3rd edn. Ontario: B.C. Decker 2001; 103–188

139. Sharief N, Crawford OF, Dinwiddie R. Fibrosing alveolitis and desquamative interstitial pneumonitis. Pediatr Pulmonol 1994; 17: 359–365

140. Stillwell P, Norris DG, O'Connell EJ, Rosenow EC, Weiland LH, Harrison EG. Desquamative interstitial pneumonitis in children. Chest 1980; 77: 165–171

141. Tal A, Maor E, Bar-Ziv J, Gorodischer R. Fatal desquamative interstitial pneumonia in three infants siblings. J Pediatr 1984; 104: 873–876

142. Amir G, Ron N. Pulmonary pathology in Gaucher's disease. Hum Pathol 1999; 30: 666–670

143. Waters KA, Bale P, Isaacs D, Mellis C. Successful chloroquine therapy in a child with lymphoid interstitial pneumonitis. J Pediatr 1991; 119: 989–991

144. Nicholson AG. Lymphocytic interstitial pneumonia and other lymphoproliferative disorders. Sem Resp Crit Care Med 2001; 22: 409–422.

145. MacDonald SLS, Rubens MB, Hansell DM, Copley SJ, Desai SR, du Bois RM *et al*. Non-specific interstitial pneumonia and usual interstitial pneumonia: comparative appearances and diagnostic accuracy of high resolution computed tomography. Radiology 2001; in press.

146. Du Bois RM. Diffuse lung disease: an approach to management. Br Med J 1994; 309: 175–179

147. Tung KT, Wells AU, Rubens MB, Kirk JM, du Bois RM, Hansell DM. Accuracy of the typical computed tomographic appearances of fibrosing alveolitis. Thorax 1993; 48: 334–338

148. Primack SL, Hartman TE, Ikezoe J, Akira M, Sakatani M, Muller NL. Acute interstitial pneumonia: radiographic and CT findings in nine patients. Radiology 1993; 188: 817–820

149. Katoh T, Andoh T, Mikawa K, Tanizawa M, Tanigawa M, Suzuki R *et al*. Computed tomographic findings in non-specific interstitial pneumonia/fibrosis. Respirology 1998; 3: 69–75

150. Colby TV, Swensen SJ. Anatomic distribution and histopathologic patterns in diffuse lung disease: correlation with HRCT. J Thorac Imag 1996; 11: 1–26

151. Primack SL, Hartman TE, Hansell DM, Muller NL. End-stage lung disease: CT findings in 61 patients. Radiology 1993; 189: 681–686

152. Hunninghake GW, Zimmerman MB, Schwartz DA, King Jr TE, Lynch J, Hegele R *et al*. Utility of a lung biopsy for the diagnosis of idiopathic pulmonary fibrosis. Am J Respir Crit Care Med 2001; 164: 193–196

4

Joint disease and the pathologist

A.J. Freemont

Joints allow bones to move relative to one another. Their structure varies with site and is dependent upon the degree of movement required between the two bones. When they work normally they are highly efficient; when they do not the patient experiences anything from minor to severe morbidity.

TYPES OF JOINTS

There is a hierarchy of joints, defined by the structure and range of movement allowed at the joint. All have in common the interposition between the bone ends of a non-osseous connective tissue.

FIBROUS JOINTS

Fibrous joints are exemplified by the symphysis pubis, the skull sutures and the joints binding the distal ends of the paired long bones of the limbs. These joints allow the smallest range of movements and are characterised structurally by the two bone ends being closely and tightly bound to one another by dense fibrous tissue.

CARTILAGINOUS JOINTS

These joints are effectively restricted to the sternum and its associated bones. The distance between the bone ends is invariably greater than with fibrous joints. This, coupled with the physical properties of cartilage, allows a greater degree and range of movements than do fibrous joints, including bending and twisting.

SYNOVIAL JOINTS

These are the joints we immediately think of when talking about joint disease. They are characterised by having a space between the two bone ends. Each bone end is covered by articular cartilage, which also forms part of the lining of the

A.J. Freemont BSc MD FRCP FRCPath, Professor of Osteoarticular Pathology, University of Manchester, Manchester, UK

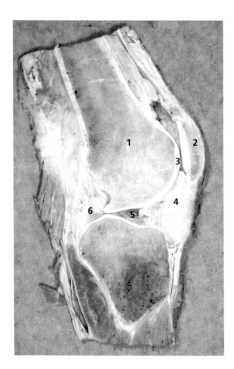

Fig. 4.1 A longitudinal section through a human knee. The various components of this, the most complex joint in the body, are labelled. 1 – Femur, 2 – patella, 3 – articular cartilage, 4 – synovium, 5 – joint space, 6 – capsule.

joint space. Synovium lines the remainder of the space. The space contains synovial fluid (SF) (Fig. 4.1).

THE NATURE OF SYNOVIUM

Synovium is an intriguing tissue. It lines not just synovial joints but also tendon sheaths and bursae. Indeed wherever spaces occur within mesenchymal connective tissue, usually as a consequence of the development of sliding planes, synovium forms. Lubrication of connective tissue sliding planes is by hyaluronan-rich fluids (mucins), and it is hardly surprising, therefore, to find one of the two types of cells on the synovial surface. The type B synoviocyte has the ability to synthesise hyaluronans. The other type of synoviocyte (type A) is derived from the macrophage and has the dual functions of phagocytosis and bioregulation through synthesis of cytokines. In human synovium, the synoviocyte layer is incomplete, leaving SF in contact with the matrix of synovium, which is usually either adipose or fibrous tissue. In this context it is worth noting that:

(a) there is no cell layer on the surface of cartilage. Thus there is no cell layer to modify movement of molecules into and across the joint as there is in other body cavities;

(b) as cartilage and SF are effectively avascular, the synovial blood vessels are key to the nutrition and fluid balance within the joint.

SYNOVIAL JOINT STABILITY

Having two bone ends capable of independent movement makes the joint inherently unstable. Stability is achieved by encasing the joint in a dense fibrous tissue capsule that attaches to the bones either side of the joint. In the directions in which physical loads are greatest within the joint, the capsule is strengthened with thickenings (ligaments) and in some joints, such as the knee and hip, ligaments are also present inside the joint. The capsule and the muscles acting across the joint effectively pull the two bone ends together, a pull resisted by the articular cartilage. These opposing forces give the joint stability. Should the capsule become 'lax' through trauma, through genetic defects in synthesis of its components, such as type I collagen or should the physical size or properties of the cartilage change (as in osteoarthritis (OA)), the joint will become 'unstable' and subject to injury both chronic, low grade and acute.

OTHER JOINTS

Other joints, such as the intervertebral disc, are variants of these three main types.

THE SPECTRUM OF JOINT DISEASE

It is widely held that joints are susceptible to two major groups of disorders – inflammatory and non-inflammatory. While this is true, were this description to be used, perfectly legitimately, to describe the diseases of the brain for instance, the lack of precision (in the context of the brain the non-inflammatory disorders would include intracranial haemorrhage, neoplasms, infarction, penetrating and blunt trauma, etc.) would result in its falling into disuse very rapidly. The reason that the same has not happened for diseases of joints is as much for the diseases that are not seen as for those that are.

NEOPLASIA AND JOINTS

Primary neoplasms are very rare within joints. Four of the most common disorders that have pseudo-neoplastic titles, benign synovioma (villonodular synovitis), synovial chondromatosis, lipoma arborescens and synovial haemangioma are all reactive or metaplastic lesions, and synovial sarcoma has as much to do with joints as does glioblastoma multiforme. So rare are true neoplasms of joints that they still make case reports.[1,2] Metastases are also exceptionally rare within joints. Haemic neoplasms are the one the pathologist is most likely to encounter within joints.[3] As myeloma is included in this group of neoplasms, and the inflammation within synovium may consist almost entirely of plasma cells, when faced with a plasma cell (as opposed to a lymphoplasmacytic) infiltrate in the synovium it is always worth excluding plasma cell malignancy by immunohistochemical investigation of light chain restriction.

Para-articular neoplasms of bone and soft tissue may mimic joint disease.[4,5] If the articular pathology seems to be out of proportion to the symptoms, it is advisable to draw the attention of the referring clinician to this and perhaps suggest he/she widens their search for a pathology.

There is one disorder, multicentric reticulohistiocytosis, in which malignancy elsewhere within the body is associated with an infiltrate of periodic acid Schiff (PAS) positive macrophages, some very large (megalocytes) in the synovium and SF.[6] Similar changes are also seen in the skin. Multicentric reticulohistiocytosis may predate the onset of symptoms from the malignancy by some time. We have one example, where the synovial changes antedated the diagnosis of meso-thelioma by almost 2 years.

INCIDENCE AND NATURE OF JOINT DISEASES

Joint disease is very common. Inflammatory disorders, such as gout and rheuma-toid disease, affect approximately 0.3% and 2.5% of the population, respectively. Non-inflammatory disorders, such as OA and discal degeneration, will have affected 90% and 100% of the population, respectively, by the age of 40. Table 4.1 lists the important diseases of synovial and non-synovial joints. There are two aspects of the pathology that require a little enlargement upon. The first is the concept of an enthesopathy. The enthesis is the point where fibrous tissue (joint capsule, annulus fibrosus, ligament or tendon) inserts into bone. The

Table 4.1 Diseases of joints

Trauma
This is usually internalised but may be penetrating. Damage may occur to: bone, cartilage, synovium (including infarction of the synovium-covered fat pad of the knee), ligaments, capsule, menisci, entheses, etc. Often associated with haemarthrosis (haemarthrosis also seen in bleeding diatheses, inflammatory arthropathies and OA).

Inflammation
Infective
Crystal induced
Primary inflammatory
  Seropositive
    Rheumatoid disease (RA)
  Seronegative
    Seronegative spondylarthropathies
      Ankylosing spondylitis (AS)
      Psoriatic arthritis
      The arthritis associated with inflammatory bowel disease
      Infection associated – e.g. reactive arthritis, Reiter's syndrome, Poncet's
        disease (TB-associated arthritis)
      Behcet's disease
      Juvenile chronic (idiopathic) arthritis (JCA or JIA)
  Others
    'Seronegative rheumatoid disease'
    Systemic sclerosis
    Systemic lupus erythematosus (SLE)
    Polyarteritis nodosa
Inflammatory enthesopathy

Non-inflammatory
OA
Joint instability
Loose bodies – e.g. avascular bone necrosis, following trauma, synovial chondromatosis (snowstorm knee variant).

Others
Pigmented villonodular synovitis (PVNS)
Synovial chondromatosis
Lipoma arborescens
Rare metabolic disorders – e.g. ochronosis, hyperlipidaemia
Synovial haemangioma
Multicentric reticulohistiocytosis

pathology at this biomechanically compromised interface is described as an enthesopathy. Enthesopathies may be traumatic (i.e. avulsion or tearing), inflammatory (e.g. enthesitis of AS) or metabolic (e.g. undermining osteoclasts in hyperparathyroidism).[7]

The second is the way in which the inflammatory arthropathies are classified. There are inflammatory disorders secondary to an 'exogenous' agents, such as an infective organism (e.g. septic arthritis) or crystals (e.g. gout), within the joint. The remaining arthritides are referred to as primary inflammatory arthropathies. They are categorised in a number of ways. In Table 4.1, they have been classified on the basis of the syndrome with which they are associated (e.g. rheumatoid disease, systemic lupus erythematosus or the seronegative spondylarthropathies (a group of apparently disparate disorders characterised by a peripheral oligoarthropathy of synovial joints and spinal enthesitis, identical to that of AS)). The important point here is that almost all primary inflammatory arthropathies are syndromes, that is, disorders recognised on the basis of a selected group of symptoms, signs and test results. The features that define these syndromes are agreed by consensus[8] and therapeutic regimes are based on them.

THE MAJOR CLINICAL DILEMMAS OF JOINT DISEASE

All types of 'front line' clinician (e.g. orthopaedic surgeon, rheumatologist, accident and emergency (A&E) physician, general physician and general practitioner) face the same problems with diagnosing and treating joint disease and most refer to diseases of synovial joints. Very simply the questions they have difficulty in answering are:

1. Is a joint infected? Within our current understanding, most infective arthritis is septic (i.e. caused by pus forming bacteria). Making this diagnosis is very difficult because SF is bacteriostatic and yet making the diagnosis is very important as irreversible joint damage occurs in the first 1–3 days following the onset of symptoms.
2. Is my patient's arthropathy inflammatory or non-inflammatory? It can be surprisingly difficult to tell these two broad groups of disorders apart clinically (and pathologically). OA can present with a red, hot joint, whereas SLE can present with joint swelling and very little evidence of 'inflammation'. Orthopaedic surgeons are increasingly frequently submitting joint tissue because, at the time of surgery, often joint replacement, in a patient they were sure had OA, they found red 'inflamed' looking synovium.
3. What syndrome underlies an inflammatory oligoarthropathy? A major problem with diagnosis and treatment based on recognition of a syndrome is what happens when a patient presents with a spectrum of signs, symptoms etc. that do not amount to a recognised syndrome. The management of acute rheumatoid disease and early Reiter's disease is very different. There is an increasing literature showing that aggressive treatment of early rheumatoid disease may have beneficial long-term effects and considerably reduce morbidity,[9] but some of the regimens are toxic and totally inappropriate for other inflammatory arthropathies.[10] A distressing mono- or oligoarthritis can be the first presentation of almost any inflammatory arthropathy and without more

specific features to indicate a syndrome, there is a reluctance on the part of clinicians to prescribe anything other than 'generic' anti-inflammatory therapy.

4. Has the nature of a joint problem changed? Many joint diseases are chronic and significantly alter the biology of the joint such that other joint diseases can supervene. The best example is rheumatoid disease. This is a chronic disorder punctuated by relapses and remissions. The inflamed synovium causes significant damage to the cartilage and capsule, leading to instability and secondary OA. Furthermore, the local and systemic immunity is altered rendering the patient more prone to immune complex deposition and infection within the joint. The patient, who complains of sudden onset of a painful, red joint may, therefore, have an acute rheumatoid flare (usually demanding active treatment with disease modifying agents, which like gold or steroids, have significant side effects), OA, a reactive arthritis or septic arthritis. Clearly distinguishing between these disorders is important.

THE PATHOLOGISTS ROLE IN THE MANAGEMENT OF JOINT DISEASE

It is widely accepted that a key clinical role of the pathologist is the diagnosis of disease. As all the scenarios outlined above require a diagnosis to be made to advance patient management, diagnosis of joint disease would seem a very valid area of pathological endeavour particularly considering how common joint disorders are. However, pathologists have a reputation amongst clinicians for contributing little in this area: consequentially relevant clinicians tend not to send tissue to us and we become less experienced, and the myth is perpetuated and strengthened.

We do not help ourselves. If you examine the clinical workload of any district general hospital (DGH) (and most Teaching Trusts), the balance between patients seen for joint disease and those seen for connective tissue tumours is weighted significantly towards joint disease. By contrast, the national orthopaedic pathology external quality assurance (EQA) scheme quality assures orthopaedic pathologists almost exclusively on their ability to diagnose bone and soft tissue tumours or tumour-like lesions. Is this a tacit admission that as pathologists we accept we have nothing to offer in the diagnosis of joint disease?

Our experiences in Manchester are quite the opposite. Of the 2500 osteoarticular specimens reported in this laboratory a year, 125 (5%) are soft tissue tumours (the local teaching trust is a regional centre for the surgical treatment of soft tissue tumours), 125 (5%) are biopsies taken for the diagnosis of metabolic bone disease (this is an international referral centre for bone histomorphometry), 75 (3%) are bone lesions (e.g. fractures, neoplasms and infection), 125 (5%) are soft tissue lesions (e.g. ganglia, skin lumps and Morton's neuromata), and all the rest (82%) are from joints.

Clearly, our experience from offering a diagnostic service in joint disease indicates a real clinical need for pathology to contribute more to the diagnosis and management of arthropathies. Why this should be at variance with the view of many clinicians and specialist pathologists is a matter of reflection. Almost certainly, a major reason has been that we have developed or refined tests specifically focused on addressing the important clinical questions outlined above. Two stand out as representing a significant progress in the diagnosis of articular disease. They are SF analysis and improvements in diagnosing intra-articular infection.

BIOPSIES TAKEN FOR EXAMINATION BY HISTO/CYTOPATHOLOGY

The clinical limitations of conventional biopsy interpretation underpin the need for new diagnostic tests. Various components of joints are biopsied conventionally and sent to the histopathologist for diagnosis. These include:

ARTICULAR SURFACES

Articular surfaces are usually removed at the time of joint replacement surgery and rarely for diagnostic purposes. It is important to examine them, as occasionally they reveal an unexpected diagnosis, such as avascular bone necrosis or ochronosis.

LIGAMENTS, TENDONS AND MENISCI

Ligaments and tendons are only rarely biopsied for diagnostic purposes, the more usual reason being to exclude an inflammatory disorder (typically rheumatoid disease). The major pathology of these dense fibrous tissues is a response to trauma, characterised by loss of the normal collagen fibre organisation and vascular ingrowth.

Menisci are biopsied either to confirm tears or myxoid change or to establish the nature of white deposits on or in the tissue. These almost invariably turn out to be crystals of calcium pyrophosphate, which is best made by making a smear from the tissue and viewing it between crossed polarisers.

Entheses are occasionally biopsied to make the diagnosis of enthesopathy. The pathology of the enthesopathies has been detailed recently.[7]

SYNOVIUM AND TENOSYNOVIUM

There is little doubt that synovial biopsy can yield important diagnostic information that can be established in no other way.[11] The key situations in which it is particularly valuable are detailed in Table 4.2. However, even in experienced hands, synovial biopsy is unreliable at distinguishing inflammatory from non-inflammatory arthropathies and in separating different types of inflammation, although gouty tophi and rheumatoid nodules can sometimes be identified within synovium and the presence of a particularly prominent neutrophil component to the inflammation is characteristic of a seronegative spondylarthropathy (but false positive and negatives make it useful only for a speculative diagnosis).

MATERIAL REMOVED AT JOINT REVISION SURGERY

Increasingly, there is pressure on orthopaedic surgeons to revise failing prosthetic implants. In one local orthopaedic hospital, 75% of all orthopaedic prosthetic surgery is for revisions. Loosening of the prosthesis is a common cause for revision including that caused by low-grade infection at the prosthetic–bone interface.

Joint disease and the pathologist

85

Table 4.2 Situations in which synovial biopsy is indicated

Infections, particularly granulomatous infection
Granulomatous inflammation
PVNS and other forms of villonodular synovitis (e.g. giant cell tumour of tendon sheath)
Synovial chondromatosis
Lipoma arborescens
Synovial haemangioma
Detritic synovitis caused by damage to prostheses
Suspected neoplastic involvement of the synovium or multicentric reticulohistiocytosis
Metabolic disorders (e.g. hyperlipidaemia, tophaceous gout, amyloid)
Unusual forms of arthritis (e.g. plant thorn arthritis in children, ochronosis)
Any situation in which SF analysis is impossible or has proved unhelpful

At this interface a fibro-vascular membrane develops. It often comes to surround the entire intra-osseous component of the prosthesis and to become continuous with the synovium surrounding the artificial joint. At revision surgery, this can be biopsied. Usually, it contains only debris from the prosthesis[12] (e.g. high-density polyethylene, metal particles and cement) but the pioneering work of Athanasou in Oxford has shown that by careful observational analysis of intra-operative frozen sections, it is possible to diagnose infection in a significant proportion of cases.[13,14] This is exceptionally important because the greatest fear of the revision surgeon is implanting into the site of infection, as this always leads to failure of the implant. Diagnosing infection prior to surgery can be exceptionally difficult. If infection is diagnosed intra-operatively the surgery changes from a one-stage revision (where the old implant is removed and a new prosthesis implanted) to a two-stage procedure (in which the old implant is removed, the surgery terminated and the patient started on aggressive local and systemic anti-microbial chemotherapy). Surgery is completed months, sometimes years, later when the infection is considered to have been eradicated.

Athanasou, amongst others, has shown that if on careful examination of frozen sections of the membrane polymorphs are seen at a density of >1 per high-power ($\times 400$) field, infection can be diagnosed with some confidence.[15] The higher the polymorph count, the more confident can the pathologist be in diagnosing infection.

Unless some process for pre-operative diagnosis of infection can be devised, the importance of Athanasou's observations are likely to impinge increasingly on the workload of diagnostic histopathologists. At a practical level, we perform intra-operative frozen sections in conjunction with a Gram stain of a smear from the membrane. The evidence base that the latter adds to the diagnostic process is less than convincing, but performing it is reassuring for the surgeon!

SYNOVIAL FLUID ANALYSIS

SF analysis is still only practiced patchily, and then often by microbiologists who on seeing neutrophils report 'pus cells seen', which can cause consternation and concern. Over the last 10 years, the potential of SF analysis as a diagnostic tool has been much more clearly defined.[16] Interestingly, it transpires that most of the data needed to address the clinical dilemmas outlined above can come from simple analyses that can be conducted in any laboratory equipped for cytopathology.

NORMAL SYNOVIAL FLUID

SF is a transudate of plasma supplemented with high-molecular weight, saccharide-rich molecules (notably hyaluronans) produced by type B synoviocytes. The fluid is kept free of debris by macrophage-derived type A synoviocytes. Formation of SF is balanced by its removal via synovial lymphatics. It contains few cells (typically $<200/mm^3$ ($<200\,000/ml$)), mainly chondrocytes and synoviocytes shed from the tissues lining the joint, together with migratory defence cells.[17]

SYNOVIAL FLUID IN DISEASED JOINTS

Variation in the volume and composition of SF reflects pathological processes within the joint. Due to unusual relationship between the tissues within the joint, chemically-mediated events, such as inflammation and enzyme-mediated degradation, within the synovium and cartilage are reflected in changes in the chemical composition of SF. These changes include the production of factors responsible for the accumulation of different cell types within the fluid. In addition intra-articular disease processes result in the presence of particles in the fluid, which have morphological characteristics under the microscope that are helpful diagnostically. In terms of their diagnostic utility, both chemical and cytological changes in the SF have been studied. Chemical changes have shown differences between cohorts of patients, but microscopy can yield data of use in diagnosing disease in individual patients.

THE BASIC APPROACH TO SYNOVIAL FLUID MICROSCOPY

There are a number of elements to SF microscopy,[17] which require relatively simple equipment: a microscope with polarisers and a quarter wave plate, a haemocytometer chamber and a cytocentrifuge.

For its analysis, SF aspirated from joints, bursae and tendon sheaths have to be sent to the laboratory unfixed and, as such, in transit and in the laboratory should be treated with the same level of awareness of health and safety issues as any other fresh body fluid. In addition, because they are unfixed, SF deteriorates rapidly, even if kept refrigerated, and so should be examined within 24 h of aspiration. Since, SF from inflamed joints has a tendency to clot it should be anti-coagulated. The best anticoagulant is lithium heparin.

Examination of anti-coagulated SF is in four parts:

- visual analysis
- measurement of the nucleated cell count
- microscopic analysis of a 'wet preparation'
- microscopic analysis of a cytocentrifuge preparation

VISUAL ANALYSIS

SF should be examined for colour, clarity and viscosity, as each gives information about the nature of the underlying disorder.

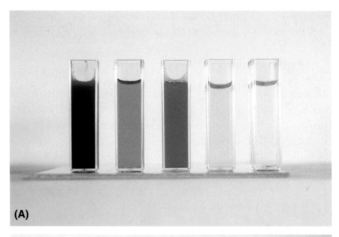

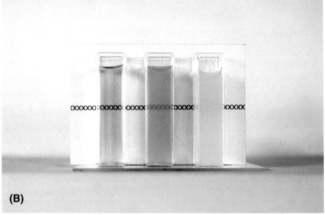

Fig. 4.2 The visual analysis of SF. (A) This shows the various colours the fluid can be. From left to right they represent: ochronosis, xanthochromia (resolving haemarthrosis), haemarthrosis, normal colour, clear fluid (usually indicates the fluid has been diluted during aspiration). (B) This shows how the turbidity can vary. That on the right has the highest density of cells or crystals.

Colour

Normally, SF is pale yellow. In haemarthroses, it will be red or orange (Fig. 4.2A) and in inflammatory arthropathies, cream or white. In septic arthritis, it may be coloured by bacterial chromogens.

Clarity

Normal SF is clear, but with increasing numbers of particles and/or cells it becomes cloudy (Fig. 4.2B).

Viscosity

SF is viscid because of the complex saccharides it contains. In inflammatory joint disease, the viscosity of the fluid falls due to enzymatic digestion and altered saccharide synthesis. This is easily demonstrated by simply allowing a small amount to trickle out of a glass pipette. In cases of inflammatory joint disease, the low-viscosity SF will form individual droplets whereas, in non-inflammatory arthropathies with more viscid fluid, a 'stringing' effect is seen.

NUCLEATED CELL COUNT

For simplicity and speed, the nucleated cell count is best performed manually using a haemocytometer chamber. It is possible to automate cell counting using a Coulter counter or similar instrument, but care has to be taken not to induce precipitation of SF hyaluronans within the capillary tubing of the instrument by using an acid-based carrier medium. In addition, hyaluronidase treatment may be necessary, if an automated counter is employed to count cell numbers in viscous fluids.

For the convenience of handling the numbers, the nucleated cell count of SF is expressed as cells/mm^3. Normal SF contains <200 cells/mm^3 (<0.2×10^9/l). In inflammatory joint disease, the cell count is >1000 cells/mm^3 (1×10^9/l) and in non-inflammatory arthropathies it is lower. Cell counts in excess of 50 000 cells/mm^3 (50×10^9/l) are virtually restricted to three clinical conditions: rheumatoid disease, septic arthritis and reactive arthritis.

WET PREPARATION

SF aspirates often contain visible particles. In making the 'wet preparation', the specimen is agitated and a small aliquot, containing as many of these particles as possible, is placed on a microscope slide. It is then gently squeezed flat beneath a cover slip and viewed unstained with a conventional microscope. For optimal results, the condenser diaphragm is partially closed to produce diffuse light in which the unstained cells and particles are more clearly seen. This preparation is examined for one cell type, the ragocyte,[18] and several different classes of crystals and other non-cellular particulate material. For better results Nomarski phase optics can be used.

Classes of crystalline material

Several classes of crystalline materials are found in the joints.[19] Their detection is not as straightforward as is sometimes believed.[20] The two most common are monosodium urate and calcium pyrophosphate dihydrate (Fig. 4.3). Monosodium urate monohydrate (urate) crystals are needle-shaped, 5–30 μm in length, and highly negatively birefringent. They can be distinguished from other crystals by their properties in polarised light. For ease, it is useful to have a microscope preparation made by smearing the contents of a superficial gouty tophus onto a slide by the microscope, as this known sample of urate crystals can then be used to standardise the optics of the microscope. When viewed between crossed polarisers with an interposed quarter wave plate the background of the microscope image is red and the urate crystals appear either yellow or blue, depending upon the direction of their long axis. Other crystals, notably calcium pyrophosphate dihydrate ('pyrophosphate') crystals, will also be yellow and blue but because they are positively birefringent, the yellow crystals will be orientated in the opposite direction to the yellow appearing urate crystals (i.e. with their axes in the same direction as the blue appearing urate crystals). Urate crystals, especially when intracellular (Fig. 4.4), are diagnostic of gout.

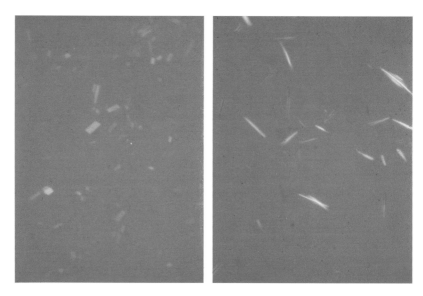

Fig. 4.3 The two most common types of intra-articular crystal viewed between crossed polarisers with an interposed quarter wave interference plate (unstained 'wet prep' ×300). The left hand image shows calcium pyrophosphate crystals – note the crystals are less bright than on the right, more cuboidal and the yellow coloured crystals have their long axes running from top right to bottom left. The right hand image is of urate crystals – note the crystals are brighter, more needle-shaped and the yellow crystals have long axes running from top left to bottom right.

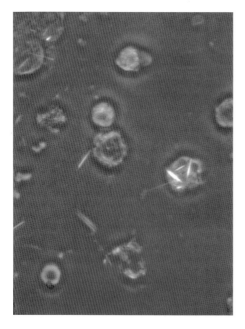

Fig. 4.4 Urate crystals within cells in a sample of SF (unstained polarised 'wet prep' ×350).

Pyrophosphate crystals accumulate within joints with advancing age and in some circumstances constitute an irrelevant finding. If pyrophosphate crystals are associated with a high nucleated cell count, the diagnosis of acute pseudogout can be made. The presence of calcium pyrophosphate crystals in association with

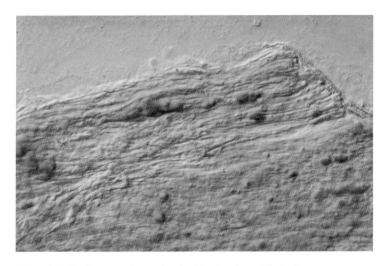

Fig. 4.5 Crystals of hydroxyapatite stained with alizarin red (×500).

otherwise typical features of OA characterises hypertrophic OA, the form of OA typified by large osteophytes and subarticular bone sclerosis.

Hydroxyapatite within SF indicates damage to calcified cartilage or underlying subarticular bone. Loss of cartilage, sufficient to expose these structures, is seen most commonly in OA and rheumatoid disease. The crystals are too small and amorphous to be seen with the light microscope, but staining with alizarin red produces a birefringent red product that is easily visualised (Fig. 4.5). A specific arthropathy, 'Milwaukee shoulder' (and its equivalent in other joints), is associated with larger apatite microspheroids.[21]

Lipids enter SF from the blood in inflammatory joint disease and haemarthroses, and from bone marrow and synovial fat in trauma. They are usually present as droplets with either a Maltese cross pattern (liquid spherical crystal) or as needle-shaped crystals within a droplet. Sometimes these crystals may be associated with inflammation.[22] Following intra-articular injection of depot corticosteroids, lipid crystalloids remain within the joint for up to 10 weeks and may be confused with pyrophosphate crystals if their true nature is not recognised.

Other crystals are found within SF, but are too numerous and rare to describe here. For a further description, see Freemont and Denton.[17]

Non-crystalline particles

Alteration to the physical structure of articular cartilage, intra-articular ligaments, menisci and synovium by primary disease or trauma leads to small fragments appearing free within the SF. Most common are fragments of articular cartilage or, specifically in the knee, internal ligament and fibrocartilage.[23]

Articular cartilage has a silken sheen in polarised light. In OA, the most common disorder in which cartilage is found free in the joint, fragments typically show clustered chondrocytes (Fig. 4.6) and the 'crimped' pattern of collagen from fibrillated cartilage, both typical of OA.

Fragments of meniscal fibrocartilage can be recognised by the curved arrays of collagen fibres and flattened chondrocytes they contain. They are typically found within traumatised knee joints.

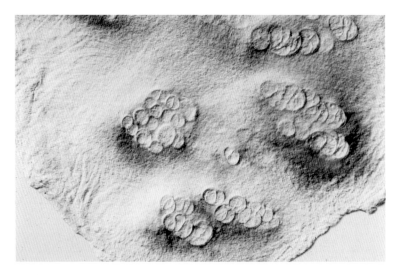

Fig. 4.6 A fragment of osteoarthritic cartilage from an SF 'wet prep'. Note the clustered chondrocytes diagnostic of OA. Unstained, Nomarski phase optics (×300).

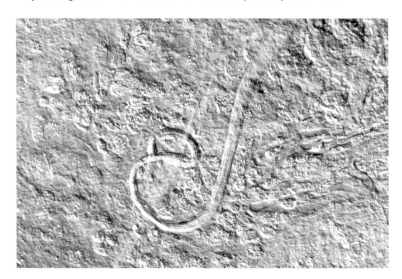

Fig. 4.7 The typical appearance of a fragment of cruciate ligament in an SF 'wet prep' (×500).

Both in traumatised joints and in rheumatoid disease, small fragments of ligament may be found within SF. They consist of long, thin twisted fibrils of no more than a dozen collagen fibres (Fig. 4.7).

There are various types of synovial chondromatosis. In one variant, cartilaginous or chondro-osseous bodies may appear in the SF in huge numbers. There is sometimes nothing to see in the synovium and the articular cartilage appears normal other than being a little soft. Due to the appearance of these white bodies within the joint inflated for arthroscopy, this has been called 'snowstorm knee'.[24] Although most common in the knee, this disorder is not restricted to this joint.

With the advent of prosthetic surgery, and particularly as the number of aging prostheses increases, wear of implanted material leads to foreign material within

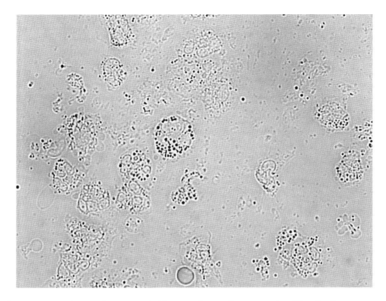

Fig. 4.8 Ragocytes in a SF 'wet prep'. These cells can be recognised by the large intracytoplasmic granules (much larger than polymorph granules), which depending on the plane in which they are viewed vary between black (as here) and apple green (×400).

the joint.[25] Many modern plastics, such as high-density polyethylene, used in prostheses, methylmethacrylate cement and biomaterial composites, such as Dacron and carbon fibre, mimic crystals if they fragment and can cause diagnostic problems.[26] Metal debris from metal-based prostheses, particularly aluminium–titanium–vanadium alloys, appears as tiny black particles. Although difficult to recognise these may be important harbingers of imminent prosthetic failure.

Occasionally, peculiar extraneous material, such as plant fibres or other foreign bodies, introduced accidentally are found within SF.

Ragocytes (Fig. 4.8) are cells of various lineages characterised by the presence of cytoplasmic refractile granules larger than conventional granulocyte granules. Ragocytes were first described in rheumatoid disease[18] (hence the name), in which they have been shown to contain immune complexes. They are not restricted to rheumatoid disease, being a constant feature of all inflammatory arthropathies, so that their diagnostic value is somewhat limited. However, with the exception of rheumatoid disease, septic arthritis, gout and pseudogout, ragocytes rarely account for more than 50% of all nucleated cells. If a crystal arthropathy is excluded, ragocyte counts above 70% are characteristic of rheumatoid disease, and above 95% of septic arthritis. The latter is diagnostic even in the absence of detectable organisms.

CYTOCENTRIFUGE PREPARATION

SF cytoanalysis can only be adequately conducted on cytocentrifuge preparations. Optimal preparations are made by diluting the fluid to 400 cells/mm^3 (0.4×10^9/l) with isotonic saline before centrifuging. The preparation is best stained with Jenner–Giemsa stain.

Staining for organisms

The one exception to the use of this dilution is when septic arthritis is suspected, when the greatest likelihood of identifying organisms is afforded by diluting the fluid to 1200 cells/mm^3 (1.2 × 10^9/l) and staining with Gram stain, most infective arthritis being caused by Gram-positive organisms.[27] Careful microscopic examination of SF allows micro-organisms to be identified in approximately 85% of instances of clinical infective arthritis. The greatest problems in diagnosing septic arthritis are: recognition of Gram-negative organisms and organisms rendered Gram-negative by incomplete antibiotic therapy; and distinguishing contaminating organisms from true pathogens.

There is an increasing incidence of non-suppurative infectious arthritis, especially in immuno-suppressed patients. Particularly common organisms include Mycobacteria and fungi. Special stains (such as Ziehl–Neelsen and periodic acid–Shiff and techniques such as lectin histochemistry, immunohistochemistry and electron microscopy) may need to be employed under these circumstances.

The significance of the cell type

Many different cell types are found within SF, reflecting the pathogenesis of the various joint diseases (Fig. 4.9). In SF microscopy, an increased diagnostic data yield comes from counting the cells and expressing them as a proportion of nucleated cells or other specific cell types. Generally, cell types are recognised on the basis of their morphology and/or tinctoral properties in the Jenner–Giemsa stain.

Polymorphs: In inflammatory arthropathies, polymorphs dominate the cytological picture (typically 60–80% of nucleated cells). They are also found in intra-articular haemorrhage (but here accompanied by significant numbers of red blood cells). However, if in an inflammatory fluid polymorphs are not the predominant cell (i.e. <50% of the cells are polymorphs) and the patient is not taking methotrexate, which specifically reduces polymorph numbers in the SF, a diagnosis of a seronegative arthropathy can be made (in this context seronegativity is meant

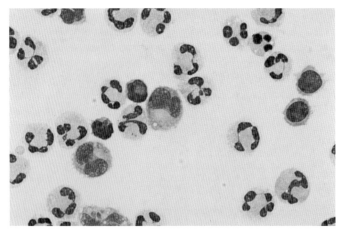

Fig. 4.9 SF cells in a Jenner–Giemsa stained cytocentrifuge preparation. Polymorphs, lymphocytes and macrophages are seen (×200).

to indicate that the patient does not have rheumatoid disease). This diagnosis incorporates the seronegative spondylarthropathies and other inflammatory arthropathies including systemic lupus erythematosus, polyarteritis nodosa and systemic sclerosis. Unfortunately, only about 50% of SFs removed from patients with a seronegative arthropathy have a seronegative pattern. In addition, about 9% of cases of rheumatoid disease will also have a seronegative pattern, but these patients also have a much-improved local prognosis in terms of interval from onset of symptoms to the need for joint replacement surgery.[28]

Septic arthritis is the only disorder in which neutrophils regularly account for more than 95% of nucleated cells. A diagnosis of septic arthritis can be made with confidence, even in the absence of identifiable organisms on Gram stain, if the sample has the following characteristics:

- total nucleated cell count $>10\,000\,\mathrm{cells/mm^3}$
- >95% of cells in the SF are neutrophils
- >95% of nucleated cells are ragocytes

Other cells: In non-inflammatory arthropathies, macrophages, lymphocytes and synoviocytes are the most commonly encountered cells.

- Lymphocytes: In inflammatory arthropathies, the presence of a cell profile of >80% lymphocytes should alert one to the possibility of SLE or tuberculous arthritis.
- Macrophages: Macrophages are the predominant cell in viral arthritis, Milwaukee shoulder and prosthetic debris-induced arthropathy. Cytophagocytic mononuclear cells (CPM) are macrophages that have phagocytosed apoptotic polymorphs (Fig. 4.10). They are found in crystal arthritis and the seronegative spondylarthropathies.[29] If CPM are seen in the absence of a crystal arthritis a confident diagnosis of a seronegative spondylarthropathy can be made, even in patients in whom the full clinical syndrome has not manifested itself. In rheumatoid disease, apoptosis occurs in the absence of CPM formation, a feature of such universal occurrence that it can also be used diagnostically.
- Mast cells: SF mast cells are seen in a number of arthropathies.[29,30] However, if they are seen on an inflammatory background (i.e. total nucleated cell count $>1000/\mathrm{mm^3}$) they are diagnostic of a seronegative spondyloarthropathy.

THE DIAGNOSTIC YIELD OF SYNOVIAL FLUID ANALYSIS

SF microscopy can provide useful data at a number of diagnostic levels, all of which have some relevance to the clinician receiving the report. In one survey, detailed microscopic analysis of SF was undertaken blinded to all clinical data on 2005 sequential specimens arriving at our laboratory over a period of 15 months. We were able to:

- make an exact diagnosis in 44% (predominantly cases of crystal arthritis, rheumatoid disease, OA and septic arthritis)
- give a relevant and clinically significant differential diagnosis in a further 22% (mainly distinguishing seronegative spondylarthropathies from rheumatoid disease in newly presented mono- and oligoarthropathies)

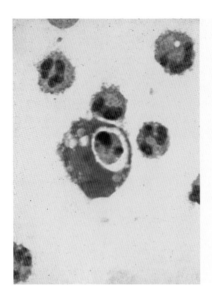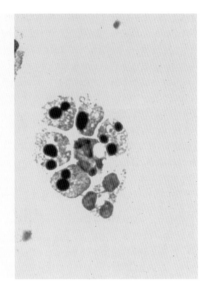

Fig. 4.10 A CPM. This characteristic cell consisting of a macrophage that has phagocytosed an apoptotic polymorph is diagnostic of the seronegative spondylarthropathies and crystal arthritis (×300).

- in a further 29% it was possible to distinguish inflammatory from non-inflammatory arthropathies
- in only 4% of cases was it not possible to give any diagnostic information

The false positive rate of SF microscopy is very low (typically <5%).[31] With clinical data, the relevant information gleaned from examination of the SF specimens is even greater.

THE PLACE OF SYNOVIAL FLUID MICROSCOPY IN DIAGNOSIS

Synovial biopsy is the investigation of choice in the disorders listed in Table 4.2. However, even experienced histopathologists can find difficulty distinguishing inflammatory from non-inflammatory arthropathies and between different members of these two groups of arthropathies on synovial biopsy.

SF microscopy on the other hand can address both these issues very well (Table 4.3). In terms of answering the questions that most concern clinicians SF microscopy is particularly useful. Most of the specimens we are sent come from clinicians who have used the service for years and are fully aware of its potential and limitations. The majority of samples are from patients with:

1. Acute inflammatory monarthropathies to exclude/diagnose infection or crystal deposition disease.
2. Acute oligoarthropathies as part of the workup of pre-syndromic inflammatory arthritis.
3. A swollen joint to distinguish inflammatory from non-inflammatory arthropathies (these requests come mainly from GPs and orthopaedic surgeons).
4. Patients with an established arthropathy (usually rheumatoid disease) who suddenly develop a 'flare'.

Table 4.3 The situations in which SF analysis is indicated

Inflammatory versus non-inflammatory arthropathy
Differential diagnosis of:
Inflammatory arthritis
Non-inflammatory arthropathies
Identification of the different types of injury within a traumatised knee
The rapid diagnosis of septic arthritis
Crystal arthritis
Oligoarthropathies
Juvenile arthritis

Synovial biopsy and SF microscopy are complementary investigations. Used together they give a very powerful tool for the diagnosis of joint disease.

THE POTENTIALLY INFECTED JOINT

So important is the subject of the infected joint that it is worth returning to it once more; first to repeat the diagnostic value of conventional histological/ cytological investigations and to introduce the potential of diagnostic molecular pathology in this area of diagnosis.

CONVENTIONAL HISTOLOGICAL/CYTOLOGICAL TESTS

Septic arthritis can be diagnosed very rapidly (within 2 h of receipt of the specimen in the laboratory) on SF microscopy, particularly if the infective organism is either a Gram-positive bacterium or a virus.

Synovial biopsy is the optimal test for diagnosing granulomatous infection particularly the more unusual organisms, such as fungi and atypical mycobacteria,[32] which infect joints surprisingly commonly.

Frozen sections of revision membranes can be used for the intra-operative diagnosis of infected orthopaedic prostheses.

Despite having this armamentarium of diagnostic tests, the clinical perspective (which is probably true) is that the pickup rate for bacterial infections, both by histopathologists and microbiologists, within joints is low.

DIAGNOSTIC MOLECULAR BIOLOGY

Recently, there has been considerable interest in the possibility of using PCR-based technology to detect organisms within joints. This has taken three directions.

IDENTIFICATION OF ORGANISMS PUTATIVELY INVOLVED IN 'PRIMARY INFLAMMATORY ARTHROPATHIES'

Since the realisation that infection in someone with a specific genetic predisposition might lead to a primary inflammatory arthropathy, potential pathogens have been sought in arthritides, such as rheumatoid disease. Using primers designed against either sequences specific to single organisms or 'pan-bacterial' sequences, synovium from cases of rheumatoid disease, etc. have been probed for evidence of bacteria. The results have been confusing in that a proportion of (but not all) cases of different types of arthritis have shown the presence of bacteria, as have some controls.[33,34] Some have interpreted their findings as indicating that the organisms have a role in initiating the arthropathy and others have described these as non-specific findings due to the joint being a site in which bacteria become sequestrated.

IDENTIFICATION OF SPECIFIC PATHOGENIC ORGANISMS

A greater success has been had by those seeking organisms believed to cause specific arthropathies. PCR-based technologies have been applied to synovium and SF to confirm a clinical diagnosis by identifying within the joint an organism known to be causally involved. Such organisms and diseases include Chlamydia in reactive arthritis[35] and Borrelia borgdorferi in Lyme disease.[36]

DIAGNOSING BACTERIAL INFECTION WITHIN A JOINT

This technology is potentially the most exciting. It employs pan-bacterial sequences, particularly to 16S ribosomal RNA, as a way of diagnosing an infective arthritis[37] or an infected prosthesis.[38] Reports are mixed. Some say that this is a highly refined and sensitive test, while others believe it is no better than standard microbiology culture, particularly if the sample has been sonicated prior to culture in order to increase the yield of viable organisms.

CONCLUDING REMARKS

With the advent of Diagnostic Molecular Pathology units as part of the process of pathology modernisation, the debate about the various merits and demerits of molecular approaches to tissue diagnosis will engage histopathologists in the future. Our current techniques will be assessed against these new technologies and we will be asked to provide material for molecular analysis.

It is worth considering SF in this context. Microscopic SF analysis is a very simple, cheap and effective diagnostic tool, which could be undertaken in any histo/cytopathology laboratory. At the same time, SF itself could be one medium that would lend itself to molecular diagnostic techniques particularly for diagnosing intra-articular infection and infection-associated prosthetic loosening, two very serious and currently diagnostically taxing disorders.

REFERENCES

1. Blokx WA, Rasing LA, Veth RP, Pruszczynski M. Late malignant transformation of biopsy proven benign synovial chondromatosis: an unexpected pitfall. Histopathology 2000; 36: 564–566
2. Thienpont E, Geens S, Nelen G. Angioleiomyoma of the knee: a case report. Acta Orthop Belg 2002; 68: 76–78
3. Jamieson KA, Beggs I, Robb JE. Synovial presentation of non-Hodgkin's lymphoma. Br J Radiol 1998; 71: 980–982

4. Kaufmann J, Schulze E, Hein G. Monoarthritis of the ankle as a manifestation of a calcaneal metastasis of bronchogenic carcinoma. Scand J Rheumatol 2001; 30: 363–365

5. Georgoulis AD, Papageourgiou CD, Moebius UG, Rossis J, Papadonikolakis A, Soucacos PN. The diagnostic dilemma created by osteoid osteoma that presents as knee pain. Arthroscopy 2002; 18: 32–37

6. Freemont AJ, Jones CJP, Denton J. The synovium and synovial fluid in multicentric reticulohistio-cytosis – a light microscopic, electron microscopic and cytochemical analysis of one case. J Clin Path 1983; 36: 860–866

7. Freemont AJ. Enthesopathies. Curr Diagnos Pathol 2002; 8: 1–10

8. The Rheumatoid Arthritis Criteria Subcommittee of the Diagnostic and Therapeutic Criteria Committee of the American Rheumatism Association. The American Rheumatism Association 1987 revised criteria for the classification of rheumatoid arthritis. Arth Rheum 1988; 31: 315–324

9. Lard LR, Visser H, Speyer I, van der Horst-Bruinsma IE, Zwinderman AH, Breedveld FC, Hazes JM. Early versus delayed treatment in patients with recent-onset rheumatoid arthritis: comparison of two cohorts who received different treatment strategies. Am J Med 2001; 111: 446–451

10. Menninger H, Herborn G, Sander O, Blechschmidt J, Rau R. A 36 month comparative trial of methotrexate and gold sodium thiomalate in the treatment of early active and erosive rheumatoid arthritis. Br J Rheumatol 1998; 37: 1060–1068

11. O'Connell JX. Pathology of the synovium. Am J Clin Pathol 2000; 114: 773–784

12. Athanasou NA. The pathology of joint replacement. Curr Diagnos Pathol 2002; 8: 26–32

13. Athanasou NA, Pandey R, de Steiger R et al. Diagnosis of infection by frozen section during revision arthroplasty. J Bone Joint Surg 1995; 77B: 28–33

14. Pandey R, Drakoulakis E, Athanasou NA. An assessment of the histological criteria used to diagnose infection in hip revision arthroplasty tissues. J Clin Pathol 1999; 52: 118–123

15. Byers RJ, Cox AJ, Freemont AJ. The pathology of the infected joint replacement. Curr Orthop 2000; 14: 243–249

16. Freemont AJ. Synovial fluid analysis. In Kippel J, Dieppe P (Eds) Rheumatology, 2nd edn, Section 2.11, New York: Mosby-Wolfe 1998

17. Freemont AJ, Denton J. Atlas of Synovial Fluid Cytopathology. Dordrecht: Kluwer Academic Publishers 1991

18. Hollander JL, McCarty DJ, Astorga G, Castro-Murillo E. Studies of the pathogenesis of rheumatoid joint inflammation. 1. The 'RA cell' and a working hypothesis. Ann Int Med 1965; 62: 271–280

19. Dieppe P, Swan A. Identification of crystals in synovial fluid. Ann Rheum Dis 1999; 58: 261–263

20. Von Essen R, Holtta AM, Pikkarainen R. Quality control of synovial fluid crystal identification. Ann Rheum Dis 1998; 57: 107–109

21. McCarty DJ, Halverson PB, Carrera GF, Brewer BJ, Kozin F. Milwaukee shoulder: association of microspheroids containing hydroxyapatite crystals, active collagenase, and neutral protease with rotator cuff defects. II. Synovial fluid studies. Arthritis Rheum 1981; 24: 474–483

22. Freemont AJ. Clinical conundrum – What is the significance of synovial fluid lipid crystals in a patient with an isolated monoarthritis? Br J Rheumatol 1992; 31: 183–184

23. Freemont AJ, Denton J. Synovial fluid finding early in traumatic arthritis. J Rheum 1988; 15: 881–882

24. Kay P, Freemont AJ, Davies DRA. The aetiology of multiple loose bodies: snowstorm knee. J Bone Joint Surg 1989; 71: 501–504

25. Bullough P, Carlo E, Hansraj K, Neves MC. Pathologic studies of total joint replacement. Orthop Clin North Am 1988; 19: 611–625

26. Clark CR, Bauer T. Routine pathological examination of operative specimens from primary total hip and total knee replacement: another look. J Bone Joint Surg Am 2000; 82-A: 1529–1530

27. Ryan MJ, Kavanagh R, Wall PG, et al. Bacterial joint infections in England and Wales: analysis of bacterial isolates over a four year period. Br J Rheumatol 1997; 36: 370–373

28. Davis MJ, Denton J, Freemont AJ et al. Comparison of serial synovial fluid cytology in rheumatoid arthritis: delineation of subgroups with prognostic implications. Ann Rheum Dis 1988; 47: 559–562

29. Freemont AJ, Denton J. The disease distribution of synovial fluid mast cells and cytophagocytic mononuclear cells in inflammatory arthritis. Ann Rheum Dis 1985; 44: 312–315

30. Dean G, Hoyland JA, Denton J, Donn RP, Freemont AJ. Mast cells in the synovium and synovial fluid in osteoarthritis. Br J Rheum 1993; 32: 671–675

31. Johnson JS, Freemont AJ. A ten year retrospective comparison of the diagnostic usefulness of synovial fluid and synovial biopsy examination. J Clin Pathol 2001; 54: 605–607

32. Harrington JT. Mycobacterial and fungal arthritis. Curr Opin Rheumatol 1998; 10: 335–338

33. Gerard HC, Wang Z, Wang GF et al. Chromosomal DNA from a variety of bacterial species is present in synovial tissue from patients with various forms of arthritis. Arthritis Rheum 2001; 44: 1689–1697

34. Kempsell KE, Cox CJ, McColm AA et al. Detection of Mycobacterium tuberculosis group organisms in human and mouse joint tissue by reverse transcriptase PCR: prevalence in diseased synovial tissue suggests lack of specific association with rheumatoid arthritis. Infect Immun 2001; 69: 1821–1831

35. Li F, Bulbul R, Schumacher HR et al. Molecular detection of bacterial DNA in venereal-associated arthritis. Arthritis Rheum 1996; 39: 950–958

36. Limbach FX, Jaulhac B, Piemont Y, Kuntz JL, Monteil H, Sibilia J. One-step reverse transcriptase PCR method for detection of Borrelia burgdorferi in mouse Lyme arthritis tissue samples. J Clin Microbiol 1999; 37: 2037–2039

37. Jalava J, Skurnik M, Toivanen A, Toivanen P, Eerola E. Bacterial PCR in the diagnosis of joint infection. Ann Rheum Dis 2001; 60: 287–289

38. Mariani BD, Tuan RS. Advances in the diagnosis of infection in prosthetic joint implants. Mol Med Today 1998; 4: 207–213

5

Liquid-based cytological preparations in gynaecological and non-gynaecological specimens

K.A. Atkins

Since the introduction and widespread use of the Papanicolaou (Pap) smear as a cervical screening test over the last 50 years, the incidence of cervical cancer in the US and Europe has declined drastically.[1] In many developing countries, cervical screening is still not commonly utilised and approximately 500 000 new cases of invasive cervical carcinoma are diagnosed each year worldwide. Although many factors play a role in the decreased incidence of invasive squamous cell carcinoma of the cervix in industrialised countries, cervical screening is probably one of the biggest contributors to the downward trend.[2] As with most screening tests, the Pap smear suffers from imperfect sensitivity and specificity. False positive results are typically a result of over-interpretation, while false negative diagnoses often are attributable to sampling and detection problems.[3] Although a clinician may have excellent collection and sampling technique, only approximately 20% of the cells collected are smeared on the glass slides in conventional Pap smears. Few advances in collection and preparation in gynaecological cytopathology in the past decades match the widespread acceptance, use and improvement in quality obtained from cytological liquid-based cytological preparation (LBC) techniques. Many studies have shown that with proper training, LBC results in a higher diagnostic yield than traditional cervical smears.[3] In the US, the Food and Drug Administration (FDA) has approved two techniques – ThinPrep (Cytyc Co., Marlborough, MA, USA) and SurePath Prep, formerly called AutoCyte (TriPath Inc., Burlington, NC, USA) – for evaluation of gynaecological and non-gynaecological cytological samples by LBC. Each technique has a unique method for producing a single monolayer of cells on a single slide while minimising blood, inflammation and proteinaceous debris. Numerous studies have evaluated diagnostic outcomes and compared the LBC techniques to conventional smear preparations and found equal or better accuracy in diagnosis using the LBC smears.[4,5]

Kristen A. Atkins MD, Assistant Professor of Pathology, Virginia Commonwealth University, Richmond, VA, USA

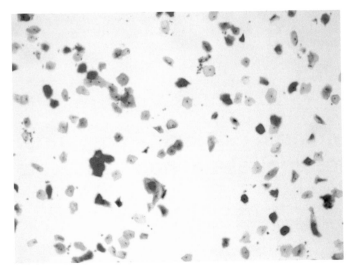

Fig. 5.1 Cytological LBC of a cervical smear at scanning power. The LBC slides generally have less inflammation, blood and mucus. Due to the processing, the cells are arranged predominantly in a single cell pattern with less clumping of cells (ThinPrep, Pap stain, ×10).

By decreasing the amount of mucus, inflammation and blood in a preparation, less clumping of the epithelial cells occur (Fig. 5.1). Mature squamous cells arrange in a single cell pattern with distinct cell borders. Both ThinPrep and SurePath Prep techniques yield a single slide that enables the cytologist to view cells with little clumping, drying artefact or other preservation problems. The gynaecological LBCs are amenable to image analysis and may promote increased utilisation of computer-generated screening techniques, which may further improve diagnostic accuracy.

LBC also lends itself nicely to testing for various human papilloma virus (HPV) strains and other sexually transmitted diseases, since the remaining sample can be utilised for testing by molecular techniques. Although the necessity and appropriateness of HPV testing is still controversial, clinicians are requesting and pathologists are utilising *in situ* hybridisation and hybrid capture techniques in questionable cases.

Although LBC is primarily used for gynaecological specimens, thin-layer preparations can also be made from fine needle aspiration biopsies (FNABs). LBCs of FNABs have both advantages and disadvantages, depending on the method employed. While the cell preservation and nuclear detail are of high quality, much of the background material and architecture is lost, which excludes a necessary component in interpretation in some circumstances. When performed in conjunction with conventional smears for Diff Quik and Pap stains, LBC may prove to be a helpful additional preparation technique.

LIQUID-BASED PREPARATION METHODS

Gynaecological specimens for LBC can be processed with traditional spatula and brush techniques, but numerous companies have made unique brushes/brooms for collecting the cervical sample. The traditional method of cervical smear procurement relies on the use of a smooth, concave spatula and separate endocervical brush. LBC collection brushes are made of numerous bristles that come to a long central point. The point is inserted into the cervical os/endocervical canal and the peripheral bristles come in contact with the ectocervix. The brush/broom is rotated, thus, sampling the ectocervix and endocervix simultaneously. The brush is then placed into either an ethanol or methanol-based liquid medium (depending on the system employed by the particular laboratory) rather than smeared on a slide, as done with traditional cervical smears. In the ThinPrep system, the brush is vigorously rinsed into the vial and then discarded. In the SurePath Prep system, the brush has a detachable head that is sent in the vial of preservative solution to the laboratory. This sampling method is easier for the clinician, who does not have to prepare the smears. Since the brush is immediately placed in fixative, less drying artefact occurs. The processing of ThinPrep and SurePath Prep cervical smear samples is different, but both produce quality slides with little cellular overlap, inflammation or obstructing debris.[6]

ThinPrep LBC is relatively fast (<30 min) and requires minimal technician time. The sample is collected in a methanol-based media, CytoLyt, and centrifuged. Two to three drops of the cell pellet are transferred to a second methanol-based preservative, PreserveCyt. The vial is then put in the ThinPrep processor. A filter-lined cylinder rotates within the vial causing a small current that breaks up mucus, debris and blood. A slight vacuum is then created and cells collect on the exterior of the filter membrane. The cylinder with the filter is removed, inverted and gently pressed against a ThinPrep slide. Air pressure ensures that the cells adhere to the slide. At this point, the slide is removed from the processor and stained by the technician according to the laboratory's protocol. The ThinPrep 3000 processor is a fully automated machine that is able to process up to 80 ThinPrep cervical smear samples at one time (four batches per 8-h shift), reducing technician time considerably.

SurePath Prep LBC takes approximately 60 min to produce the slides and requires more technician intervention. However, the machine also performs the Pap stain, thus relieving the technician of that procedure. The sample is collected in an ethanol-based media (CytoRich) that is then centrifuged. The supernatant is removed and the cell pellet is resuspended in distilled water and centrifuged a second time. After the supernatant is removed, the cell pellet is put into the SurePath system. The cells settle on a poly-L-lysine coated slide and the slides are automatically stained by the instrument.

LIQUID-BASED PREPARATIONS COMPARED TO CONVENTIONAL CERVICAL SMEARS

Numerous studies have been undertaken that compare each type of LBC with traditional smears. There is some evidence that LBC yields a reduction in the number of inadequate smears, improves sensitivity and possibly reduces interpretation time.[7] One problem in evaluating and comparing different gynaecological cytological preparations is the need for a gold standard or a means of assessing in an un-biased manner. Although surgical biopsy is the most viable option, simple biopsy does not always capture the lesion identified on the cervical smear and the pathological interpretation itself is sometimes fraught with poor interobserver agreement, particularly, at the low end of the atypical spectrum. However, tissue biopsy is the closest routine specimen available to establish such a standard. Some of the findings are based on 'split' sample-matched studies in which a traditional smear is taken first followed by LBC collection (Fig. 5.2). Although some problems with split-sample studies include reviewer bias, decreased cellularity in both samples (since a single collection is used for both preparations), most of these studies have shown a 10–20% improvement over conventional Pap smears in the detection of dysplasia.[5,6,8–11]

A multicentre trial incorporating eight different laboratories by Bishop et al. evaluated 8983 split samples.[8] Conventional smears were made and the brush with the remaining cells was placed in PreserveCyt. Approximately, 87% of the

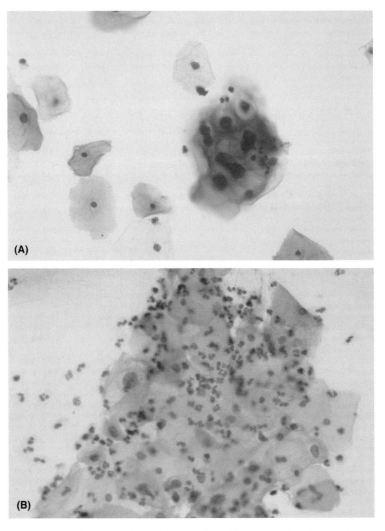

Fig. 5.2 Split sample showing (A) LBC (ThinPrep) and (B) conventional smear in a patient with low grade squamous intra-epithelial lesions (LGSIL). Note the increased inflammation in the conventional smear (Pap stains, ×40).

cases had similar diagnoses, and there was no difference in the detection of infectious organisms. Bishop *et al.* found a 46% increase in the detection of low-grade squamous intra-epithelial lesions (LGSIL) and a 6% increase in the identification of high-grade squamous intra-epithelial lesions (HGSIL)/cervical intra-epithelial neoplasia grades 2 and 3 (CIN 2 and 3) in the LBC.

LBC seems to be more sensitive and specific over conventional Pap smears. Some studies have identified a significant number (>75%) of biopsy-confirmed LGSIL/CIN 1 in the LBC that were not diagnosed in the matched conventional smear.[10,11]

The few studies that have compared detection rates of glandular dysplasia in conventional and LBC Pap smears demonstrate at least equivalent diagnostic rates. Wang *et al.* found that cases of atypical glandular cells of undetermined significance (AGUS) diagnosed by LBC and conventional Pap smears had the same rate of significant pathology on subsequent histological study. As would be expected, most of the AGUS cases had negative follow-up biopsies or were the result of a squamous intra-epithelial lesion. Although a diagnosis of 'AGUS, favour neoplastic' had more positive follow-up biopsies, neither conventional nor LBC Pap smears were more sensitive in picking up the 'favour neoplastic' diagnoses (similar positive predictive values).[12] Some investigators have found an increased sensitivity in identifying adenocarcinoma *in situ* (AIS) by LBC.[13] Vassilakos *et al.* evaluated two large patient groups controlled for age and socio-economic status in which one group was evaluated by conventional cervical smears and the other by SurePath Prep LBC. The study was designed to avoid potential bias of split-sample studies.[14] The researchers found a three-fold increase in the detection of squamous dysplasia and squamous cell carcinoma in the LBC group. They also found that the number of ambiguous diagnoses, such as atypical squamous cells of uncertain significance (ASCUS) and AGUS, was decreased in LBC.

PITFALLS IN LIQUID-BASED PREPARATIONS

Benign cellular changes and infectious organisms, such as *Candida* spp. and *Trichomonas vaginalis*, have similar features on conventional and LBC. Since the inflammation is negligible in the ThinPrep LBC and more dispersed and less concentrated in the TriPath LBC, the balls of neutrophils commonly seen in *Trichomonas* spp. infections are often minimised. However, since the cells are more discohesive and less obscuring inflammation is present, the organisms are often easier to see on LBC once the cytologist is trained to depend less on the background environment. In addition, the organism's detail is enhanced on LBC including the flagella of *T. vaginalis*.

LGSIL is often easier to detect by both LBC techniques. The squamous cells in the TriPath LBC sometimes have rounded, curled edges, which can simulate HPV-halo effect. The lack of nuclear changes (nucleomegaly, hyperchromasia) aids in avoiding overcalling LGSIL. Otherwise, the cytological features of LGSIL are identical in LBC and conventional smears (Fig. 5.3).

Perhaps the most difficult area in gynaecological LBC is detecting HGSIL. The cells of HGSIL tend to be smaller in LBC than in conventional cervical smears and can occur as single rare cells. Although the squamous cells with HGSIL can

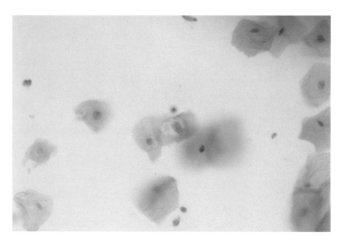

Fig. 5.3 SurePath preparation in a patient with LGSIL. Since this technique relies on a density gradient in the slide preparation, some cell overlap is seen (SurePath Prep, Pap stain, ×20).

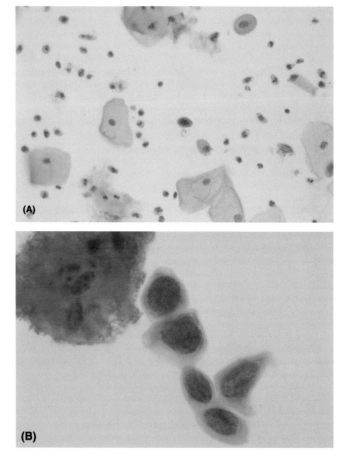

Fig. 5.4 (A) HGSIL by LBC. Due to the processing of the material by SurePath Prep technique, squamous cells with HGSIL are more often found as single cells or small clusters (Pap stain, ×20); **(B)** Due to the processing of the material by ThinPrep technique, squamous cells with HGSIL are more often found as single cells or small clusters (Pap stain, ×1000).

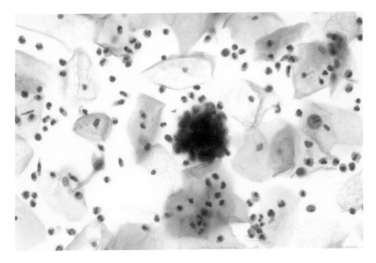

Fig. 5.5 Endometrial cells in an LBC. The nuclear contours of glandular cells are often sharper than seen in conventional smears (SurePath Prep, Pap stain, ×40).

be few in number, they often group together on a conventional Pap smear. Since the cells are centrifuged and homogenised in LBC, it is not uncommon for HGSIL to present as single-dispersed abnormal cells (Fig. 5.4).

Endocervical atypia and carcinoma look similar on LBC and conventional smears. Benign endocervical and endometrial cells can be alarming initially because the cell borders are so crisp and the nuclei appear more hyperchromatic (Fig. 5.5). The maintenance of nuclear polarity is helpful in avoiding over-interpretation of reactive endocervical cells on LBC. As with any new test, adequate training and experience are paramount to good diagnostic acumen.

HUMAN PAPILLOMA VIRUS DETECTION ON LIQUID-BASED PREPARATIONS

Most low- and high-grade dysplasias and squamous cell carcinoma have been linked to the HPVs, a group of deoxyribonucleic acid (DNA) viruses belonging to the papovaviridae family. This virus easily invades into differentiating host squamous epithelial cells and inserts its DNA into the host DNA. Most women infected with this virus have subclinical manifestations. A small percentage of women, however, will develop cervical squamous cell carcinoma. In large multicentre studies, over 99% of cervical cancers have been associated with one of the high-risk HPV strains: HPV 16, 18, 31, 33, 35, 39, 45, 51 and 52.[15] Other genital tract carcinomas including vaginal and vulval carcinoma have also been associated with these high-risk HPV strains. The low-risk strains, HPV 6, 11, 42, 43 and 44, are usually indolent and often regress.[16]

Identifying the strains of HPV known to be associated with squamous cell carcinoma (high-risk strains) has been the focus of much research in the past decade. The main way HPV has been detected commercially is either through a consensus primer PCR system or through RNA probes. The US FDA has approved the Hybrid Capture, an example of RNA probes, developed by Digene Diagnostics (Silver Spring, MD, USA). The Hybrid Capture II, utilises numerous RNA sequences constructed to identify the most prevalent high- and low-risk HPV DNA types in infected cells. The fluid remaining from the liquid-based media is centrifuged and the DNA is extracted/denatured from the resultant cell pellet. The RNA is then hybridised with the DNA. Any RNA/DNA hybrids are captured in a solid phase. Multiple antibodies are added that will specifically conjugate with targeted hybrids. A chemiluminescent signal will be detected by the antibody labelled RNA/DNA hybrid. This system can also be utilised for other sexually transmitted disease detection, such as chlamydia and gonorrhoea. Studies have found that the Hybrid Capture II is extremely sensitive in detecting high-risk HPV types in all invasive carcinomas and most high-grade lesions but is less specific than cytological evaluation.[17] A second method of HPV detection by *in situ* hybridisation has been developed by Ventana Medical Systems (Tuscon, AZ) called Inform HPV. This is an automated slide-based test that utilises high- and low-risk probes by *in situ* hybridisation, allowing the pathologist to visualise the infected cells. The advantage of LBC in both of these techniques is the original Pap slide can be preserved, while additional material is used for HPV testing.

Even with the refined procurement and interpretation techniques that are developing, some squamous lesion diagnoses will still fall into an uncertain category. The recently revised Bethesda System of classification of Pap smears divides this diagnosis into two main categories: atypical squamous cells (ASC) and atypical squamous cells, high grade not excluded (ASC-H). Many patients with a diagnosis of ASC undergo either early repeat Pap smear or colposcopy and biopsy. The follow-up biopsies vary from reactive changes or immature squamous metaplasia to CIN 1 or, most importantly, CIN 3. Some researchers advocate HPV testing to triage the uncertain cases for early repeat cervical smear or colposcopy and biopsy depending on the identification of high-risk virus. Others have advocated doing HPV testing on all abnormal smears to see if the patient has high-risk strain of HPV and, therefore, is at risk of developing more severe lesions in the future.[18]

One of the largest studies of ASCUS in the US is the ASCUS, Low-grade Triage Study (ALTS) trial. This is a randomised, multicentre study designed to evaluate and compare three strategies in detecting high-grade cervical dysplasia in patients with a cervical smear diagnosis of ASCUS or LGSIL. The preliminary findings by the ALTS trial is that HPV testing on women with LGSIL offers improved sensitivity, but not specificity, over conventional cytology. In the patients with a diagnosis of ASCUS, the Hybrid Capture II was extremely sensitive in identifying those patients with high grade lesions.[19] One problem with the patient HPV Hybrid Capture II outcomes is a high rate of high-risk HPV detected in young women with LGSIL and ASCUS; the need for increased specificity without compromise to sensitivity was noted in the preliminary findings. Smaller studies have concluded that it is not cost effective in triaging patients with ASCUS or LGSIL by HPV testing.[20,21] It is still uncertain whether other large-scale trials in other countries, such as the Trial of Management of Borderline and Other Low-grade Abnormalities (TOMBOLA) by the UK Medical Research Council/National Health Service, will find similar outcomes.

Recently, the European Society for Infectious Disease in Obstetrics and Gynaecology issued new guidelines for cervical cancer screening that included HPV testing as an alternative to the Pap smear. In the US, trials of combined Pap smear and HPV testing in women over the age of 30 are being instituted to measure the cost and health benefit of combined screening. This may prove to be an effective, sensitive and specific means of primary screening, since the rate of HPV infection drops drastically in women over the age of 30. Further studies are needed that evaluate the utility of HPV high- and low-risk probes, in cases of ASCUS, where the differential diagnosis is between HGSIL and immature squamous metaplasia.

AUTOMATED SCREENING

The principal obstacles to early image analysis of cervical smears included cell overlap, lack of cells in a single plane and obstructing debris and blood in conventional smears. LBC has minimised these problems. Different systems exist but all work on the general principle of identifying the most atypical cells. The machine screens the cytological LBC (or in some cases conventional Pap smear slides) and identifies the most abnormal cells on the slide.

The AutoPap System (TriPath Imaging, Inc, Burlington, NC, USA) and PapNet test (Neuromedical Systems, Suffern, NY, USA) were approved by the US FDA in 1996 for quality assurance and adjunct rescreening of negative cervical smears. One study from Switzerland evaluated 8688 cervical samples by usual screening and AutoPap.[11] In that report, the system ranked all cases of HGSIL in a high-risk category, with 85% in the "most suspicious for dysplasia" rank, demonstrating a high sensitivity for HGSIL. In rescreening smears originally diagnosed as 'within normal limits', most studies have found a small percentage of cases (<10%) get reclassified as abnormal, and most of the reclassification is to ASCUS. O'Leary et al. found one additional abnormal smear (usually ASCUS) per 913 cases (from a total of 5478 cervical smears originally diagnosed as normal). Based on these findings, it was calculated that the cost range for each additional ASCUS or AGUS detected by PapNet was $5825 to $33 781.[22] The consensus so far has been that it is not cost effective to perform 100% rescreening of negative cervical smears (i.e. adjunct rescreening).[22]

Image analysis systems are not yet generally part of cytology laboratories. However, in 1998, the US FDA approved the AutoPap System for primary screening of cases with a threshold of eliminating 25% of the cases for 'no further review'. More information is needed to know if the imaging systems will become more prevalent in laboratories and utilised as initial screening tools, and whether the use of automated screening will enhance detection of abnormal smears and alleviate some of the human error inherent in the current manual screening system. It is also unclear how cost effective the instruments will be and whether better initial screening will improve detection of high-grade lesions and aid in the decrease in cervical cancer.

LIQUID-BASED CYTOLOGICAL PREPARATIONS COMPARED TO CONVENTIONAL FINE NEEDLE ASPIRATION BIOPSY (FNAB) SMEARS AND OTHER NON-GYNAECOLOGICAL SAMPLES

The literature presents mixed reviews and outcomes of LBC compared to conventional FNAB smears. For the most part, Pap-stained FNAB slides prepared

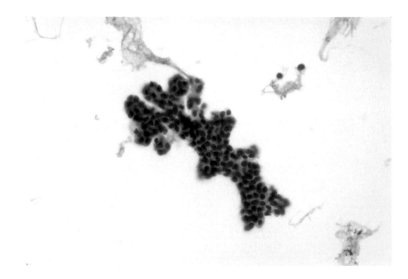

Fig. 5.6 Breast aspirate of a fibroadenoma prepared by LBC. In this aspirate, the staghorn arrangement of benign duct cells is intact; however, the background myoepithelial and stromal cells are inconspicuous (ThinPrep, Pap stain, ×40) (case courtesy of Dr Christina Kong, Stanford Medical Center, California, USA).

by the LBC have similar cellular features as conventional FNAB slides (Figs 5.6 and 5.7). The biggest problem seems to be the loss of background stroma and cell architecture pattern. One study found these differences more marked in the ThinPrep technique than TriPath.[6] This may be due to the increased preservation of architecture and background material in TriPath prepared slides due to the mechanics of the processing. Papillary clusters and glands tend to be more intact using the TriPath technique. However, other studies have found excellent preservation of cell arrangements by using ThinPrep LBC and have not found the increased cell dispersion a handicap in making accurate interpretations.[23] Since ThinPrep has been FDA approved longer, most of the literature evaluating FNAB and LBC involves this monolayer method. When the most frequent palpable aspiration sites are evaluated, conventional smears seem to outperform the LBC in overall specificity,[24] although some have found an increase in specificity of malignant diagnoses.[25]

In aspirates in which the architecture and background are particularly important, LBC has been reported as superior, equivalent and suboptimal to conventional smears.[6,23,25,26] This discrepancy is particularly notable in breast aspirates. Perez-Reyes et al. split their breast aspirates: half of the sample was used for conventional smears and half of the aspirate was prepared by LBC. They found that they could definitively diagnose only four out of 21 cases of fibroadenoma (diagnosed by the conventional smear) because of discohesion of the cells and lack of stroma and background 'naked nuclei'.[27] Conversely, Biscotti et al. found that cellularity and nuclear detail of breast aspirates was better on LBC and that the difference in specificity between LBC and conventional smears was not statistically significant.[26] Bedard and Pollette evaluated 21 193 conventional breast aspirate smears and 7903 LBC breast aspirates and found a small decrease in specificity of LBC (96.5% LBC versus 98.6% conventional smear) or negative-predictive value (88.0% LBC versus 91.1% conventional) but

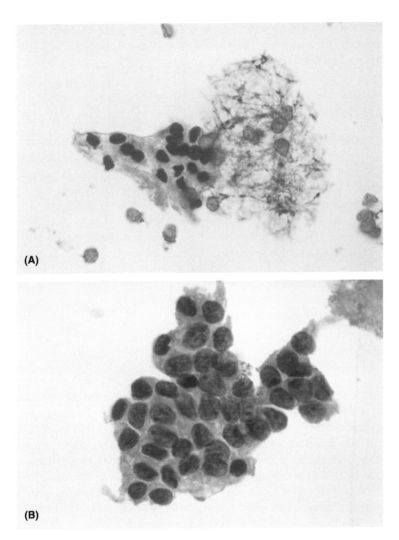

Fig. 5.7 Thyroid aspirates prepared by ThinPrep LBC. (A) Non-neoplastic thyroid demonstrating a rare cluster of benign follicular cells (Pap stain, ×20). (B) Papillary carcinoma showing nucleomegaly and nuclear grooves (Pap stain, ×40) (cases courtesy of Dr Christina Kong, Stanford Medical Center, California, USA).

no significant change in sensitivity and positive predictive value. They also found better cellularity in the LBC.[28]

Non-gynaecological, non-FNAB samples (such as bronchial washes and brushes prepared by LBC) seem equivalent in quality and diagnostic outcome to cytospins.[23,29]

IMMUNOCHEMISTRY AND LIQUID-BASED CYTOLOGICAL PREPARATIONS

LBCs are as amenable to immunochemistry evaluation as conventional smears.[30] An added advantage is the lack of non-specific background staining due to decreased debris. The quality of immunochemistry has been found to be equivalent in LPB and cytospins from effusion material, with cell block material yielding the best results.[31]

LASER SCANNING CYTOMETRY

Laser scanning cytometry (LSC) is a method that allows for detection of antibodies through multicolour fluorescence, light scatter and location of a cell adherent to a slide. It combines features of flow cytometry as well as static image analysis. LSC can evaluate DNA ploidy and is amenable to fluorescence *in situ* hybridisation (FISH) and antigen retrieval and quantitation. It can be used with conventional smears and has been shown to be effective with ThinPrep LBC.[32] Wojcik *et al.* utilised the laser scanning techniques to evaluate DNA ploidy from bladder specimens. They used the ploidy results in conjunction with the cytology to assess for recurrence of urothelial carcinomas. They noted that DNA ploidy analysis was more rapid using ThinPrep slides, but produced histograms that were more difficult to interpret, when compared to cell suspension flow cytometry histograms.

CONCLUSION

LBC has aided in cervical smear collection and the detection of dysplasia. With cervical samples, both ThinPrep and SurePath Prep techniques have equivalent interpretation rates as well as increased detection of LGSIL and HGSIL. In addition, LBC has provided an improved method for exploring other means of cervical screening, such as automated screening techniques. The additional sample that remains in the collection fluid is a great resource for HPV testing and other sexually transmitted diseases. The specific use of HPV testing is still being explored to determine which diagnoses (ASCUS, ASCUS-H, LGSIL) will benefit from HPV subtyping. As with traditional smears, the LBC cervical preparation is a screening test and, despite the increase in sensitivity in detecting dysplasia in LBC, public education to ensure maximal coverage is still critical in all countries to ensure the downward trend in the incidence of cervical carcinoma.

The LBC can be utilised for FNAB material, although there are mixed reviews in the literature pertaining to the architecture and background material in the slides. It may prove to be useful for clinicians or pathologists who do not perform FNABs frequently and as an adjunct to traditional smears. As more cytologists gain experience in utilising LBC, refined diagnostic criteria may arise to supplement the changes seen in these preparations.

REFERENCES

1. Cramer DW. The role of cervical cytology in the declining morbidity and mortality of cervical cancer. Cancer 1974; 34: 2018–2027
2. Jenkins D. Diagnosing human papillomaviruses: recent advances. Curr Opin Infect Dis 2001; 14: 53–62
3. Ferenczy A, Franco E. Cervical cancer screening beyond the year 2000. Lancet Oncol 2001; 2: 27–32

4. Sprenger E, Schwarzmann P, Kirkpatrick M *et al*. The false negative rate in cervical cytology. Comparison of monolayers to conventional smears. Acta Cytol 1996; 40: 81–89

5. Hessling JJ, Raso DS, Schiffer B, Callicott Jr J, Husain M, Taylor D. Effectiveness of thin-layer preparations vs. conventional Pap smears in a blinded, split-sample study. Extended cytologic evaluation. J Reprod Med 2001; 46: 880–886

6. Michael CW, McConnel J, Pecott J, Afify AM, Al-Khafaji B. Comparison of ThinPrep and TriPath PREP liquid-based preparations in nongynecologic specimens: a pilot study. Diagn Cytopathol 2001; 25: 177–184

7. Payne N, Chilcott J, McGoogan E. Liquid-based cytology for cervical screening. Cytopathology 2000; 11: 469–470

8. Bishop JW, Bigner SH, Colgan TJ *et al*. Multicenter masked evaluation of AutoCyte PREP thin layers with matched conventional smears. Including initial biopsy results. Acta Cytol 1998; 42: 189–197

9. Minge L, Fleming M, VanGeem T, Bishop JW. AutoCyte Prep system vs. conventional cervical cytology. Comparison based on 2,156 cases. J Reprod Med 2000; 45: 179–184

10. Tench W. Preliminary assessment of the AutoCyte PREP. Direct-to-vial performance. J Reprod Med 2000; 45: 912–916

11. Vassilakos P, Schwartz D, de Marval F *et al*. Biopsy-based comparison of liquid-based, thin-layer preparations to conventional Pap smears. J Reprod Med 2000; 45: 11–16

12. Wang N, Emancipator SN, Rose P, Rodriguez M, Abdul-Karim FW. Histologic follow-up of atypical endocervical cells. Liquid-based, thin-layer preparation vs. conventional Pap smear. Acta Cytol 2002; 46: 453–457

13. Johnson T, Maksem JA, Belsheim BL, Roose EB, Klock LA, Eatwell L. Liquid-based cervical-cell collection with brushes and wooden spatulas: a comparison of 100 conventional smears from high-risk women to liquid-fixed cytocentrifuge slides, demonstrating a cost-effective, alternative monolayer slide preparation method. Diagn Cytopathol 2000; 22: 86–91

14. Vassilakos P, Griffin S, Megevand E, Campana A. CytoRich liquid-based cervical cytologic test. Screening results in a routine cytopathology service. Acta Cytol 1998; 42: 198–202

15. Kjellberg L, Wiklund F, Sjoberg I *et al*. A population-based study of human papillomavirus deoxyribonucleic acid testing for predicting cervical intra-epithelial neoplasia. Am J Obstet Gynecol 1998; 179: 1497–1502

16. Moscicki AB. Genital infections with human papillomavirus (HPV). Pediatr Infect Dis J 1998; 17: 651–652

17. Clavel M, Bory J, Putaud I *et al*. Hybrid capture II-based human papillomavirus detection, a sensitive test to detect routine high-grade cervical lesions: a preliminary study on 1518 women. Br J Cancer 1999; 80: 1306–1311

18. Cox JT, Lorincz AT, Schiffman MH, Sherman ME, Cullen A, Kurman RJ. Human papillomavirus testing by hybrid capture appears to be useful in triaging women with a cytologic diagnosis of atypical squamous cells of undetermined significance. Am J Obstet Gynecol 1995; 172: 946–954

19. Solomon D, Schiffman M, Tarone R. Comparison of the three management strategies for patients with atypical squamous cells of undetermined significance: baseline results from a randomized trial. J Natl Cancer Inst 2001; 93: 293–299

20. Kaufman RH, Adam E, Icenogle J *et al*. Relevance of human papillomavirus screening in management of cervical intra-epithelial neoplasia. Am J Obstet Gynecol 1997; 176: 87–92

21. Kaufman RH, Adam E, Icenogle J, Reeves WC. Human papillomavirus testing as triage for atypical squamous cells of undetermined significance and low-grade squamous intra-epithelial lesions: sensitivity, specificity, and cost-effectiveness. Am J Obstet Gynecol 1997; 177: 930–936

22. O'Leary TJ, Tellado M, Buckner SB, Ali IS, Stevens A, Ollayos CW. PAPNET-assisted rescreening of cervical smears: cost and accuracy compared with a 100% manual rescreening strategy. JAMA 1998; 279: 235–237

23. Leung CS, Chiu B, Bell V. Comparison of ThinPrep and conventional preparations: nongynecologic cytology evaluation. Diagn Cytopathol 1997; 16: 368–371

24. Florentine BD, Wu NC, Waliany S, Carriere C, Hindle W, Raza A. Fine needle aspiration (FNA) biopsy of palpable breast masses: comparison of conventional smears with the Cyto-Tek MonoPrep system. Cancer 1999; 87: 278–285

25. Lee KR, Papillo JL, St John T, Eyerer GJ. Evaluation of the ThinPrep processor for fine needle aspiration specimens. Acta Cytol 1996; 40: 895–899
26. Biscotti CV, Shorie JH, Gramlich TL, Easley KA. ThinPrep vs. conventional smear cytologic preparations in analyzing fine-needle aspiration specimens from palpable breast masses. Diagn Cytopathol 1999; 21: 137–141
27. Perez-Reyes N, Mulford DK, Rutkowski MA, Logan-Young W, Dawson AE. Breast fine-needle aspiration. A comparison of thin-layer and conventional preparation. Am J Clin Pathol 1994; 102: 349–353
28. Bedard YC, Pollett AF. Breast fine-needle aspiration. A comparison of ThinPrep and conventional smears. Am J Clin Pathol 1999; 111: 523–527
29. Nasuti JF, Mehrotra R, Gupta PK. Diagnostic value of fine-needle aspiration in supraclavicular lymphadenopathy: a study of 106 patients and review of literature. Diagn Cytopathol 2001; 25: 351–355
30. Leung SW, Bedard YC. Immunocytochemical staining on ThinPrep processed smears. Mod Pathol 1996; 9: 304–306
31. Fetsch PA, Simsir A, Brosky K, Abati A. Comparison of three commonly used cytologic preparations in effusion immunocytochemistry. Diagn Cytopathol 2002; 26: 61–66
32. Wojcik EM, Saraga SA, Jin JK, Hendricks JB. Application of laser scanning cytometry for evaluation of DNA ploidy in routine cytologic specimens. Diagn Cytopathol 2001; 24: 200–205

6

The diagnosis of cervical glandular intra-epithelial neoplasia

L.J.R. Brown

Adenocarcinoma of the cervix is increasing, representing up to 24% of invasive cervical tumours.[1,2] The importance of recognising the pre-invasive stage, cervical glandular intra-epithelial neoplasia (CGIN) at a point where it can be easily treated cannot be over-emphasised. By analogy with the corresponding squamous lesion (cervical intra-epithelial neoplasia, CIN), CGIN forms a spectrum of changes classified as low- and high-grade CGIN (L-CGIN and H-CGIN), ranging from normal through mild aberrations of nuclear size, shape, staining and orientation to adenocarcinoma *in situ* (AIS). These changes have previously been called cervical glandular atypia and cervical intra-epithelial glandular neoplasia (CIGN) by workers, who initially classified the lesions as low- and high-grade cervical glandular atypia and cervical intrepithelial glandular neoplasia (CIGN) Grades I–III, respectively.[3,4]

AIS has been known since 1894.[5] The first detailed descriptions of AIS dating from 1953 by Freidell and Mackay,[6] have been supplemented by many subsequent authors.[3,7–18] H-CGIN is indistinguishable from AIS, but also includes the highly atypical end of a spectrum that extends through moderate atypia to L-CGIN. The abnormal cytology of AIS and less severe changes can be detected by cytology[19] and confirmed by morphometry.[13] In common with columnar cell neoplasia at other sites,[20] it is even more difficult than with CIN to reproducibly recognise three grades of CGIN. Consequently, CGIN is divided into H-CGIN and L-CGIN. This classification has been adopted by the Royal College of Pathologists 'Histopathology Reporting in Cervical Screening'[21] (Table 6.1).

Table 6.1 The relationship of the different classifications of CGIN

L-CGIN	→→→→→→→→→→→→→→→→→		H-CGIN
CIGN I	CIGN II	CIGN III	ACIS
Glandular atypia		EGD	AIS

Laurence J.R. Brown BSc MB BS FRCPath, Consultant Histopathologist and Honorary Senior Lecturer, Leicester Royal Infirmary, Leicester, UK

In the US and elsewhere in the world, the terminology proposed by the World Health Organization (WHO) is more commonly used. This nomenclature features AIS, endocervical glandular dysplasia (EGD) and glandular atypias less severe than EGD.[22] Although it can be difficult to distinguish reactive glandular proliferations from L-CGIN under some conditions, I feel the increasing recognition of reactive hyperplasias and the range of further techniques available has helped to isolate CGIN as a more definable lesion. Furthermore, the intra-epithelial terminology defined in CGIN is consonant with other sites.

In the original descriptions of CGIN, Brown and Wells[3] identified seven examples of H-CGIN and nine of L-CGIN accompanying 105 examples of CIN 3 and 100 normal controls. This translated to a 15% incidence for CGIN in CIN 3 compared to 2% in the controls, although one of these controls had undergone a previous excision for CIN.

Gloor and Hurlimann[4] defined three grades in 23 cases of cervical intra-epithelial glandular neoplasia (CIGN) utilising histochemistry and lectins. Endocervical type A lesions contain neutral mucins, sulphomucins and sialomucins similar to normal endocervical mucosa. Intestinal type B lesions feature small intestinal goblet cells lacking sulphomucins.

Other work has documented H-CGIN co-existing with CIN 3 in a ratio of between 1:26[9] and 1:239.[8] Approximately, 50% of cases showing CGIN also feature CIN.[23] L-CGIN is harder to detect but has been found with 55–63% of squamous lesions.[24,25] L-CGIN commonly accompanies H-CGIN, typically distributed around the periphery, but may rarely be seen in isolation where it may represent the only explanation for 'atypical glandular cells' detected by cervical cytology. Due to the common association with squamous intra-epithelial lesions, the CIN may dominate the histological appearance and beguile the pathologist into overlooking the CGIN.[26]

HISTOLOGY OF CERVICAL INTRA-EPITHELIAL GLANDULAR NEOPLASIA

The classification of CGIN outlining the distinction between high and low grades is determined by the degree of nuclear stratification, mitotic activity, hyperchromasia, nuclear/cytoplasmic ratio and preservation or type of mucin production. This range of changes is similar to mucinous ovarian tumours and the adenoma/carcinoma sequence of the colon.[3,4,25]

LOW-GRADE CERVICAL INTRA-EPITHELIAL GLANDULAR NEOPLASIA

The changes in L-CGIN may be subtle, the most arresting feature being increased hyperchromasia in an area or strip of epithelium appreciable at low power (Fig. 6.1). On closer examination, this hyperchromasia is accompanied by mild nuclear enlargement, mild variation in nuclear size, slight loss of polarity, mitotic activity (usually no more than one or two per crypt profile) and abnormal chromatin. The nuclei are generally limited to the basal two-thirds of the epithelial height. The epithelium is usually columnar but may be cuboidal,

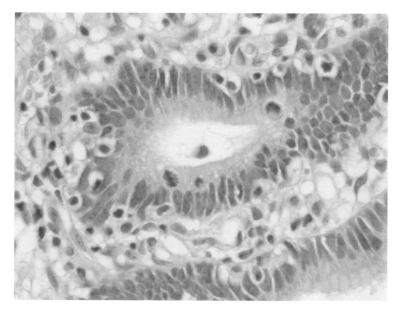

Fig. 6.1 L-CGIN exhibiting nuclear enlargement, hyperchromasia and pleomorphism with variable chromatin patterns. There are occasional mitoses but polarity is generally preserved. Some mucin loss is apparent.

pseudostratified or tufted. Mucin production may be aberrant with intestinal-type vacuoles, reduced or absent. The glands may retain a normal profile or be crowded, branched or budded. The epithelium may line a whole or part of a crypt with a characteristically abrupt border between the normal and adjacent abnormal epithelium. L-CGIN is most common around the margins of areas of H-CGIN, but may be found in isolation. In my experience, it has sometimes been the only finding to explain abnormal cervical cytology.[3,176]

HIGH-GRADE CERVICAL INTRA-EPITHELIAL GLANDULAR NEOPLASIA INCLUDING ADENOCARCINOMA *IN SITU*

In a similar fashion to CIN 3 incorporating squamous cell carcinoma *in situ*, H-CGIN includes AIS, but also encompasses a spectrum of appearances ranging from the less severe features of L-CGIN. In the most atypical variants, the cells are indistinguishable by conventional microscopy and by morphometry from invasive adenocarcinoma, but naturally without invasion of the underlying stroma.[10,11] The involved glands appear obviously hyperchromatic at low power displaying normal, branched or budded profiles (Fig. 6.2). As with L-CGIN, there may be an abrupt junction between normal and neoplastic epithelium. The degree of glandular complexity may be greater than seen in L-CGIN and may include cribriform foci (Fig. 6.3). Some authors (see below on identification of early invasion) consider cribriform areas to be a marker of stromal invasion, but similarly complex cribriform areas can be seen in benign conditions (such as microglandular hyperplasia) and should not, by themselves, be diagnostic of invasion.

H-CGIN is also separated from lesser grades by the combination of increased nuclear staining, by more abnormal, densely granular chromatin and stratification of nuclei above two-thirds of the epithelial height. Signs of increased cell turnover include frequent mitoses, some abnormal mitoses (Fig. 6.3) and apoptotic bodies.[27,28] Apoptotic bodies may be more obvious than in invasive adenocarcinoma and help to distinguish CGIN from reactive conditions.[28] Other features of cell proliferation include epithelial budding with intraluminal projections, occasionally lacking stromal cores.

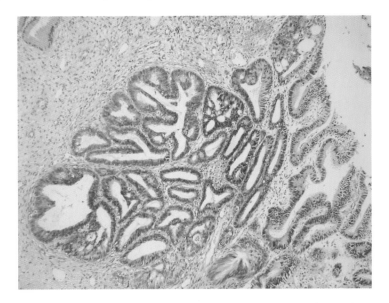

Fig. 6.2 H-CGIN. This medium power view displays the marked hyperchromasia associated with H-CGIN. Although there are some cribriform areas, the glands are limited to the normal glandular field and there is no stromal reaction to indicate invasion. Compare the appearances with a normal gland in the upper left-hand corner.

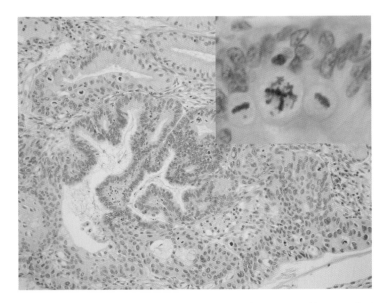

Fig. 6.3 This high power view of H-CGIN shows the loss of polarity and increased mitotic activity with numerous apoptotic bodies typical of H-CGIN. The inset shows bizarre mitoses.

In most examples of H-CGIN (96%), the epithelium is endocervical in type, and endometrioid a rare sub-type. Rarely, counterparts of intestinal, serous, clear-cell or adenosquamous carcinomas are also seen.[11,12,15,17]

Glands involved by CGIN are limited to the normal glandular field extending to maximum depth of 7.8 mm[29] and may extend up to 30 mm along the endocervical canal. There is some evidence that CGIN arises at the transformation zone through a process of atypical reserve cell hyperplasia and grows in continuity along the surface epithelium of the endocervical canal, replacing the normal epithelium of underlying crypts extending under squamous epithelium, being multifocal only occasionally.[7,8,30] Others have observed multifocal and skip lesions[3,4,11,14,17,31] involving the superficial cervix, deep endocervical canal, groups of glands or separate cervical quadrants. These disparate views may be resolved by considering the effect of tangential cutting through complex crypts and lesions bordering the endocervical canal.[32] Disputes about the growth pattern and the difficulties of recognising the changes colposcopically[24,33] have lead to various strategies for treatment.

INTESTINAL METAPLASIA

The original report of intestinal metaplasia in endocervical epithelium illustrated goblet mucin secreting cells with absorptive and argentaffin cells in epithelium that was said to be otherwise normal but which most workers would now consider to show signs of CGIN. Paneth cells may also be present.[34] This type of metaplasia is a reliable marker of CGIN or adenocarcinoma and is rarely (if ever) seen in non-neoplastic epithelium.[11,14]

This link is so constant that any focus of intestinal metaplasia is an excellent indicator of CGIN[35] (Fig. 6.4).

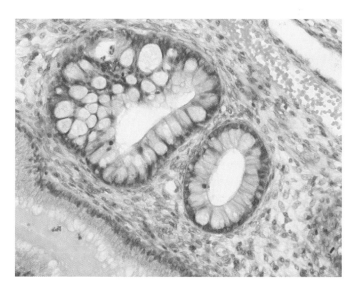

Fig. 6.4 These crypts display large intestinal-type metaplasia with L-CGIN. There is mild nuclear hyperchromasia and loss of polarity.

STRATIFIED MUCINOUS INTRA-EPITHELIAL LESION

This resembles CIN but with mucin vacuoles distributed in cells throughout the whole height of the dysplastic epithelium. The lesions may form a spectrum of malignant transformation with atypical reserve cell hyperplasia and may show a similar surface layer of normal columnar cells. In contrast to benign reserve cell hyperplasias, stratified mucinous intra-epithelial lesion (SMILE) exhibits dysplastic nuclear characteristics and a high proliferative index with MIB 1. In the series of 18 cases reported, 15 were associated with CIN or H-CGIN. All the co-existing nine invasive lesions featured glandular areas. This consistent association with intra-epithelial or invasive glandular lesions has lead the authors to conclude that SMILE represents a marker of epithelial phenotypic instability in the progression to adenocarcinoma, calling for more extensive sampling of the cervix if detected by biopsy.[36]

CILIATED CERVICAL INTRA-EPITHELIAL GLANDULAR NEOPLASIA

The dysplastic cells of CGIN may occasionally be ciliated. Fortunately, this is very rare as it causes considerable difficulty in the distinction from tubo-endometrioid metaplasia and those inflamed metaplastic epithelia that display appreciable atypia.[37] The glandular architecture may be more complex than usually seen in tubo-endometrioid metaplasia with complex branched or cribriform areas. Ciliated CGIN is also said to exhibit more mitotic activity, stratification of the whole epithelial height and mucin loss. The most helpful distinguishing features are nuclear irregularity, hyperchromasia and loss of polarity. A recent study has added a note of caution by showing that 10 ciliated atypias were negative for human papilloma virus (HPV) and had low MIB 1 indices,[35] suggesting a benign behaviour. However, these authors concede the existence of ciliated AIS.

IS CERVICAL INTRA-EPITHELIAL GLANDULAR NEOPLASIA A PRECURSOR OF CERVICAL ADENOCARCINOMA?

Most workers accept that CGIN is a pre-malignant, non-invasive lesion. The histological appearance of the epithelium is similar and the lesions are found in the same distribution as adenocarcinoma. Areas of both L-CGIN and H-CGIN may abut foci of invasive adenocarcinoma.[3,25,38] Eighteen percent of microinvasive adenocarcinomas feature associated L-CGIN.[25]

It is widely accepted that H-CGIN may progress. If H-CGIN is ignored or inadequately treated either by wedge excisions[39] or large loop excision of the transformation zone (LLETZ),[40] invasion can occur as early as 1–7 years[10] or by 14 years on average.[8]

There is evidence of a progression to invasive adenocarcinoma through L-CGIN and H-CGIN. Kurian and Al-Nafussi[25] report 121 cases with an almost equal ratio of intra-epithelial to invasive disease. The mean age increased from

39 years for L-CGIN, through 43 for H-CGIN and microinvasive adenocarcinoma to a mean of 48 years for the invasive cases. Other studies have shown a more rapid progression to invasion than in squamous lesions. Progression from L-CGIN to H-CGIN is 1–4 years and from H-CGIN to invasion of 9–22 years. The mean ages for L-CGIN are 34–40 years, H-CGIN 34–43 years, microinvasive carcinoma 43–44 years and 48–57 years for more deeply invasive tumours.[3,4,19,24,41,42] In a large series of 5845 patients, the mean age of AIS was 38.8 years and 51.7 years for invasive adenocarcinoma.[1] In this study, progression from AIS to invasion took 13 years compared to nearly 18 years for squamous cell carcinoma, although this difference may be a result of cervical screening detecting CIN at an earlier stage. This fact may be salient as combined squamous and glandular lesions can be detected in younger women that when CGIN alone is present.[4]

CGIN is often associated with atypical reserve cell hyperplasia and, sometimes, with SMILEs, supporting the origin of both glandular and squamous intra-epithelial lesions arising from a common precursor.[9,15,36,43–45] Glandular neoplasia, subcolumnar reserve cells and scattered stromal precursors all react for CD44 endorsing this hypothesis.[96]

A contrary view is expressed by some American workers,[32] who do not recognise intra-epithelial neoplasia of lesser severity than H-CGIN (AIS in their terminology). They acknowledge that the morphological distinction from normal is difficult and highlight pseudostratified nuclei in normal epithelium, without indicating that this is a well-accepted appearance related to the physiological influence of progestagens.[21,46] Some of their illustrations of AIS would be diagnosed as examples of L-CGIN in the UK. I agree that some cases of L-CGIN (EGA, endocervical glandular atypias in their terminology) may be reactive[3] implying that their inclusion in a category of AIS may result in overtreatment.

FURTHER SUPPORT FOR CERVICAL INTRA-EPITHELIAL GLANDULAR NEOPLASIA AS A PRE-MALIGNANT LESION

Immunohistochemical and molecular studies furnish additional evidence for the link between CGIN and adenocarcinoma.[47]

MOLECULAR ALTERATIONS

H-CGIN and adenocarcinoma both exhibit reductions in cytoplasmic lactoferrin and lactoferrin mRNA. Both show reduced p53 and sex steroid receptors with increased Ki-67 counts.[48]

Telomerase activation was detected in all of nine H-CGIN, each of 12 adenocarcinomas and the only adenosquamous carcinoma tested.[49,50] This is probably an early event in carcinogenesis in this site.[51]

PROLIFERATION

Ki-67 and MIB 1 indicate significantly higher proliferation in adenocarcinoma and H-CGIN than in normal endocervical epithelium, tubo-endometrioid metaplasia,[42] endocervicitis and microglandular hyperplasia.[53] Labelling indices of over 16% for Ki-67 and over 30% for MIB 1 are highly suggestive of neoplasia. Invasive and non-invasive glandular neoplasia cannot be distinguished by these markers as there is some overlap between groups, and they may not help in an individual case. However, high Ki-67 counts, p53 expression and carcinoembryonic antigen (CEA) reactivity strongly suggests glandular neoplasia.[54] A recent study failed to show HPV or increased MIB1 in all their glandular atypias implying that this may be a heterogeneous group lacking universal pre-malignant potential.[35]

CHROMOSOME STUDIES

Some work has shown aneuploidy and triploidy in adenocarcinoma correlating with decreased survival, although this may not relate to the risk of recurrence.[57] Two of three cases of H-CGIN[26] were tetraploid and one was diploid.

LECTIN HISTOCHEMISTRY

Luminal binding with several different lectins can be detected in 90% of adenocarcinomas, 92% of cases of H-CGIN and 63% of cases of L-CGIN.[58]

CARCINOEMBRYONIC ANTIGEN

The normal crypts are negative for CEA, but 59–100% of cervical adenocarcinomas express CEA.[59–65] H-CGIN expresses CEA in 63–67%.[63,66]

MUCIN HISTOCHEMISTRY

Normal endocervical glands produce both acidic and neutral mucins during the course of physiological menstrual cyclical changes.[67] Decreased sulphomucins and increased sialomucins[68] have been shown in intra-epithelial and invasive glandular lesions of the cervix.[69] The mucicarmine stain has helped to identify SMILE as a pre-malignant glandular lesion.[36]

NUCLEOLAR ORGANISER REGIONS

Both H-CGIN and adenocarcinoma feature no significant difference in the numbers of silver-stained nucleolar organiser regions (AgNORs). Furthermore, glandular neoplasias contain more AgNORs than normal glands or microglandular hyperplasia.[70–73] AgNOR counts do not correlate with proliferation[74] but do increase with grade of intra-epithelial neoplasia.[75]

EPITHELIAL MEMBRANE ANTIGENS

All but one of 14 adenocarcinomas and 15 of 17 examples of H-CGIN[76] showed dense cytoplasmic reactivity for HMFG1 compared to a linear luminal reaction in all but two of 28 normal and reactive glands. In one study, epithelial membrane antigen (EMA) reacted strongly and reliably with the cytoplasm of neoplastic glands but reactions with AGF4:48 were less reliable. Both antibodies gave a luminal reaction in normal glandular epithelium but could not distinguish tubo-endometrioid metaplasia from neoplastic glandular epithelium. Neither antibody reacted with microglandular hyperplasia.[38] An epithelial-specific antigen (ESA) directed against a cell surface glycoprotein showed basal and heavy cytoplasmic reactivity in both H-CGIN and invasive adenocarcinoma contrasting with the basal reactivity in normal endocervical epithelium. A further six of 10 'glandular dysplasia's also showed this pattern.[77]

OTHER CARBOHYDRATE TUMOUR MARKERS

AIS and invasive adenocarcinoma showed granular cytoplasmic reactivity with absence of luminal reactivity for CA125 contrasting with the luminal surface and apical cytoplasm of normal glands.[78] Other studies have confirmed reactivity for 1C5 with 18 of 20 adenocarcinomas and showed reactivity with three of four cases of AIS and all six cases of adenosquamous carcinoma.[79]

ONCOGENE PRODUCTS

Thirteen of a series of 14 cases of H-CGIN and L-CGIN and each of 17 cases of adenocarcinoma showed pancellular expression for the c-*myc* oncogene product.[80] Out of 14 normal endocervices, 11 did not express the gene, but three cases showed nuclear and/or slight basal cytoplasmic expression.

DIFFERENTIAL DIAGNOSIS OF CERVICAL GLANDULAR INTRA-EPITHELIAL NEOPLASIA

Intra-epithelial glandular lesions of the cervix must be distinguished from a range of benign and reactive conditions, superficially invasive adenocarcinoma and minimal deviation (well-differentiated) adenocarcinoma (MDA) (Table 6.2).

Table 6.2 The differential diagnosis of CGIN

Normal cyclical changes
Tubo-endometrioid metaplasia
Prostatic metaplasia
Sebaceous metaplasia
Tunnel clusters
Microglandular hyperplasia
Lobular endocervical hyperplasia
Laminar endocervical hyperplasia
Endocervicosis
Mesonephric hyperplasia
Arias–Stella change
Atypical endocervical oxyphilic metaplasia
Florid cystic endosalpingiosis
Papillary cervicitis
Radiation atypia
Endocervical adenomyoma
Microinvasive (FIGO Stage 1A) adenocarcinoma
Minimal deviation adenocarcinoma (adenoma malignum)

NORMAL CYCLICAL CHANGES

In women of reproductive age, the endocervical canal is lined by a single layer of columnar cells that covers up to 100 oblique folds, clefts or villi that appear as crypts in histological sections.[46] This epithelium includes mucin cells producing acidic and neutral glycoproteins interspersed with ciliated cells that transport secretions towards the vagina. The cyclical variation of the hormones of the menstrual cycle alters the relative ratio of sialo- and sphingomucins in the cervical mucus,[67,81] facilitating sperm passage though watery sialomucin-rich secretion in the periovulatory phase. As the mucin producing cells progress through a cycle of synthesis, secretion and exhaustion the nuclei may rise to occupy a higher position in the columnar cells, simulating a stratified or pseudo-stratified appearance. This may cause confusion with CGIN. The most reassuring feature is the uniformity of staining of the epithelial nuclei. The preservation of nuclear polarity and the lack of pleomorphism, abnormal chromatin, hyperchromasia or mitotic activity also distinguish these normal cyclical changes from intra-epithelial neoplasia.

TUBO-ENDOMETRIOID METAPLASIA

This condition was first recognised as the benign condition most likely to cause confusion with CGIN in 1986,[3] but was not formally described until 1990.[82] The crypts are lined with tubal or endometral-type epithelium (Fig. 6.5). Tubal

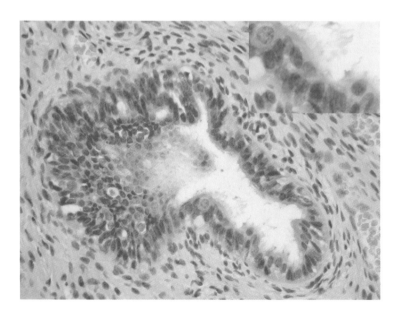

Fig. 6.5 In tubo-endometrioid metaplasia, the glandular epithelium may present a worryingly hyperchromatic and pleomorphic appearance at low power but higher magnification (inset) reveals the typical ciliation and cellular heterogeneity of tubal-type epithelium. Ciliated cells, mucus secreting cells and intercalated (resting) cells account for the variegated appearance. There are no nuclear features of malignancy.

epithelium produces amylase[83] and features ciliated, secretory or inactive cells incorporating basal T-lymphocytes.[3,84] The epithelium may involve the whole or part of the gland with a high nuclear cytoplasmic ratio and may be worryingly hyperchromatic at low power. The glands usually display a normal outline but may be branching, rarely extending into the outer third of the cervical wall.[85] The border of the epithelium is smooth and when pseudostratified resembles endometrial epithelium more closely. Normal mitotic figures may be observed, and there may be apoptotic bodies, but both of these are far fewer than in CGIN.[28] This heterogeneity of cell types is particularly worrying as it may impart a variegated appearance to the epithelium causing confusion with the nuclear and cellular pleomorphism of CGIN. However, CGIN features atypical mitoses, coarse nuclear chromatin, stratification, many apoptotic bodies and loss of polarity while tubo-endometrioid metaplasia does not.

Occasionally, the immediately adjacent stroma may resemble endometrial stroma, reacting with CD10[86] and demonstrating investment of individual cells by reticulin fibres[87] sometimes with haemorrhage, as in endometriosis. The stroma may appear hypercellular but the absence of desmoplasia helps to exclude an invasive lesion.[17,85]

Atypical tubal metaplasia[37] may feature solid, reticular or pseudoinfiltrative patterns with occasional signet cells that can be extremely difficult to separate from CGIN or adenocarcinoma by morphology. The epithelium features enlarged hyperchromatic nuclei and varying degrees of pseudostratification. The most difficult differential is from ciliated CGIN.[37] The best diagnostic features are the lack of plentiful mitoses, scanty apoptotic bodies and preserved polarity in the pseudostratified areas of tubo-endometrioid metaplasia.[28]

Tubo-endometrioid metaplasia can be distinguished from CGIN by diffuse cytoplasmic reactivity for bcl2.[89,95] Tubo-endometrioid metaplasia gives a luminal reaction with HMFG contrasting with the heavy cytoplasmic reactivity seen in CGIN.[76] A MIB 1 labelling index of greater than 30% and a Ki67 index greater than 16% favour CGIN.[53,90] Cameron et al.[90] have recently found MIB 1 reactivity of less than 10% of cells in tubo-endometrioid metaplasia. Concurrently, Pirog et al.[91] found considerable overlap in counts between CGIN and benign conditions, especially in inflamed tubo-endometrioid metaplasia, but determined a MIB 1 reaction of less than 10% was benign and a reaction of greater than 50% was neoplastic. This is supported by Cameron et al.'s finding[90] that 10% or more cells in CGIN were MIB 1 positive.

Tubo-endometrioid metaplasia contains vimentin but reacts for CEA in only 39% contrasting with more extensive CEA expression (up to 67%) and the absence of vimentin in H-CGIN.[63,66]

Any cervical trauma, such as LLETZ, cervical surgery or prolapse,[92] can cause tubo-endometrioid metaplasia. There does not appear to be any association with the menstrual cycle or other pathology. Similar metaplasia can be seen in the skin.[93] This can be particularly worrying when local surgery for CGIN causes an area of tubo-endometrioid metaplasia at the resection margin or residual tubo-endometrioid metaplasia in a hysterectomy specimen. Under these circumstances, it is vital not to confuse benign lymph node inclusions of endosalpingiosis with metastatic adenocarcinoma when examining radical surgery specimens.

PROSTATIC METAPLASIA

There have been rare reports of prostatic tissue in the cervix, exhibiting typical acini or ducts sometimes with areas of squamous metaplasia. The glands may form papillary or cribriform areas and are probably of metaplastic origin.[94,97] The tissue is positive for prostate specific antigen and prostatic acid phosphatase.

SEBACEOUS METAPLASIA

Sebaceous glands, similar to those in the vulva may rarely develop in the cervix following trauma, surgery or chronic inflammation. Pilosebaceous units have not been reported. The glands may be metaplastic or may represent embryonal rests.[98,99]

TUNNEL CLUSTERS

Fluhmann[100] classified proliferations of endocervical glands as type A or type B according to the degree of dilatation of the crypt profiles. In type A, the crypts are hyperplastic, branched, budded or lobular and not dilated, sometimes around a prominent central duct. In type B, there are collections of crypts exhibiting varying degrees of dilatation and that appear as exuberant collections of variably sized Nabothian follicles (mucin-filled cysts) (Fig. 6.6). Both conditions are benign and are usually incidental, common findings in women over 30. These collections of glands may result from involution of glands that have become hyperplastic following hormone use or pregnancy, but often there

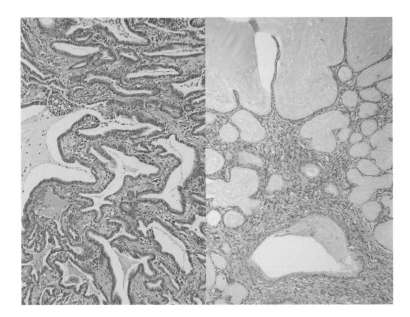

Fig. 6.6 Type A tunnel clusters (left) form tightly-packed collections of branching glands or acini. Type B tunnel clusters (right) form collections of dilated glands. The lining epithelium is banal with no nuclear characteristics of malignancy.

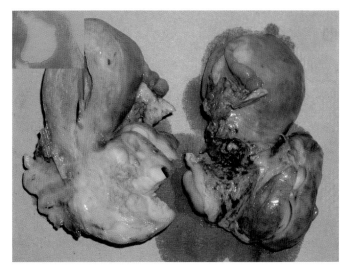

Fig. 6.7 Deep Nabothian cysts have caused massive expansion of the cervix to give a tumour-like mass. The inset at scanning magnification shows a typical crypt dilated to form a Nabothian follicle.

is no recognisable aetiology.[101] Gross enlargement of the cervix by cystic tunnel clusters, especially where Nabothian follicles extend deeply into the cervical stroma, can be confused on clinical or macroscopic examination with advanced cervical malignancy[102] (Fig. 6.7).

A significant danger is the risk of confusion between type A tunnel clusters and adenoma malignum (well-differentiated endocervical adenocarcinoma). Atypia in the epithelium of tunnel clusters (usually due to inflammation) may also be misdiagnosed as CGIN especially when the borders of the clusters are irregular or feature a pseudoinfiltrative pattern. Such tunnel clusters do not commonly show mitotic activity, coarse chromatin or apoptotic bodies.[103]

MICROGLANDULAR HYPERPLASIA

Microglandular hyperplasia most probably results from florid reserve cell hyperplasia forming small glands and leads to a proliferation of tightly packed, small endocervical glands supported by hyperplastic reserve cells that have a characteristic lacy appearance. Cuboidal, columnar or flattened epithelial cells may form acini or solid sheets. The cells may feature supranuclear and subnuclear mucin vacuoles, occasionally resembling signet ring cells. Areas of squamous metaplasia may be present. The epithelium and gland lumina are typically permeated by neutrophils and there may be mixed acute and chronic inflammatory cells in the stroma (Fig. 6.8). This hyperplasia may be multifocal and exist within crypts or on the surface of the endocervical canal as a non-polypoid area, a sessile polyp or form a more elongated, protrusion into the canal. A large polyp may be mistaken for carcinoma clinically.

Microglandular hyperplasia is usually encountered incidentally, but a patient may complain of post-coital, intermenstrual or postmenopausal bleeding.

Worrying features, such as signet ring cells, hobnail cells, solid areas, clear cells, stromal hyalinisation, pseudoinfiltration or mitotic activity (usually no more than 1/10hpf) may lead to confusion with adenocarcinoma.[104,105] The absence of numerous or abnormal mitoses, lack of significant apoptotic activity,[28] absence of more than mild focal nuclear atypia and the close association with more obvious areas of microglandular hyperplasia help to distinguish the condition from malignant conditions. In contrast to clear cell carcinoma, microglandular hyperplasia lacks cytoplasmic glycogen and contains cytoplasmic mucin.

Although microglandular hyperplasia is usually seen within the reproductive years, it is well recognised in up to 6% of postmenopausal women.[106] Microglandular hyperplasia is often associated with exogenous hormone use or pregnancy, although this aetiological connection has been disputed.[107]

The finding of a small fragment of endocervix displaying microglandular hyperplasia may explain postmenopausal bleeding when seen in an endometrial biopsy containing little other than scanty inactive postmenopausal endometrium. Under these circumstances one must be aware of the potential for misdiagnosis with microglandular adenocarcinoma of the endometrium.[108,175] Lacy subcolumnar reserve cells are more typical of microglandular hyperplasia and the presence of endometrial stroma supports a diagnosis of endometrial carcinoma. Immunohistochemistry may be helpful with luminal reactivity for HMFG1 and anti-CA125 and lack of significant reaction for CEA, contrasting with cytoplasmic reactions with all these antibodies in most adenocarcinomas. Microglandular adenocarcinoma of the endometrium exhibits cytoplasmic and

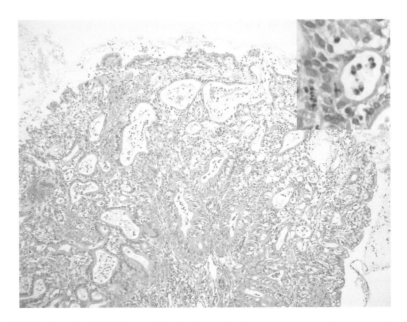

Fig. 6.8 In microglandular hyperplasia the lacy subcolumnar reserve cells, permeation by neutrophils and tightly-packed acini forming occasional cribriform areas all present a typical appearance. The inset gives a high power detail of neutrophils within acini formed by back to back epithelium. There are no nuclear characteristics of malignancy.

apical reactions for CEA and TAG72.[61,76,78] Not all adenocarcinomas are CEA positive. Thus this reagent must be used with care.[109]

These morphological and immunohistochemical differences with adenocarcinoma are inconsistent with the suggestion that microglandular hyperplasia is a pre-malignant condition[110] and support the findings of clinical studies indicating that microglandular hyperplasia is not a pre-malignant condition.[111]

LOBULAR ENDOCERVICAL HYPERPLASIA

Lobular endocervical glandular hyperplasia is characterised by a well-demarcated proliferation of simple tubular glands forming lobules through the cervical stroma. Lobular hyperplasia may extend into the outer half of the cervical wall with penetration to 12 mm, but in most cases the proliferation is limited to the inner half of the wall. It is usually an incidental finding that first alarms the pathologist. Some cases may present with a mucoid discharge and cervical enlargement where there may be no gross morphological features that would help to distinguish this lesion from adenocarcinoma. However, the glands are lined by a single layer of tall or cuboidal, epithelium producing pyloric-type mucin[112] lacking nuclear atypia and with indistinct nucleoli. Mitoses are rare with up to 2/10 hpf. There is no vascular space or perineural invasion and although some inflammation may be present around glands, no desmoplastic stromal response is present (Fig. 6.9).

The most important differential diagnosis of lobular endocervical hyperplasia is adenoma malignum. The two conditions can be distinguished by the

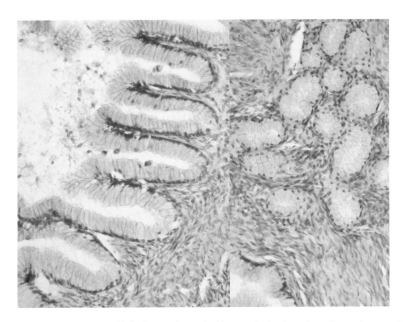

Fig. 6.9 These two views of lobular endocervical hyperplasia show banal, mucin secreting epithelium, forming quite distinct lobules. This hyperplastic process may extend deeply into the outer third of the cervical wall but no cytological atypia, desmoplastic stromal reaction or vascular space involvement is seen. These features help to distinguish the condition from well-differentiated adenocarcinoma (adenoma malignum).

irregular, deep stromal infiltration by crab-like or claw-shaped glands in adenoma malignum and by the absence of a desmoplastic stromal response, lymphovascular space involvement and focal atypia in lobular hyperplasia. In further contrast to adenoma malignum, the glands are negative for CEA and display a luminal reaction with HMFG1 in lobular hyperplasia, supporting a benign diagnosis.[113]

LAMINAR ENDOCERVICAL HYPERPLASIA

Jones and co-workers[114] described a well-demarcated proliferation of endocervical glands sharply delineated from the deeper two-thirds of the cervical stroma occurring in women of reproductive age. As with lobular endocervical hyperplasia, the focus of diagnostic confusion is with adenoma malignum. The lack of nuclear atypia, desmoplastic stromal response, irregular invasion, mitoses or apoptotic bodies all help to establish a benign diagnosis.[28] This condition is usually an incidental finding, but may be associated with a vaginal discharge.[115]

ENDOCERVICOSIS

Endocervicosis of the bladder is the presence of a proliferation of endocervical-type glands in the bladder wall and may represent mucinous differentiation in endometriosis.[116] Similar cysts or variably shaped glands lined by banal endocervical or flattened epithelium lacking a stromal response may be found in the outer half of the cervical wall or extend into the paracervical tissues. The diagnosis depends on the identification of a zone of uninvolved stroma between the normal glandular field and the deep glands.[117] There is a theoretical potential for neoplastic transformation in the cervix, as seen in an adenocarcinoma arising in a vaginal deposit.[118]

GARTNER'S DUCT REMNANTS/MESONEPHRIC HYPERPLASIA

The mesonephric ducts form parts of the efferent ducts of the testis in the male and the analogous epoophoron in the female. Remnants may persist in the lateral portions of the uterus and cervix as Gartner's ducts. Hyperplasia of these remnants is usually asymptomatic but may cause cervical enlargement or bleeding leading to clinical confusion with carcinoma.[88,119] The lesion is seen as ramifying ductular outgrowths extending beyond the lateral portions of the cervix to involve any quadrant. Hyperplasia produces lobular or diffuse growth patterns, and the latter may be difficult to distinguish from adenoma malignum.[120] The glands form simple groups of acini formed by low columnar or cuboidal cells incorporating pale vesicular nuclei. The glands lack papillae, cribriform areas, branching or budding (Fig. 6.10). This absence of glandular complexity helps to distinguish the proliferation from well-differentiated neoplasia[81] or clear cell adenocarcinoma.[105] Continuity with a vestigial duct is another helpful feature. A stromal response is absent.

The gland lumen characteristically encloses a brightly eosinophilic often hyaline secretion that is PAS positive and diastase resistant, staining with Alcian blue (pH 2.5) and mucicarmine.[121] The epithelium is mucin negative, gives a

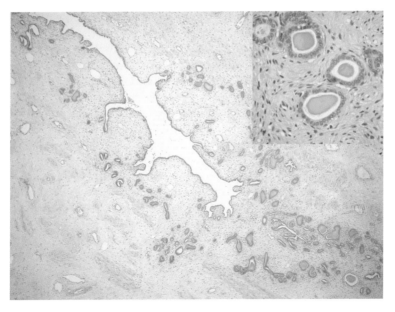

Fig. 6.10 Gartner's duct (mesonephric) hyperplasia, a lobular proliferation forms small acini lined by columnar cells enclosing an eosinophilic luminal secretion (inset). A central vestigial mesonephric duct can be seen.

luminal reaction with HMFG1[76] and is negative for CEA helping to distinguish from adenoma malignum. Thirty per cent are positive for vimentin.[122]

There are rare reports of mesonephric (Wolffian) adenocarcinoma,[88,123,124] and malignant mesonephric tumours supported by malignant stroma[125] developing from mesonephric hyperplasia. However, mesonephric hyperplasia is a common lesion and probably does not present a significant risk of malignancy. It does not appear to recur once excised.[120,126]

MINIMAL DEVIATION ADENOCARCINOMA (MDA)

In MDA or adenoma malignum of the cervix, abnormally shaped, branched, budded, slit-shaped or claw- or crab-like glands invade deeply into the cervical stroma. This condition can be extremely difficult to diagnose on biopsy because the glandular morphology and epithelium may be very well differentiated and it is obviously impossible to detect deep invasion on biopsy. However, the cervix is usually enlarged or friable and the patient may complain of a profuse vaginal discharge. Other clinical associations are with Peutz–Jeghers syndrome (where there is loss of heterozygosity on chromosome 19p[127]), sex cord tumours with annular tubules and mucinous ovarian tumours.[128–130] This is a rare condition representing around 1% of cervical adenocarcinomas.[131] Although it has been claimed that the prognosis is poor,[132] it is important to make an early diagnosis as this appears to improve survival.[133,134] However, these statistics may include benign conditions, such as various glandular hyperplasias and pyloric metaplasia that have only recently been described.[135]

The glands are lined by endocervical-type epithelium that for the most part displays a low nuclear–cytoplasmic ratio, no mitoses, inconspicuous nucleoli and no atypia. However, extensive sampling may reveal a few small foci of atypia where there is nuclear enlargement, mitotic activity and loss of polarity.[81,136] The main diagnostic difficulty with CGIN is where MDA (adenoma malignum) features areas of nuclear atypia.

MDA must also be separated from benign conditions (such as tunnel clusters, diffuse laminar endocervical glandular hyperplasia, lobular endocervical glandular hyperplasia, florid deep glands, deep Nabothian cysts, mesonephric hyperplasia, endocervical adenomyomas, endocervicosis and pyloric metaplasia).[112–114,131,135,137,138] A particularly difficult distinction is from Flumann's type A non-cystic tunnel clusters ramifying deeply into the cervix.[103]

Endometrioid variants of MDA can be encountered and these may be more easily confused with CGIN, tubo-endometrioid metaplasia and endometriosis because of the endometrial-like epithelial pseudostratification.[139,140]

The most helpful diagnostic features are the low and medium power histological appearance of bizarrely shaped glands extending beyond the middle third of the cervical wall. Invasive glands, in common with other types of cervical tumour, excite a stromal reaction of periglandular condensation, fibrosis or oedema, but this may only be seen focally. Nevertheless, it is important to remember that normal glands may also, occasionally, provoke a stromal reaction by inflammation or mucin extravasation.[114,141] The glands of MDA may be seen next to medium-sized arterioles (usually only seen deep in the cervical wall) and the finding of lymphatic or perineural invasion, obviously, confirms a malignant diagnosis. The benign condition of lobular endocervical hyperplasia may also extend beyond the inner third of the cervical wall, but, in contrast, MDA does not show a lobular growth pattern.

Immunohistochemistry may help to diagnose MDA. Dense cytoplasmic reactions for CEA are usually seen, contrasting with the fine luminal reaction of normal glands, but these may not be sufficiently uniform for diagnosis in a small biopsy. Adenoma malignum lacks diffuse CA125 positivity or oestrogen or progesterone receptors, in contrast to benign lesions and normal glands.[130,138,141]

Recently chemical, immunohistochemical and ultrastructural similarities with gastric pyloric mucosa have been reported.[130,142] MDA displays cytoplasmic reactivity with an antibody to pyloric gland mucin, HIK 1083, in contrast to the usual forms of endocervical adenocarcinoma and normal glands.[143] Other features of intestinal differentiation include increased numbers of argyrophilic endocrine cells containing serotonin or peptide hormones.[4,81,136,144] The cells produce PAS positive, sialomucin predominant, neutral gastric mucin with absent sulphomucins.[13,145] This is a useful contrast to the sulphomucin containing normal or hyperplastic endocervical glandular epithelium that gives a mixed acidic and neutral purple/violet with alcian blue and PAS.[146] Pyloric metaplasia may exhibit a similar phenotype and must be distinguished from MDA by the lack of malignant morphological characteristics but note that HIK1083 positive cells are also present in lobular endocervical hyperplasia.[112,147]

ARIAS–STELLA CHANGE

In up to 9% of pregnancies the endocervical glands, foci of tubo-endometrioid metaplasia or endometriosis may adopt the typical hypersecretory changes of the Arias–Stella change.[148] The nuclei may appear banal or may exhibit a spectrum of hyperchromasia and pleomorphism, but mitoses are very rare and there is no loss of polarity in stratified areas. Rare nuclear inclusions may be observed. The cytoplasm is usually vacuolated, but may show regressing secretory changes if the pregnancy has failed.

Arias–Stella change may show a combination of clear cell and hobnail cell areas and this may be similar to clear cell adenocarcinoma.[105] However, in Arias–Stella change the nuclei do not possess the prominent nucleoli of clear cell carcinoma and do not show diffuse atypia.[149] The best discriminatory aid is a willingness to consider Arias–Stella change in a pregnant patient before diagnosing adenocarcinoma.[101]

ATYPICAL ENDOCERVICAL OXYPHILIC METAPLASIA

In a change that is similar to apocrine metaplasia, the endocervical epithelium may become more eosinophilic and display apical blebbing (Fig. 6.11). This benign alteration causes no cervical enlargement and is invariably an incidental finding. It usually occurs in inflamed areas.[150] Scope for confusion with CGIN may arise from the appearance of the nuclei that may be enlarged, hyperchromatic or polylobated. In contrast to CGIN, there is no stratification or mitotic activity.

FLORID CYSTIC ENDOSALPINGIOSIS

This is a proliferation of cysts lined by tubal-type epithelium[151] that causes enlargement of the outer part of the cervical wall. It may be associated with similar deposits of endosalpingiosis on the serosa of the uterus and on the ovaries.

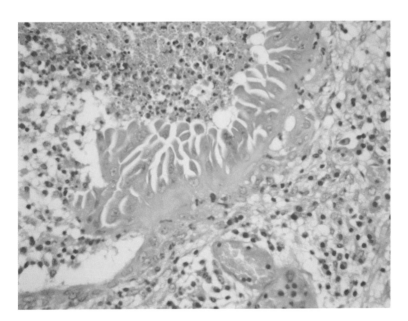

Fig. 6.11 In atypical oxyphilic metaplasia of the endocervical epithelium, there may be prominent apical snouting associated with nuclear enlargement. However, nuclear features of malignancy are absent and the metaplasia is usually associated with inflammation.

Although there is scope for confusion with endometrioid adenocarcinoma and MDA, the diagnosis can be made by the lack of atypia or stromal response.

PAPILLARY CERVICITIS

An accentuation of the normal crypt pattern forms blunt-tipped papillae projecting into the endocervical canal. The tips of the papillae become congested, haemorrhagic and inflamed, contributing to post-coital or intermenstrual bleeding. The condition can be distinguished from papillary adenocarcinomas or villoglandular carcinoma by the absence of dysplastic nuclear changes and the lack of epithelial proliferation.[152]

RADIATION ATYPIA

After radiation therapy, the cervix may be hard and fibrotic containing endocervical glands that may be atrophic. The glandular epithelium may appear atypical, but this is usually limited to a slight increase in nuclear cytoplasmic ratio and loss of polarity (Fig. 6.12). Nuclear hyperchromasia is rare.[153] The presence of atypical stromal fibroblasts may indicate the aetiology. It is important to note that the epithelium may show cytoplasmic reactivity for CEA.

ENDOCERVICAL ADENOMYOMA

This benign lesion has been reported as a cervical mass up to 23 cm in diameter. It grossly resembles a cervical leiomyoma and features a proliferation of smooth muscle bundles, but it also incorporates endocervical glands. There is potential

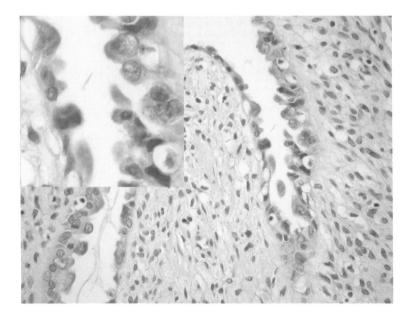

Fig. 6.12 In radiation atypia, there may be marked variation of the epithelial nuclei (inset) but hyperchromasia is focal and limited and mitosis are rare. The stromal cells may show typical alterations associated with irradiation.

for confusion with glandular neoplasia, especially MDA (adenoma malignum) or its mimics.[138] The glandular epithelium lacks any signs of atypia and characteristically lines lobular glands.

MICROINVASIVE (STAGE 1A) GLANDULAR LESIONS

Invasion of the cervical stroma clearly delineates CGIN from adenocarcinoma. Unfortunately, the smallest invasive foci can be extremely difficult to identify. The extension of neoplastic glands beyond the normal glandular field is a clear marker of invasion, but several benign conditions (such as lobular endocervical hyperplasia, deep Nabothian follicles and endocervicosis) also feature deep glands. Invasion within the range of the depth of normal glands represents the most superficial encroachment into the stroma, but this can be very difficult to spot.

Stage 1Ai adenocarcinoma, like squamous cell carcinoma, is defined as invasion to less than 3 mm depth, less than 7 mm width. Stage 1Aii adenocarcinoma is greater than 3 mm but less than 5 mm depth and less than 7 mm width. Vascular space invasion does not alter the stage (FIGO, 1995). Some authors[15,16,154] have limited microinvasion to less than 2 or 5 mm deep or a volume of less than 500 mm^3.[155]

A stromal response of oedema, loose fibrosis and inflammation often signifies invasion but many normal crypts are accompanied by a stromal reaction and inflammation may be absent in carcinoma.[154,156,157] Normal crypts do not extend beyond 7.8 mm from the surface,[29] but tangential sectioning of the cervical canal can make measurement of the depth of invasion and assessment of the extent of the normal endocervix difficult. The earliest stage of invasion is usually within the normal glandular area where small buds of eosinophilic, squamoid epithelium encroach into the superficial adjacent stroma (type 6 below). These are extremely helpful pointers of invasion, if identified, but they can be very easy to overlook or misinterpret.

Cribriform glands may be found in well-characterised AIS of other sites, such as breast or colon, and so cannot be said to be diagnostic of invasion in the endocervix. Furthermore, hyperplastic areas of the endocervix, such as microglandular hyperplasia, may display cribriform architecture.

The detection of basement membrane breaks using immunohistochemistry for laminin and type IV collagen has detected early invasion,[158] but invasive glands may continue to produce an intact basement membrane.[159,160]

In 2000, Ostor[156] described seven types of microinvasive adenocarcinoma:

1. Tiny foci of squamoid differentiation, the smallest invasive foci, usually less than 1 mm in diameter, similar to the earliest stages of squamous cell carcinoma.[68,161]
2. Large irregular crab-shaped glands.
3. Solid areas resembling adenosquamous carcinoma.
4. Invasion along a broad front.
5. Cribriform glands.
6. Small glandular foci within the normal endocervical field.
7. Naked invasion, lacking a stromal response.

Measuring the depth of invasion may be problematical. There is no difficulty in quantifying the depth and width of stromal involvement where tiny buds invade the stroma (type 1 above). The lesion is measured from the point of origin in the basement membrane of the epithelium or crypt, as with squamous carcinoma. However, where there is stromal invasion by glandular acini or sheets, the depth of invasion is less easy to measure than in squamous lesions and the point of origin may be impossible to determine. If this is the case, and there is doubt about the point of origin, tumour thickness should be measured from the surface of the invasive area. Ostor has acknowledged that depth of invasion measurement may be less reproducible than tumour thickness.[156] It is helpful to give the method of measurement in the report.

PROGNOSIS OF CERVICAL GLANDULAR INTRA-EPITHELIAL NEOPLASIA

The mainstays of local surgery for CGIN are LLETZ and cold knife cone biopsy. As the diathermy artefact that LLETZ causes may obscure the margins, cold knife cone has been recommended for excision of CGIN.[40]

Local surgery may not be curative. Luesley et al.[162] noted residual disease in hysterectomy specimens in one of two cases where cone margins were not involved and in four of eight cases where the margins were involved. Hopkins et al.[163] showed eight instances of residual disease (with one fatal case) in 12 cases where the cone margins were involved. AIS was found in two of the subsequent hysterectomies in 32 cases where the margins were not involved.

One of nine cases of AIS with negative margins had residual disease at hysterectomy.[164] Of 11 patients with negative margins after LLETZ, four had residual H-CGIN in subsequent hysterectomy, yet two of six patients with involved margins had no residual neoplasia at hysterectomy.[165] In one study of 19 positive margin cone biopsies,[166] 10 had residual disease at hysterectomy including five that were invasive. Seven of the 21 with negative margins had residual disease of which three were invasive. Deheny et al.[167] found residual neoplasia in eight of 10 where there were positive margins and four of seven with negative margins.

Rare case reports detail in situ[168] or invasive adenocarcinoma appearing in the upper vagina even after simple or radical hysterectomy for H-CGIN.[162,163,169]

Most now accept that involved margins are unreliable predictors of residual disease. There is a 33–50% risk with negative margins and up to 80% risk with involved margins.[7,14,30,33,42,162,163,165,167,170,171] In a review of 13 studies[174] 23% of 142 cases with uninvolved margins and 56% of 110 cases with involved margins had residual disease.

Thus, follow-up using cytology and possibly endocervical curettage is necessary. Nevertheless, despite claims to the contrary,[33,166] there is evidence that curettage does not detect a sufficiently high proportion of cases.[167,172]

The behaviour of L-CGIN is less clear. There was residual disease in 43% of L-CGIN with positive margins or with a disease-free margin of less than 3 mm by LLETZ.[25] Treatment by pin and ball diathermy left residual disease in one of nine examples of 'glandular dysplasia less than AIS'.[24] Three patients who had margins involved by H-CGIN had residual L-CGIN at hysterectomy.[24] None of 24 cases of CGIN less than AIS developed invasive malignancy on 12-year follow-up.[173] In an other series, all of 12 cases of glandular atypia less than AIS were negative on cytological follow-up after cone ($n = 7$) or hysterectomy ($n = 5$).[162]

With our present knowledge it is reasonable to treat L-CGIN, when rigorously diagnosed, by complete excision followed by cytological surveillance.

REFERENCES

1. Plaxe SC, Saltzstein SL. Estimation of the duration of the pre-clinical phase of cervical adenocarcinoma suggests that here is ample opportunity for screening. Gynecol Oncol 1999; 75: 55–61
2. Miller BE, Flax SD, Arheart K, Photopulos G. The presentation of adenocarcinoma of the uterine cervix. Cancer 1993; 72: 1281–1285
3. Wells M, Brown LJR. Glandular lesions of the cervix: the present state of our knowledge. Histopathology 1986; 10: 777–792
4. Gloor E, Hurlimann J. Cervical intraepithelial glandular neoplasia (adenocarcinoma in-situ and glandular dysplasia). Cancer 1986; 58: 1272–1280
5. Hauser G. Zur Histogenese des Krebes. Virchows Archiv fur Pathologische Anatomie 1894; 134: 482–498
6. Friedell GH, McKay DG. Adenocarcinoma in-situ of the endocervix. Cancer 1953; 6: 887–897
7. Qizilbash AH. In-situ and microinvasive adenocarcinoma of the uterine cervix. Am J Clin Pathol 1975; 64: 155–170
8. Christopherson WM, Nealson N, Gray LA. Non-invasive precursor lesions of adenocarcinoma and mixed adenosquamous carcinoma of the cervix uteri. Cancer 1979; 44: 975–983
9. Boon ME, Kirk RS, Scheffers-Rieveld PEM. The morphogenesis of adenocarcinoma in-situ – a complex pathological entity. Histopathology 1981; 5: 565–577
10. Boon ME, Baak JPA, Kurver PJH, Overdiep SH, Verdonk GW. Adenocarcinoma in-situ of the cervix: an underdiagnosed lesion. Cancer 1981; 48: 768–773
11. Gloor E, Ruzicka J. Morphology of adenocarcinoma in-situ of the uterine cervix: a study of 14 cases. Cancer 1982; 49: 294–302
12. Noda K, Kimura K, Ikeda M, Teshima K. Studies on the histogenesis of cervical adenocarcinoma. Int J Gynecol Pathol 1983; 1: 336–346
13. van Roon E, Boon ME, Kurver PJH, Baak JPA. The association between pre-cancerous columnar and squamous lesions of the cervix: a morphometric study. Histopathology 1983; 7: 887–896
14. Ostor AG, Pagan R, Davoren RAM, Fortune DW, Chanen W, Rome R. Adenocarcinoma in-situ of the cervix. Int J Gynecol Pathol 1984; 3: 179–190
15. Teshima S, Shimosata Y, Kishi K, Kasamatou T, Ohmi K, Uei Y. Early stage adenocarcinoma of the uterine cervix: histopathologic analysis with consideration of histogenesis. Cancer 1985; 56: 167–172
16. Betsill WG, Clark AH. Early endocervical glandular neoplasia. I. Histomorphometry and cytomorphology. Acta Cytol 1986; 30: 115–126
17. Jaworski RC, Pacey NF, Greenberg ML, Osborn RA. The histologic diagnosis of adenocarcinoma in-situ and related lesions of the cervix uteri. Cancer 1988; 61: 1171–1181
18. Tobon H, Dave H. Adenocarcinoma in-situ of the cervix. Int J Gynecol Pathol 1988; 7: 139–151
19. Bousefield L, Pacey F, Young Q, Krumins I, Osborn R. Extended cytologic criteria for the diagnosis of adenocarcinoma in-situ of the cervix and related lesions. Acta Cytol 1980; 24: 283–295
20. Dixon MF, Brown LJR, Gilmour HM et al. Observer variation in the assessment of dysplasia in ulcerative colitis. Histopathology 1988; 13: 385–398
21. Fox H, Buckley CH. Histopathology reporting in cervical screening National Health service cervical screening program. 1999; 10: 16–26
22. Clement PB, Young RH. Atlas of Gynecological Surgical Pathology. Philadelphia: WB Saunders 2000; 5: 112
23. Cullimore JE, Luesley DM, Rollason TP, Byrne P, Buckley CH, Anderson M, Williams DR, Waddell C, Hudson E, Shafi MI. A prospective study of conization of the cervix in the

management of cervical intraepithelial glandular neoplasia (CIGN) – a preliminary report. Br J Obstet Gynaecol 1992; 99: 314–318

24. Casper GR, Ostor AG, Quinn MA. A clinicopathologic study of glandular dysplasia of the cervix. Gynecol Oncol 1996; 64: 166–170

25. Kurian K, Al-Nafussi A. Relation of cervical glandular intraepithelial neoplasia to microinvasive and invasive adenocarcinoma of the uterine cervix: a study of 121 cases. J Clin Pathol 1999; 52: 112–117

26. Burghardt E. Early histological diagnosis of cervical cancer. In: Friedman EA (Ed.) Major Problems in Obstetrics and Gynecology, Vol. 6. Philadelphia: Saunders, 1973; 335–362

27. Biscotti CV, Hart WR. Apoptotic bodies: a consistent morphologic feature of endocervical adenocarcinoma *in situ*. Am J Surg Pathol 1998; 22: 434–439

28. Moritani S, Ioffe OB, Sagae S, Dahmoush L, Silverberg SG, Hattori T. Mitotic activity and apoptosis in endocervical glandular lesions. Int J Gynecol Pathol 2002; 21: 125–133

29. Anderson MC, Hartley RB. Cervical crypt involvement by intraepithelial neoplasia. Obstet Gynecol 1980; 55: 546–550

30. Bertrand M, Lickrish GM, Colgan TJ. The anatomic distribution of cervical adenocarcinoma *in-situ*: implications for treatment. Am J Obstet Gynecol 1987; 157: 21–25

31. Colgan TJ, Lickrish GM. The topography and invasive potential of cervical adenocarcinoma *in situ* with and without associated squamous dysplasia. Gynecol Oncol 1990; 36: 246–249

32. Goldstein NS, Ahmad E, Hussain M, Hankin RC, Perez-Reyes N. Endocervical glandular atypia. Does a pre-neoplastic lesion of adenocarcinoma *in situ* exist. Am J Clin Pathol 1998; 110: 200–209

33. Andersen ES, Arffman E. Adenocarcinoma *in-situ* of the uterine cervix: a clinico-pathologic study of 36 cases. Gynecol Oncol 1989; 35: 1–7

34. Trowell JE. Intestinal metaplasia with argentaffin cells in the uterine cervix. Histopathology 1985; 9: 551–559

35. Lee KR, Sun D, Crum CP. Endocervical intraepithelial glandular atypia (dysplasia): a histopathologic, human papillomavirus, and MIB-1 analysis of 25 cases. Hum Pathol 2000; 31: 656–664

36. Park JJ, Sun D, Quade BJ, Flynn C, Sheets EE, Yang A, McKeon F, Crum CP. Stratified mucin-producing intraepithelial lesions of the cervix: adenosquamous or columnar cell neoplasia? Am J Surg Pathol 2000; 24: 1414–1419

37. Schlesinger C, Silverberg SG. Endocervical adenocarcinoma *in situ* of tubal type and its relation to atypical tubal metaplasia. Int J Gynecol Pathol 1999; 18: 1–4

38. Rollason TP, Byrne P, Williams A, Brown G. Expression of epithelial membrane and 3-fucosyl-N-acetyllactosamine antigens in cervix uteri with particular reference to adenocarcinoma *in situ*. J Clin Pathol 1988; 41: 547–552

39. Kashimura M, Shinohara M, Oikawa K, Hamasaki K, Sato H. An adenocarcinoma *in-situ* of the uterine cervix that developed into invasive adenocarcinoma after 5 years. Gynecol Oncol 1990; 36: 128–133

40. Kennedy AW, el Tabbakh GH, Biscotti CV, Wirth S. Invasive adenocarcinoma of the cervix following LLETZ (large loop excision of the transformation zone) for adenocarcinoma *in situ*. Gynecol Oncol 1995; 58: 274–277

41. Gloor E, Hurlimann J. Cervical intraepithelial glandular neoplasia (adenocarcinoma *in-situ* and glandular dysplasia). Cancer 1986; 58: 1272–1280

42. Muntz HG, Bell DA, Lage JM, Goff BA, Feldman S, Rice LW. Adenocarcinoma *in situ* of the uterine cervix. Obstet Gynecol 1992; 80: 935–939

43. Duggan MA, McGregor E, Benoit JL, Inoue M, Nation JG, Stuart GCE. The human papillomavirus status of invasive cervical adenocarcinoma: a clinicopathological and outcome analysis. Human Pathol 1995; 26: 319–325

44. Parazzini F, La Vecchia C. Epidemiology of adenocarcinoma of the cervix. Gynecol Oncol 1990; 39: 40–46

45. Yamakawa Y, Forslund O, Chua KL, Dillner L, Boon ME, Hansson BG. Detection of the BC 24 transforming fragment of the herpes simplex virus type 2 (HSV-2) DNA in cervical carcinoma tissue by polymerase chain reaction (PCR). Acta Pathol, Microbiol Immunol Scand 1994; 102: 401–406

46. Hafez ESE. Structural and ultrastructural parameters of the uterine cervix. Obstet Gynecol Sur 1982; 37: 507–516

47. Wells M, Brown LJ. Symposium Part IV: Investigative approaches to endocervical pathology. Int J Gynecol Pathol 2002; 21: 360–367

48. Farley J, Loup D, Nelson M. Neoplastic transformation of the endocervix associated with downregulation of lactoferrin expression. Mol Carcinogen 1997; 20: 240–250

49. Anderson S, Shera K, Uhle J et al. Telomerase activity in cervical cancer. Am J Pathol 1997; 151: 25–31

50. Yashima K, Ashfaq R, Nowak J et al. Telomerase activity and expression of its RNA component in cervical lesions Cancer 1998; 82: 1319–1327

51. Nakano K, Watney E, McDougall JK. Telomerase activity and expression of telomerase RNA component and telomerase catalytic subunit gene in cervical cancer. Am J Pathol 1998; 153: 857–864

52. McCluggage WG, Maxwell P, McBride HA, Hamilton PW, Bharucha H. Monoclonal antibodies Ki-67 and MIB1 in the distinction of tuboendometrioid metaplasia from endocervical adenocarcinoma and adenocarcinoma in situ in formalin-fixed material. Int J Gynecol Pathol 1995; 14: 209–216

53. van Hoeven KH, Ramondetta L, Kovatich AJ, Bibbo M, Dunton CJ. Quantitative analysis of MIB-1 reactivity in inflammatory, hyperplastic and neoplastic endocervical lesions. Int J Gynecol Pathol 1997; 16: 15–16

54. Cina SJ, Richardson MS, Austin RM. Immunohistochemical staining for Ki-67 antigen, carcinoembryonic antigen and p53 in the differential diagnosis of glandular lesions of the cervix. Mod Pathol 1997; 10: 176–180

55. Leminen A, Paavonen J, Forss M, Wahlstrom T, Vesterinen E. Adenocarcinoma of the uterine cervix. Cancer 1990; 65: 53–59

56. Fu YS, Hall TL, Berek JS, Hacker NF, Reagen JW. Prognostic significance of DNA ploidy and morphometric analyses of adenocarcinoma of the uterine cervix. Anal Quant Cytol Histol 1987; 9: 17–24

57. Magtibay PM, Perrone JF, Stanhope CR, Katzmann JA, Keeney GL, LiH. Flow cytometric DNA analysis of early stage adenocarcinoma of the cervix. Gynecol Oncol 1999; 75: 242–247

58. Griffin NR. Studies of glycoconjugates and amylase in the normal human cervix and in endocervical neoplasia. University of Leeds. MD Thesis, 1992

59. Wahlstrom T, Lindgren J, Korhonen M, Seppala M. Distinction between endocervical and endometrial adenocarcinoma with immunoperoxidase staining of carcinoembryonic antigen in routine histological sections. Lancet 1979; ii: 1159–1160

60. Cohen C, Shulman G, Budgeon LR. Endocervical and endometrial adenocarcinoma: an immunoperoxidase and histochemical study. Am J Surg Pathol 1982; 6: 151–157

61. Speers WC, Picaso LG, Silverberg SG. Immunohistochemical localisation of carcinoembryonic antigen in microglandular hyperplasia and adenocarcinoma of the endocervix. Am J Clin Pathol 1983; 79: 105–107

62. Ueda S, Tsubara A, Izumi H, Sasaki M, Morii R. Immunohistochemical studies of carcinoembryonic antigen in adenocarcinoma of the uterus. Acta Pathol (Japan) 1983; 33: 59–69

63. Hurlimann J, Gloor E. Adenocarcinoma in-situ and invasive adenocarcinoma of the uterine cervix: an immunohistologic study with antibodies specific for several epithelial markers. Cancer 1984; 54: 103–109

64. Cooper P, Russel G, Wilson B. Adenocarcinoma of the endocervix – a histochemical study. Histopathology 1987; 11: 1321–1330

65. Maes G, Fleuren GJ, Bara J, Nap M. The distribution of mucins, carcinoembryonic antigen and mucus associated antigens in endocervical and endometrial adenocarcinomas. Int J Gynecol Pathol 1988; 7: 112–122

66. Marques T, Andrade LA, Vassallo J. Endocervical tubal metaplasia and adenocarcinoma in situ: role of immunohistochemistry for carcinoembryonic antigen and vimentin in differential diagnosis. Histopathology 1996; 28: 549–550

67. Wakefield EA, Wells M. Histochemical study of endocervical glycoproteins throughout the normal menstrual cycle and adjacent to cervical intraepithelial neoplasia. Int J Gynecol Pathol 1985; 4: 230–239

68. Matsukuma K, Tsukamoto N, Kaku T, Matsumura M, Toki N, Toh N, Nakano. Early adenocarcinoma of the uterine cervix – its histologic and immunohistologic study. Gynecol Oncol 1989; 35: 38–43

69. Kase H, Kodama S, Tanaka K. Observations of high iron diamine-alcian blue stain in uterine cervical glandular lesions. Gynecol Obstet Invest 1999; 48: 56–60

70. Cullimore JE, Rollason TP, Marshall T. Nucleolar organiser regions in adenocarcinoma *in-situ* of the endocervix. J Clin Pathol 1989; 42: 1276–1280

71. Wood AJ, Egan MJ. The silver colloid technique applied to endocervical tissue. Histopathology 1989; 15: 306–308

72. Darne JF, Polacarz SV, Sheridan E, Anderson D, Ginsberg R, Sharp F. Nucleolar organiser regions in adenocarcinoma *in situ* and invasive adenocarcinoma of the cervix. J Clin Pathol 1990; 43: 657–660

73. Allen JP, Gallimore AP. Nuclear organiser regions in benign and malignant glandular lesions of the cervix. J Pathol 1992; 166: 153–156

74. Newbold KM, Rollason TP, Luesley DM, Ward K. Nucleolar organiser regions and proliferative index in glandular and squamous carcinomas of the cervix. J Clin Pathol 1989; 42: 441–442

75. Miller B, Flax S, Dockter M, Photopulos G. Nuclear organiser regions in adenocarcinoma of the uterine cervix. Cancer 1994; 74: 3142–3245

76. Brown LJR, Griffin NR, Wells M. Cytoplasmic reactivity with the monoclonal antibody HMFG1 as a marker of cervical glandular atypia. J Pathol 1987; 151: 203–208

77. Umezaki K, Sanezumi M, Okada H, Okamura A, Tsubra A, Kanazaki H. Distribution of epithelial-specific antigen in uterine cervix with endocervical glandular dysplasia. Gynecol Oncol 1997; 66: 393–398

78. Nanbu Y, Fujii S, Konishi I, Nonogaaki H, Mori T. Immunohistochemical localisation of Ca125, carcinoembryonic antigen and Ca 19–9 in normal and neoplastic glandular cells of the uterine cervix. Cancer 1988; 62: 2580–2588

79. Kudo R, Sasano H, Koizumi M, Orenstein JM, Silverberg SG. Immunohistological comparison of new monoclonal antibody 1C5 and carcinoembryonic antigen in the differential diagnosis of adenocarcinoma of the uterine cervix. Int J Gynecol Pathol 1990; 9: 325–336

80. Polacarz SV, Darne J, Sheridan EG, Ginsberg R, Sharp F. Endocervical carcinoma and precursor lesions: *c-myc* expression and demonstration of field changes. J Clin Pathol 1991; 44: 896–899

81. Gilks CB, Young RH, Aguirre P, DeLellis RA, Scully RE. Adenoma malignum (minimal deviation adenocarcinoma) of the uterine cervix: a clinicopathological and immunohistochemical analysis of 26 cases. Am J Surg Pathol 1989; 13: 717–729

82. Suh KS, Silverberg SG. Tubal metaplasia of the uterine cervix. Int J Gynecol Pathol 1990; 9: 122–128

83. Bruns DE, Mills DE, Davory J. Amylase in fallopian tube and serous ovarian neoplasms. Immunohistochemical localization. Arch Pathol Lab Med 106: 17–20

84. Peters WM. 1986 Nature of 'basal' and 'reserve' cells in oviductal and cervical epithelium in man. J Clin Pathol 1982; 39: 306–312

85. Oliva E, Clement PB, Young RH. Tubal and tubo-endometrioid metaplasia of the uterine cervix. Unemphasized features that may cause problems in differential diagnosis: a report of 25 cases. Am J Clin Pathol 1995; 103: 618–623

86. Toki T, Shimizu M, Takagi Y, Ashida T, Konishi I. CD10 is a marker for normal and neoplastic endometrial stromal cells. Int J Gynecol Pathol 2002; 21: 41–47

87. Kim KR. Utility of trichrome and reticulin stains in the diagnosis of superficial endometriosis of the uterine cervix. Int J Gynecol Pathol 2001; 20: 173–176

88. Ferry JA, Scully RE. Mesonephric remnants, hyperplasia, and neoplasia in the uterine cervix. Am J Surg Pathol 1990; 14: 1100–1111

89. McCluggage G, McBride H, Maxwell P, Bharucha H. Immunohistochemical detection of p53 and bcl-2 proteins in neoplastic and non-neoplastic endocervical glandular lesions. Int J Gynecol Pathol 1997; 16: 22–27

90. Cameron RI, Maxwell P, Jenkins D, McGluggage WG. Immunohistochemical staining with MIB1, bcl2, and p16 assists in the distinction of cervical glandular intraepithelial neoplasia from tuboendometrial metaplasia, endometriosis and microglandular hyperplasia. Histopathology 2002; 41: 313–321

91. Pirog EC, Isacson C, Szabolcs MJ, Kleter B, Quint W, Richart RM. Proliferative activity of benign and neoplastic endocervical epithelium and correlation with HPV DNA detection. Int J Gynecol Pathol 2002; 21: 22–26

92. Ismail SM. Cone biopsy causes cervical endometriosis and tubo-endometrioid metaplasia. Histopathology 1991; 18: 107–114

93. Varma SK, Rayner SS, Brown LJR. Cutaneous ciliated cyst: case report and literature review. Plas Recontruct Surg 1991; 86: 344–346

94. Nucci MR, Ferry JA, Young RH. Ectopic prostatic tissue in the uterine cervix: a report of four cases and review of ectopic prostatic tissue. Am J Surg Pathol 2000; 24: 1224–1230

95. McCluggage WG, Maxwell P. bcl-2 and p21 immunostaining of cervical tubo-endometrioid metaplasia. Histopathology 2002; 40: 107–108

96. Ibrahim E, Blackett AD, Tidy JA, Wells M. CD44 is a marker of endocervical neoplasia. Int J Gynecol Pathol 1999; 18: 101–108

97. Larraza-Hernandez O, Molberg KH, Lindberg G, Albores-Saavedra J. Ectopic prostatic tissue in the uterine cervix. Int J Pathol 1997; 16: 291–293

98. Fichera G, Santanocito A. Pilo-sebaceous cystic ectopy of the uterine cervix. Clin Exp Obstet Gynecol 1989; 16: 21–25

99. Robledo MC, Vazquez JJ, Contreras-Mejuto F, Lopez-Garcia G. Sebaceous glands and hair follicles in the cervix uteri. Histopathology 1992; 21: 278–280

100. Fluhmann CF. Focal hyperplasia (tunnel clusters) of the cervix uteri. Obstet Gynecol 1961; 17: 206–214

101. Nucci MR. Symposium Part III: tumor-like glandular lesions of the uterine cervix. Int J Gynecol Pathol 2002; 21: 347–359

102. Segal GH, Hart WR. Cystic endocervical tunnel clusters. A clinicopathologic study of 29 cases of so-called adenomatous hyperplasia. Am J Surg Pathol 1990; 14: 895–903

103. Jones MA, Young RH. Endocervical type A (noncystic) tunnel clusters with cytological atypia. A report of 14 cases. Am J Surg Pathol 1996; 20: 1312–1318

104. Young RH, Scully R. Atypical forms of microglandular hyperplasia of the cervix simulating carcinoma. Am J Surg Pathol 1989; 13: 50–56

105. Matias-Guiu X, Lerma E, Prat J. Clear cell tumours of the female genital tract. Semin Diagnos Pathol 1997; 14: 233–239

106. Chumas JC, Nelson B, Mann WJ, Chalas E, Kaplan CG. Microglandular hyperplasia of the uterine cervix. Obstet Gynecol 1985; 66: 406–409

107. Greeley C, Schroeder S, Silverberg SG. Microglandular hyperplasia of the cervix: a true 'pill' lesion? Int J Gynecol Pathol 1995; 14: 50–54

108. Zaloudek C, Hayashi GM, Ryan IP, Powell CB, Miller TR. Microglandular adenocarcinoma of the endometrium: a form of mucinous adenocarcinoma that may be confused with microglandular hyperplasia of the cervix. Int J Gynecol Pathol 1997; 16: 52–59

109. Steeper TA, Wick MR. Minimal deviation adenocarcinoma of the uterine cervix ('adenoma malignum'). An immunohistochemical comparison with microglandular endocervical hyperplasia and conventional endocervical adenocarcinoma. Cancer 1986; 58: 1131–1138

110. Dallenbach-Hellweg G. On the origin and histological structuer of adenocarcinoma of the endocervix in women under 50 years of age. Pathol Res Pract 1984; 179: 38–50

111. Jones MW, Silverberg SG. Cervical adenocarcinoma in young women: possible relationship to microglandular hyperplasia and use of oral contraceptives. Obstet Gynecol 1989; 73: 984–988

112. Mikami Y, Hata S, Fujiwara K, Imajo Y, Kohno I, Manabe T. Florid endocervical glandular hyperplasia with intestinal and pyloric gland metaplasia: worrisome benign mimic of 'adenoma malignum'. Gynecol Oncol 1999; 74: 504–511

113. Nucci MR, Clement PB, Young RH. Lobular endocervical glandular hyperplasia, not otherwise specified: a clinicopathological analysis of thirteen cases of a distinctive pseudoneoplastic lesion and comparison with fourteen cases of adenoma malignum. Am J Surg Pathol 1999; 23: 886–891

114. Jones MA, Young RH, Scully RE. Diffuse laminar endocervical glandular hyperplasia. A benign lesion often confused with adenoma malignum (minimal deviation adenocarcinoma). Am J Surg Pathol 1991; 15: 1123–1129

115. Maruyama R, Nagaoka S, Terao K, Honda M, Koita H. Diffuse laminar endocervical glandular hyperplasia. Pathol Int 1995; 45: 283–286

116. Clement PB, Young RH. Endocervicosis of the urinary bladder. A report of six cases of a benign mullerian lesion that may mimic adenocarcinoma. Am J Surg Pathol 1992; 16: 533–542

117. Young RH, Clement PB. Endocervicosis involving the uterine cervix: a report of four cases of a benign process that may be confused with deeply invasive endocervical adenocarcinoma. Int J Gynecol Pathol 2000; 19: 322–328

118. McCluggage WG, Price JH, Dobbs SP. Primary adenocarcinoma of the vagina arising in endocervicosis. Int J Gynecol Pathol 2001; 20: 399–402

119. Jones MA, Andrews J, Tarraza HM. Mesonephric remnant hyperplasia of the cervix: a clinicopathologic analysis of 14 cases. Gynecol Oncol 1993; 49: 41–47

120. Seidman JD, Tavassoli FA. Mesonephric hyperplasia of the uterine cervix: a clinicopathologic study of 51 cases. Int J Gynecol Pathol 1995; 14: 293–299

121. Ayroud Y, Gelfand MM, Ferenczy A. Florid mesonephric hyperplasia of the cervix: a report of a case with review of the literature. Int J Gynecol Pathol 1985; 4: 245–254

122. Lang G, Dallenbach-Hellweg G. The histogenetic origin of cervical mesonephric hyperplasia and mesonephric adenocarcinoma of the uterine cervix studied with immunohistochemical methods. Int J Gynaecol Pathol 1990; 9: 145–157

123. Buntine DW. Adenocarcinoma of the uterine cervix of probable Wolffian origin. Pathology 1979; 11: 713–718

124. Valente PT, Susin M. Cervical adenocarcinoma arising in florid mesonephric hyperplasia: report of a case with immunocytochemical studies. Gynecol Oncol 1987; 27: 58–68

125. Clement PB, Young RH, Keh P, Ostor AG, Scully RE. Malignant mesonephric neoplasms of the uterine cervix. Am J Surg Pathol 1995; 19: 1158–1171

126. Shah KH, Kurman RJ, Scully RE, Norris HS. Atypical hyperplasia of mesonephric remnants in the cervix. Lab Invest 1980; 42: 149

127. Lee JY, Dong SM, Kim HS. A distinct region of chromosome 19p13.3 associated with the sporadic form of adenoma malignum of the uterine cervix. Cancer Res 1998; 58: 1140–1143

128. Young RH, Scully RE. Mucinous ovarian tumours associated with mucinous adenocarcinomas of the cervix. Int J Gynecol Pathol 1988; 7: 99–111

129. Young RH, Welsh WR, Dickersin GR, Scully RE. Ovarian sex cord tumour with annular tubules. Cancer 1982; 50: 1384–1402

130. Toki T, Shiozawa T, Hosaka N, Ishii K, Nikaido T, Fujii S. Minimal deviation adenocarcinoma of the uterine cervix has abnormal expression of sex steroid receptors. Int J Gynecol Pathol 1997; 121: 971–975

131. Hart WR. Symposium Part II: Special types of adenocarcinoma of the uterine cervix. Int J Gynecol Pathol 2002; 21: 327–346

132. McKelvey JL, Goodlin RR. Adenoma malignum of the cervix: a cancer of deceptively innocent histologic pattern. Cancer 1963; 16: 549–557

133. Silverberg SG, Hurt WG. Minimal deviation adenocarcinoma ('adenoma malignum') of the cervix: a reappraisal. Am J Obstet Gynecol 1975; 121: 971–975

134. Kaminski PF, Norris AJ. Coexistence of ovarian neoplasms and endocervical adenocarcinoma. Obstet Gynecol 1984; 64: 553–556

135. Daya D, Young RH. Florid deep glands of the uterine cervix. Anatomic Pathol 1995; 103: 614–617

136. Kaku T, Enjoji M. Extremely well differentiated adenocarcinoma ('adenoma malignum') of the cervix. Int J Gynecol Pathol 1983; 2: 28–41

137. Clement PB, Young RH. Deep nabothian cysts of the uterine cervix. Int J Gynecol Pathol 1989; 8: 340–348

138. Gilks CB, Young RH, Clement PB, Hart WR, Scully RE. Benign endocervical adenomyomas and adenoma malignum. Mod Pathol 1996; 9: 220–224

139. Rahilly MA, Williams AR, al-Nafussi A. Minimal deviation endometrioid adenocarcinoma of the cervix: a clinicopathological and immunohistochemical study of two cases. Histopathology 1992; 20: 351–354

140. Young RH, Scully RE. Minimal deviation endometrioid adenocarcinoma of the uterine cervix. A report of five cases of a distinctive neoplasm that may be misinterpreted as benign. Am J Surg Pathol 1993; 17: 660–665

141. Michael H, Grawe L, Kraus FT. Minimal deviation endocervical adenocarcinoma: clinical and histologic features, immunohistochemical staining for carcinoembryonic antigen and differentiation from confusing benign lesion. Int J Gynecol Pathol 1984; 3: 261–276

142. Ishii K, Hidaka E, Katsuyama T, Ota H, Shiozawa T, Tsuchiya S. Ultrastructural features of adenoma malignum of the uterine cervix: demonstration of gastric phenotype. Ultrastruct Pathol 1999; 23: 375–381

143. Utsugi K, Hirai Y, Takeshima N, Akiyama F, Sakurai S, Hasumi K. Utility of the monoclonal antibody HIK 1083 in the diagnosis of adenoma malignum of the uterine cervix. Gynecol Oncol 1999; 75: 345–348

144. Ferry JA. Adenoid basal carcinoma of the uterine cervix. Int J Gynae Pathol 1997; 16: 299–300

145. Bulmer JN, Griffin NR, Bates C, Kingston RE, Wells M. Minimal deviation adenocarcinoma (adenoma malignum) of the endocervix: a histochemical and immunohistochemical study of two cases. Gynecol Oncol 1990; 36: 139–146

146. Hayashi I, Tsuda H, Shimoda T. Reappraisal of orthodox histochemistry for the diagnosis of minimal deviation adenocarcinoma of the cervix. Am J Surg Pathol 2000; 24: 559–562

147. Mikami Y, Hata S, Melamed J, Fujiwara K, Manabe T. Lobular endocervical glandular hyperplasia is a metaplastic process with a pyloric gland phenotype. Histopathology 2001; 39: 364–372

148. Schneider V. Arias–Stella reaction of the endocervix: frequency and location. Acta Cytol 1981; 25: 224–228

149. Cove H. The Arias–Stella reaction occurring in the endocervix in pregnancy: recognition and comparison with an adenocarcinoma of the endocervix. Am J Surg Pathol 1979; 3: 567–568

150. Jones MA, Young RH. Atypical oxyphilic metaplasia of the endocervical epithelium: a report of six cases. Int J Gynecol Pathol 1997; 16: 99–102

151. Clement PB, Young RH. Florid cystic endosalpingiosis with tumor-like manifestations: a report of four cases including the first reported cases of transmural endosalpingiosis of the uterus. Am J Surg Pathol 1999; 23: 166–175

152. Young RH, Clement PB. Pseudoneoplastic glandular lesions of the uterine cervix. Semin Diagnos Pathol 1991; 8: 234–249

153. Lesack D, Wahab I, Gilks CB. Radiation-induced atypia of endocervical epithelium: a histological immunohistochemical and cytometric study. Int J Gynecol Pathol 1996; 15: 242–247

154. Ostor AG, Rome R, Quinn M. Microinvasive adenocarcinoma of the cervix: a clinicopathological study of 77 women. Obstet Gynecol 1997; 89: 88–93

155. Burghardt E. Microinvasive carcinoma in gynaecological pathology. Clin Obstet Gynaecol 1984; 11: 239–257

156. Ostor AG. Early invasive adenocarcinoma of the uterine cervix. Int J Gynecol Pathol 2000; 19: 29–38

157. Fu YS, Berek JS, Hilborne LH. Diagnostic problems of *in situ* and invasive adenocarcinoma of the uterine cervix. Appl Pathol 1987; 5: 47–55

158. Yavner DL, Dwyer IM, Hancock WW, Ehrmann RL. Basement membrane of cervical adenocarcinoma: an immunoperoxidase study of laminin and type IV collagen. Obstet Gynecol 1990; 76: 1014–1019

159. Toki N, Kaku T, Tsukamoto N *et al*. Distribution of basement membrane antigens in the uterine cervical adenocarcinomas: an immunohistochemical study. Gynecol Oncol 1990; 38: 17–21

160. Vogel HP, Mendelsohn G. Laminin immunostaining in hyperplastic, dysplastic and neoplastic lesions of the endometrium and uterine cervix. Obstet Gynecol 1987; 69: 794–799

161. Rollason TP, Cullimore J, Bradgate MG. A suggested columnar cell morphological equivalent of squamous carcinoma *in-situ* with early stromal invasion. Int J Gynecol Pathol 1989; 8: 230–236

162. Luesley DM, Jordan JA, Woodman CBJ, Watson N, Williams DR, Waddell C. A retrospective review of adenocarcinoma *in situ* and glandular atypia of the uterine cervix. Br J Obstet Gynaecol 1987; 94: 699–703

163. Hopkins MP, Roberts JA, Schmidt RW. Cervical adenocarcinoma *in-situ*. Obstet Gynecol 1988; 71: 842–844

164. Schorge JO, Lee KR, Flynn CE, Goodman AK, Sheets EE. Stage 1Ai cervical adenocarcinoma: definition and treatment. Obstet Gynecol 1999; 93: 219–222

165. Im DD, Duska LR, Rosenshein NB. Adequacy of conization margins in adenocarcinoma in situ of the cervix as a predictor of residual disease. Gynecol Oncol 1995; 59: 179–182

166. Wolf JK, Levenback C, Malpica A, Morris M, Burke T, Mitchell MF. Adenocarcinoma *in situ* of the cervix: significance of cone biopsy margins. Obstet Gynecol 1996; 88: 82–86

167. Deheny TR, Gregori CA, Breen JL. Endocervical curettage, cone margins and residual adenocarcinoma *in situ* of the cervix. Obstet Gynecol 1997; 90: 1–6

168. Cullimore JE, Luesley DM, Rollason TP, Waddell C, Williams DR. A case of glandular intraepithelial neoplasia involving the cervix and vagina. Gynecol Oncol 1989; 34: 249–252

169. Krivak TC, Retherford B, Voskuil S, Rose GS, Alagoz T. Recurrent invasive adenocarcinoma after hysterectomy for cervical adenocarcinoma *in situ*. Gynecol Oncol 2000; 77: 334–335

170. Weisbrot IM, Stabinsky C, Davis AM. Adenocarcinoma *in situ*. Cancer 1972; 29: 1179–1187

171. Nicklin JL, Wright RG, Bell JR, Samaratunga H, Cox NC, Ward BG. A clinicopathological study of adenocarcinoma *in situ* of the cervix. The influence of cervical HPV infection and other factors, and the role of conservative surgery. Aust NZ J Obstet Gynaecol 1991; 31: 179–183

172. Poynor EA, Barakat RR, Hoskins WJ. Management and follow-up of patients with adenocarcinoma *in situ* of the uterine cervix. Gynecol Oncol 1995; 57: 158–164

173. Hitchcock A, McDowell K, Johnson J, Johnson IR. A retrospective study into the occurrence of cervical glandular intraepithelial neoplasia (CGIN) in cone biopsy specimens resected in 1977 and 1978 with clinical follow-up. J Pathol 1990; 161: 350a

174. Goldstein NS, Mani A. The status and distance of cone biopsy excision margins as a predictor of excision adequacy for endocervical adenocarcinoma *in situ*. Am J Clin Pathol 1998; 109: 727–732

175. Tambouret R, Bell DA, Young RH. Microcystic endocervical adenocarcinomas. Am J Surg Pathol 2000; 24: 369–374

176. Jaworski RC, Jones A. DNA ploidy in adenocarcinoma *in situ* of the uterine cervix. J Clin Pathol 1990; 43: 435–436

7

Secondary neoplasms of the urinary tract and male genital tract: a differential diagnostic consideration

A.W. Bates S.I. Baithun

INTRODUCTION

When the prevalence of secondary neoplasia of the genito-urinary tract was first estimated by means of autopsy-based studies in the 1950s and 1960s, it was found to be greater than expected – up to one-third of all tumours were secondary.[1,2] The present rise in the numbers of endoscopic and percutaneous biopsies (and the decline in autopsies) places greater importance on histological identification of secondary neoplasms in smaller samples: secondary bladder tumours, for example, are biopsied about as frequently as all non-transitional-cell bladder tumours combined. Retrospective studies of secondary neoplasia in biopsy and autopsy material and reports of rare types of primary neoplasms have provided fresh information on potential pitfalls in the diagnosis of genito-urinary neoplasia. This review concentrates upon practical approaches to secondary neoplasms of the genito-urinary tract encountered by the surgical pathologist, including the role of immunohistochemistry and other special techniques in their differential diagnosis.

SECONDARY NEOPLASMS OF THE URINARY BLADDER

INCIDENCE

Secondary tumours of the bladder (or any other site) can be classified into three groups: those that reach there by direct spread, metastatic solid tumours and leukaemias/lymphomas.[3] This article is concerned with solid tumours only;

Alan W. Bates PhD, Consultant Histopathologist and Honorary Clinical Senior Lecturer in Pathology, The Royal London Hospital, London, UK

Suhaill I. Baithun MB ChB FRCPath, Senior Lecturer in Pathology and Honorary Consultant Pathologist, The Royal London Hospital, London, UK

the reader is referred to other sources for information on the differential diagnosis of genito-urinary lymphoma.[4-6] The earliest systematic reviews of secondary bladder tumours, based on autopsy material, are those of Melicow[7] and Ganem and Batal.[3] Later series include those of Goldstein[8] and Roberts.[9] Sheehan et al.[2] found that 33% of bladder tumours in a series of 5200 male autopsies were secondary in origin. This is a substantially higher proportion than that found in surgical material, a trend also seen at other genito-urinary sites. This difference is due to a variety of reasons: there is a tendency to record unusual post-mortem findings, the diagnosis of secondary tumour is more readily made at autopsy than in a small biopsy, and lesions involving the outer wall of the bladder may not be amenable to biopsy diagnosis.[10] In surgical specimens, secondary neoplasms account for some 2–14% of all malignant neoplasms of the bladder[11] and a recent retrospective study found that only 2.3% of all malignant tumours in biopsy and cystectomy specimens were demonstrably secondary, compared with 20% at autopsy.[10]

The most common primary sites of secondary bladder tumours have been consistently shown to be the colorectum, prostate, cervix, lung, breast, stomach and skin (malignant melanoma) (Table 7.1).[8,10] The predominance of colorectal, prostate and cervical primaries is due to direct spread from these sites. Stomach, skin, lung and breast are the commonest primary sites of origin of metastatic tumour.[10] The bladder is not a favoured site for metastatic disease. Although patients with metastases in the bladder almost invariably have carcinomatosis, patients with carcinomatosis seldom have bladder metastases.[10] No bladder metastases were found in an autopsy series of 585 patients with disseminated carcinoma of the breast[12,13] and there was only one bladder metastasis from 67 disseminated gastric carcinomas.[14] An exception is malignant melanoma, as some 14–18% of patients with melanomatosis have macroscopically demonstrable involvement of the bladder.[15,16] Sufficient pigment may be released to darken the urine.[17] Rare cases of tumours initially presenting as metastases to the bladder do occur: for example, gastric carcinoma,[18] breast carcinoma[19] and malignant melanoma.[20]

Table 7.1 Relative incidence of secondary tumours of the bladder by primary site[10]

Primary site/type	Number of cases	%
Colorectum	93	33
Prostate	54	20
Cervix	32	12
Ovary	17	6
Uterus	13	5
Stomach	12	4
Skin (melanoma)	11	4
Lung	8	3
Breast	7	2.5
Pancreas, kidney	3 each	1 each
Ewing's/PNET, mesothelioma	2 each	0.7 each
Bone (osteosarcoma), vulva	1 each	<1 each
Undetermined	19	7
Total	278	100

GROSS FINDINGS

Cystoscopically, secondary tumours of the bladder can be indistinguishable from primary lesions. Secondary tumour deposits, in contrast to transitional cell carcinoma or primary adenocarcinoma,[21–23] are almost always solitary (96.7%), and more than half are located in the bladder neck or trigone.[10] The site of involvement by direct spread depends upon primary site: prostatic tumours invade the neck and trigone, whereas colorectal neoplasms tend to involve the fundus.[10] Urachal adenocarcinomas at the fundus must be distinguished from invasive colonic adenocarcinomas, as the former are amenable to treatment by cystectomy.[22]

HISTOLOGY

Before the histological subtypes are considered in more detail, an important general point for the diagnosis of bladder cancer is that areas of adenocarcinoma, squamous cell carcinoma and clear cell carcinoma may be present within transitional cell carcinoma, of which they were once regarded as variants.[7] Therefore, any area of transitional cell differentiation within a bladder tumour suggests a primary origin. Extensive vascular invasion is, of course, always suggestive of secondary tumour[24] but is seldom seen in surgical biopsy specimens. The histological diversity of primary bladder tumours (Table 7.2) means that even lesions with unusual histological appearances cannot be assumed to be metastases.[10]

ADENOCARCINOMA

Adenocarcinomas present by far the greatest differential diagnostic problem in the bladder. In a review of 215 secondary bladder neoplasms, 117 were adenocarcinomas, 29 squamous cell carcinomas, three clear cell carcinomas, two adenosquamous carcinomas, two sarcomatoid carcinomas, one choriocarcinoma and one small cell (oat cell) carcinoma.[10] Primary adenocarcinomas of the bladder account for some 0.5–2% of all bladder carcinomas,[25] and, therefore, have a similar incidence to secondary adenocarcinomas.

In a recent large series, one-third of primary adenocarcinomas of the bladder were found to be urachal in origin.[26] Urachal adenocarcinoma arises directly from remnants of glandular urachal epithelium that persist near the fundus. Although squamous or even transitional cell carcinomas can arise in urachal remnants, the vast majority of urachal malignancies are adenocarcinomas of

Table 7.2 Unusual primary tumours of the bladder

Leiomyosarcoma[108]
Osteosarcoma[109,110]
PNET[111,112]
Choriocarcinoma[113,114]
Giant cell carcinoma[115]
Lymphoepithelioma-like carcinoma[116,117]
Yolk sac tumour[118]

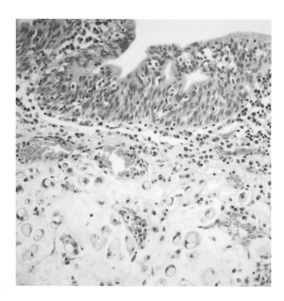

Fig. 7.1 Bladder mucosa diffusely infiltrated by signet-ring cells metastatic from a gastric adenocarcinoma. The overlying urothelium is not dysplastic.

intestinal type. As urachal remnants are in many cases situated within the bladder wall, urachal malignancy does not necessarily involve the bladder mucosa,[27] thus increasing its resemblance to secondary neoplasia. Furthermore, urachal carcinoma arises at the bladder dome, the site most prone to invasion by adenocarcinomas of the large bowel.[10]

Non-urachal primary adenocarcinomas of the bladder show a variety of histological subtypes, including mucinous, enteric, signet ring and mixed forms.[26] Histological subtype is, therefore, not useful for distinguishing primary from secondary adenocarcinoma of the bladder.[11] Signet-ring cells are found in as many as 20% of primary urachal and a third of primary non-urachal carcinomas (some of which infiltrate diffusely, so there is no macroscopically identifiable lesion) as well as in metastatic disease (Fig. 7.1).[26]

The non-neoplastic lesions of endometriosis, endocervicosis and endosalpingiosis (collectively known as 'Mullerianosis') involve the bladder in about 1% of cases,[28–32] and although the presence of a stromal component serves to distinguish them from glandular neoplasia, they can cause diagnostic confusion and should be carefully examined as adenocarcinoma occasionally arises in an endometrial focus.[33]

SQUAMOUS CELL CARCINOMA

The most commonly encountered secondary squamous cell carcinoma of the bladder is direct spread of cervical carcinoma. This typically involves the trigone and may explain the excess of primary squamous cell carcinomas once thought to arise in this region.[11] Cervical cancers that have reached this stage tend to be unresectable.[34] Primary squamous cell carcinoma accounts for some 5–7% of primary carcinomas of the bladder in the Western world,[25,35] though this proportion is much higher in areas where schistosomiasis is endemic.[36] Squamous metaplasia is a common incidental finding,[37] but is sometimes pre-neoplastic having been associated with a p16/p19 deletion also found in squamous cell carcinoma.[38] The presence of metaplastic squamous epithelium as well as squamous cell carcinoma in a specimen supports a primary origin.[39] In biopsies showing squamous cell carcinoma alone, primary and secondary lesions are histologically indistinguishable.

CLEAR CELL CARCINOMA

Many carcinomas can show clear cell change: there is a clear cell variant of transitional cell carcinoma[40] and of adenocarcinoma of the bladder.[41] Clear cell carcinoma arising in endometriosis of the bladder has been reported,[42] and another example arose in a Müllerian duct cyst.[43] Despite the numerous lesions in which it can arise, there are less than 50 cases of primary clear cell carcinoma of the bladder in the English literature (mesonephric and mesonephroid adeno-carcinoma are synonymous with clear cell carcinoma).[11] Another rare entity, nephrogenic adenoma (thought by some to be non-neoplastic and, therefore, also called nephroid/nephrogenic metaplasia) enters the differential diagnosis. This lesion has a papillary architecture and a low-mitotic count (<1/10 high-power fields), which help to distinguish it from carcinoma.[44,45] A single case of clear cell carcinoma arising in nephroid/nephrogenic metaplasia is recorded.[46]

It is important to distinguish these clear cell lesions from metastatic renal cell carcinomas. These are also relatively rare in the bladder, with some 30 case reports in the world literature,[47] only one of which was initially diagnosed from the bladder metastasis. Fortunately, metastatic renal cell carcinoma often retains its branching vascular pattern, which along with the likely history of a primary renal tumour should reveal the correct diagnosis.[47] Despite the propensity of renal cell carcinoma to metastasise early, so that some 20–30% of patients have metastases at the time of diagnosis, the bladder is not a favoured recipient and it seems likely that the few metastases that do occur travel by conventional lymphatic and vascular routes, rather than floating downstream along the urinary tract, as is sometimes suggested.[10,48]

SMALL CELL CARCINOMA

Sheehan et al.[2] described three cases of 'reserve cell carcinoma' metastatic to the bladder to which one more has since been added.[10] Surprisingly, these appear to be the only documented cases, perhaps because some older series do not describe the histological subtypes of metastatic tumours. Under-representation of secondary small cell carcinomas may also be due to misinterpretation of these lesions as primary. It is not clear, for example, what steps were taken to exclude metastases from the 18 cases of primary small cell carcinoma of the bladder described by Blomjous et al.[49] The finding of concurrent transitional cell carci-noma is a strong evidence that a small cell carcinoma is of primary origin.[50] Whether primary or secondary, the prognosis is grave; the median survival of patients with primary tumours is only 5 months.

MALIGNANT MELANOMA

The differential diagnosis between primary malignant melanoma of the bladder and metastatic disease from a distant primary (which may subsequently have regressed) has been facilitated by the clear criteria laid down by Stein and Kendall.[51] Melanomas are regarded as secondary unless all of the criteria are met:

- There is no history of a melanomatous lesion elsewhere.
- No cutaneous lesion (including depigmentation) is found after careful examination of the whole skin surface.
- The pattern of spread, if it occurs, is consistent with a bladder primary.
- The margin of the lesion contains atypical melanocytes.

A review in 1998 found only seven cases (including Stein and Kendall's original three) in which these criteria were fulfilled.[11] The stringency of the criteria is intended to identify cases that might benefit from radical surgery, though we are not aware of long-term survival in any case.

IMMUNOHISTOCHEMISTRY

In a proportion of biopsies of bladder malignancies, the pathologist will be unable to distinguish primary from secondary tumour histologically. In our experience (Table 7.1), adenocarcinoma causes most difficulty in this respect. Histochemical stains for mucins are not useful in distinguishing primary from secondary adenocarcinoma as the pattern of mucin expression is similar in both.[52] This is to be expected as glandular metaplasia in the mammalian bladder yields epithelium of 'true' colonic type.[53] Immunohistochemical staining patterns of primary and secondary adenocarcinomas are also similar. Carcino-embryonic antigen (CEA) may have some discriminatory value if negative, as a proportion of primary non-urachal adenocarcinomas do not express CEA, whereas colonic adenocarcinomas almost invariably do.[54] However, most primary vesical adenocarcinomas are CEA positive.[10]

Another common differential diagnosis is between primary vesical tumours and prostatic adenocarcinoma. Prostate-specific antigen (PSA) and prostatic acid phosphatase (PAP) immunostaining is usually but not invariably positive in prostatic adenocarcinomas. Poorly differentiated transitional cell carcinoma can also be distinguished from prostate cancer by expression of cytokeratins 7 and 20.[55] Endometrial adenocarcinomas can mimic a bladder primary but can be differentiated in more than 90% of cases by their vimentin positivity.[54]

Thyroid transcription factor-1 (TTF-1) immunostaining, normally positive in small cell lung carcinoma, has been suggested as a means of differentiating small cell lung carcinomas from other small cell carcinomas, but it does not appear to have discriminatory value in the bladder.[56,57]

SECONDARY NEOPLASMS OF THE PROSTATE

INCIDENCE

Secondary neoplasms of the prostate are usually incidental findings at autopsy: in one series 5.6% of patients who had died from neoplasia showed evidence of metastatic spread to the prostate at autopsy.[58] Secondary prostatic neoplasia is less often reported in surgical specimens, and very rarely presents clinically. In a series of over 30,000 patients undergoing treatment for malignant disease, a clinical diagnosis of prostatic secondaries was made in only three (0.01%).[59] Nevertheless, secondary neoplasms account for a similar proportion of malignant neoplasms in surgical material from the prostate (2.1%), as they do at other genito-urinary sites.[60] Zein et al.[58] reported 185 cases of secondary neoplasms of the prostate from 6000 autopsies over 25 years, all but 58 of which were leukaemias or lymphomas. Johnson et al.[59] described 18 new cases of solid tumours metastatic to the prostate and a further 25 cases from the literature. Involvement of the prostate by metastatic disease is a late occurrence: patients almost invariably have carcinomatosis[58] and symptomatic secondary prostatic tumours carry a very poor prognosis.[61]

GROSS FINDINGS

Most secondary tumours reach the prostate by direct spread, either from the bladder or rectum. Metastatic deposits can be solitary or multiple. Presenting symptoms include prostatism and haematuria.[62] The distinction between primary and secondary transitional cell carcinomas can be difficult to make as it may depend on differentiating between contiguous and non-contiguous involvement, the latter perhaps the result of 'field change'.[63] The distinction is not merely semantic: contiguous pT4a bladder cancers with prostatic invasion have a worse prognosis than if a separate primary is present in the prostate.[64]

HISTOLOGY

Transitional cell carcinoma of the prostate is the commonest histological type of secondary tumour (Table 7.3). Transitional cell carcinoma should be considered as secondary if there is prostatic invasion and a documented primary tumour arising in the bladder. Invasive transitional cell carcinoma in the presence of dysplastic urothelium in situ within prostatic ducts without evidence of a bladder lesion favours a prostatic primary. If detailed 'mapping' of the prostate is performed in cases of primary bladder cancer, 'Pagetoid' spread of tumour along prostatic duct urothelium is quite a frequent finding (9 out of 20 in one series)[65] and it is difficult to distinguish primary from secondary transitional cell carcinoma of the prostate on biopsy alone. Fortunately, the presence of stromal invasion, rather than the site of origin of the lesion, is the most important factor in determining the prognosis.[66] Oliai et al.[67] have reviewed the histology

Table 7.3 Relative incidence of secondary tumours of the prostate gland by primary site[62]

Primary site	Number of cases	%
Bladder	30	59
Lung	8	16
Rectum	6	12
Pancreas	2	4
Skin (malignant melanoma), breast, eye (malignant melanoma), adrenal cortex, gallbladder	1 each	2 each
Total	51	100

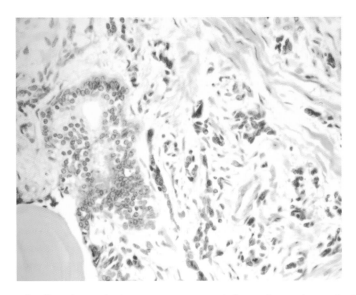

Fig. 7.2 Small cell carcinoma in the prostate metastatic from a lung primary. An 'Indian file' pattern of infiltration is apparent.

of transitional cell carcinoma of the prostate, primary and secondary, and they emphasise the importance of aggressive treatment.

Most metastatic solid tumours to the prostate do not resemble primary prostatic neoplasms histologically. An exception is small cell carcinoma (the commonest histological type of metastasis, Fig. 7.2), which may show no morphological difference with primary small cell carcinoma and which has been reported in a patient as young as 23 years.[68] The rare (0.5–2% of all prostatic carcinomas) primary small cell carcinoma is one of the most aggressive prostatic tumours, believed to derive from a putative stem cell.[69] The presence of areas of histologically typical prostatic adenocarcinoma suggests a primary origin but such areas may not be included in a small sample. Rare histological subtypes of primary prostatic adenocarcinoma, for example, mucinous, signet-ring cell and ductal endometrioid types, can mimic adenocarcinoma metastatic from other sites.

Metastatic solid tumours reach the prostate principally by intravascular spread, and intravascular tumour is a frequent finding in secondary tumours of the prostate.[62] Surprisingly, considering the prevalence of prostatic adenocarcinoma in older age groups, there are only two reported cases of prostatic adenocarcinoma as the recipient of tumour-to-tumour metastasis.[70]

IMMUNOHISTOCHEMISTRY

Primary prostatic adenocarcinomas generally show PSA and PAP positivity that distinguishes them from metastatic disease, though occasionally primary prostatic adenocarcinomas, often those that are histologically atypical, may prove PSA and PAP negative.[71] Primary small cell carcinoma of the prostate is typically PSA and PAP negative.[69] TTF-1 immunostaining, normally positive in primary lung small cell carcinoma, has been suggested as a means of differentiating small cell lung carcinomas (the commonest primary site of small cell carcinoma metastatic to the prostate) from other small cell carcinomas,[56] though it is unhelpful in separating primary from secondary prostatic small cell carcinomas as TTF-1 is expressed by at least some primary small cell prostatic carcinomas.[57]

SECONDARY NEOPLASMS OF THE KIDNEY

INCIDENCE

The kidney is the fifth most common site of metastatic malignancy following the lungs, liver, bones and adrenals.[72] At autopsy, metastases have been described in as many as 20% of patients who died of malignancies, or 1.8% of all autopsies. Although secondary tumours represent some 30% of all renal tumours at autopsy, they account for only 3% in surgical material and are only rarely a cause of diagnostic difficulties. The most common sites of origin of secondary kidney tumours are the lung (44% – hence the excess of secondary renal carcinoma in males), followed by stomach (9%), breast (6%), colon (5%) and oesophagus (4%). Case reports have described unusual primary tumours metastatic to kidney, including malignant mixed tumour of the parotid gland,[73] osteosarcoma[74] and carcinomas of the nasopharynx, nose, vulva and penis.[60]

GROSS FINDINGS

In a series of 435 secondary solid renal tumours,[60] multiple metastatic deposits were somewhat more common (53%) than solitary metastases (43%), with only 3% of secondary tumours reaching the kidney by direct spread. Most metastases (71%) were found in the cortex and half of these were subcapsular. The remaining 1% were micrometastases detected histologically and did not show macroscopical changes. Symptomatic secondary renal neoplasms usually present with haematuria or loin pain. There is almost invariably carcinomatosis.

HISTOLOGY

The most common histological type of secondary tumour was adenocarcinoma (31%), followed by squamous cell carcinoma (24%), small cell carcinoma (13%) and anaplastic large cell carcinoma (3.9%). Diagnosis is more straightforward than in other genito-urinary sites as most primary renal tumours are renal cell carcinomas, which do not, in our experience, resemble secondary tumours histologically. An exception, as at other sites, is small cell carcinoma. Most of the data on secondary renal tumours are from autopsy series as these tumours are rarely biopsied. In one series, only 16 of 435 secondary tumours were from surgical material (Table 7.4). Cytological examination of FNA specimens has been used to confirm the secondary nature of tumours visualised in the kidney[75] and a transjugular biopsy approach has also been described for sampling hilar tumours.[76]

Micrometastases, microscopical intraglomerular and extracapillary tumour deposits, have been the subject of case reports,[77] but would probably be found quite commonly in carcinomatosis if sufficient glomeruli are examined. In a recent study of kidneys with macroscopic secondary tumour deposits, additional micrometastases were found in 4 out of 42.[78] Several theories have been proposed to explain the presence of intraglomerular metastases: intravascular spread from arterial or venous emboli,[78] mechanical obstruction of circulating tumour cells due to size, selective adhesion to the glomerular basement membrane or even that neoplastic cells are in transit and not truly metastatic.[79] In our experience, the size and cohesion of the tumour cell groups (Fig. 7.3) favours the first of these hypotheses.

Xanthogranulomatous pyelonephritis can mimic carcinoma macroscopically, and it occasionally occurs adjacent to a renal cell carcinoma.[80,81] While this may be fortuitous, it is possible that xanthogranulomatous inflammation develops in response to the tumour as has been suggested in the bladder.[82] We have also encountered an ovarian carcinoma metastatic to the kidney with associated

Table 7.4 Relative incidence of secondary tumours of the kidney by primary site[60]

Primary site	Number of cases	%
Lung	192	44
Stomach	40	9
Breast	29	7
Colon	22	5
Oesophagus	20	5
Pancreas	17	4
Uterus	11	2.5
Unknown	10	2.3
Kidney	8	1.8
Skin	8	1.8
Others	77	18
Total	434	100

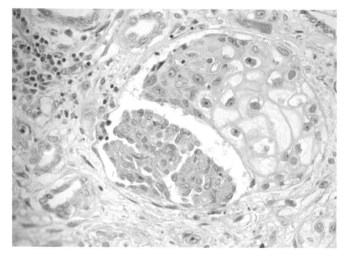

Fig. 7.3 A glomerular micrometastasis of squamous cell carcinoma from a lung primary shows cellular cohesion.

xanthogranulomatous pyelonephritis. Whatever the cause of the association, it emphasises the need for careful examination of inflammatory renal masses.

SECONDARY NEOPLASMS OF THE TESTIS, SPERMATIC CORD AND PENIS

INCIDENCE

The testis is traditionally regarded as an unusual site for secondary tumours, perhaps because of its remote anatomical location. Although the incidence of secondary neoplasms of the testis has been reported as being as low as 0.02% of all autopsies,[83] primary tumours are also comparatively uncommon and in biopsy material secondary neoplasms account for a similar proportion of the total as they do elsewhere in the genito-urinary tract. Almost all secondary testicular tumours are metastases from distant primary sites, of which lung, prostate and gastrointestinal tract are the commonest (Table 7.5).[84–86] The testicular metastasis is said to be the presenting symptom of disseminated malignancy in 6% of cases,[87] though this may be an overestimate due to bias from reports of unusual cases. Most present as a mass in the testis, though sometimes testicular pain is the presenting symptom. Melanospermia may occur due to metastatic melanoma.[88] Metastases to the spermatic cord and epididymis are even less frequent, with some 42 cases, almost all single case reports, in the world literature.[89–91] However, as primary tumours of the epididymis and spermatic cord are also rare, secondary neoplasms account for over 8% of the total at these sites.[90] Metastases to the male genital tract are usually a late event and mean survival after diagnosis is less than 12 months.[90]

Secondary testicular tumours show a bimodal distribution with respect to age of the patient. Most primary testicular germ cell tumours occur in the fourth decade, between these two peaks. In adults, there are clear histological distinctions between most primary and secondary testicular neoplasms, but the predominance of 'small round blue cell' tumours in children means that metastases should be considered in the differential diagnosis of testicular tumours. Relapse of acute lymphoblastic leukaemia is relatively common (around 5% of treated leukaemias[92]) in the testis as this area is spared during irradiation. The clinical

Table 7.5 Relative incidence of secondary tumours of the testis by primary site

Primary site	Number of cases	%
Prostate	25	29
Lung	24	28
Colon	11	13
Stomach	8	9
Kidney and ureter	8	9
Melanoma	3	3.5
Neuroblastoma, rhabdomyosarcoma	2 each	2.3 each
Bladder, salivary gland, medulloblastoma	1 each	1.2 each
Total	86	100

history should indicate the diagnosis. Other secondary testicular tumours of childhood include neuroblastoma, rhabdomyosarcoma and medulloblastoma (post-neurosurgery). In one report, 4% of males with neuroblastoma had testicular metastases.[93]

There have been only two reported series of secondary neoplasms of the penis[94,95] plus many single case reports.[89] For so vascular an organ, the penis is a rare site for secondary tumours, possibly because the penile soft tissue is a poor substrate for tumour growth. Prognosis is uniformly poor regardless of primary site and treatment, except for palliation, is not indicated.

GROSS FINDINGS

There has been some discussion of whether metastases to the testes show a side-specific distribution. In one series, there was a predominance of right-sided metastases (12 on right; 4 on left), though other series have showed no difference. Some metastases presented as solitary nodules and others were multiple; a third group involved the testis diffusely and presented with an enlarged testis without a focal lesion.[95] Bilateral metastases are uncommon, but there are now some 30 cases in the literature. Kay et al.[96] postulated that metastases may reach the testis by retrograde extension through the vas deferens. This mode of spread was favoured by Hanash et al.[83] on the grounds that metastases of prostatic adenocarcinoma to the testis are relatively frequent and that in such cases palpation of the spermatic cord often suggests tumorous involvement. The statement that prostatic adenocarcinoma metastasises to the testis along the vas is often repeated in the literature.[97] Of course, all tumour metastatic to the testis must arrive via the spermatic cord, unless there is a congenital hydrocoele, but to our knowledge no tumour has yet been shown to metastasise along the lumen of the vas and the apparent excess of prostatic secondaries, that the theory seeks to explain, may be accounted for by reporting bias: metastases are routinely sought in therapeutic orchidectomy specimens. Tumour emboli are, however, commonly seen within lymphatic and vascular channels in the vas[98] and we agree with Hunter and Hutcheson[99] that metastases reach the testes predominantly through the vascular system.

HISTOLOGY

In a series of 31 cases, the most common histological type of metastasis to the testis was adenocarcinoma and the next most common were paediatric 'small round blue cell' tumours. In general, secondary tumours of the adult testis do not resemble primary ones histologically, though on occasion misdiagnoses occur, for example of metastatic carcinoma as embryonal carcinoma,[24] of metastatic carcinoid as primary[100] or of renal cell carcinoma as seminoma.[97] Both nodular and diffuse secondary tumours tend to spare the seminiferous tubules (Fig. 7.4). A rare entity that has recently received attention is adenocarcinoma of the rete testis, which can be very difficult to differentiate from metastatic adenocarcinoma histologically.[101,102] Interpretation of paediatric tumours is more difficult owing to the prevalence of the 'small round blue cell' type. Primary neoplasms from which these must be distinguished include desmoplastic small round cell tumour[103] and retinal anlage tumour of the epididymis.[104]

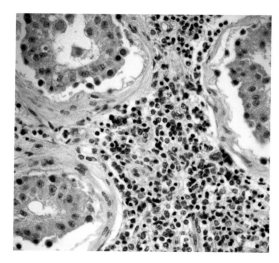

Fig. 7.4 Secondary small cell carcinoma of the testis. Diffuse infiltration with sparing of seminiferous tubules is often seen in metastases to the testis.

Secondary carcinomas of the penis are usually manifestations of end-stage disease, the histology of which is well described by Young *et al.*,[105] who emphasise the need to distinguish pagetoid spread of transitional cell carcinoma of the urinary tract from the rarer Paget's disease of the penis.

IMMUNOHISTOCHEMISTRY

This is usually indicated in paediatric testicular tumours and the possibility of metastases, as well as unusual primary tumours, commends the use of a broad immunohistochemical panel. The reader is referred to recent reviews for details of immunohistochemical and cytogenetic methods in paediatric tumour diagnosis.[106,107] The reader is also referred to Chapter 1, 'The diagnostic challenge of paediatric small round cell tumours'.

CONCLUSION

- Despite wide variations in the overall incidence of secondary tumours at different sites in the genito-urinary tract, the proportion of malignant tumours in surgical material that are of secondary origin remains about the same (1.6–3.0%).
- Direct spread accounts for most secondary neoplasms of the bladder and prostate. Secondary renal and testicular tumours are usually metastatic.
- Metastases usually occur in patients with widely disseminated malignancy and carry a poor prognosis.
- Many secondary neoplasms are histologically distinctive but some, particularly secondary neoplasms of the bladder, and of the testis in childhood, are histologically indistinguishable from primary tumours in biopsy material. Immunohistochemistry, preferably in comparison with the primary lesion, plays only a minor role. A proper clinical history and an appropriate index of suspicion may be the most important factors in suggesting the true diagnosis.

REFERENCES

1. Klinger ME. Secondary tumors of the genito-urinary tract. J Urol 1951; 65: 144–153
2. Sheehan EE, Greenberg SD, Scott R. Metastatic neoplasms of the bladder. J Urol 1963; 90: 281–284
3. Ganem EJ, Batal JT. Secondary malignant tumours of the urinary bladder metastatic from primary foci in distant organs. J Urol 1956; 75: 965–972
4. Isaacson PG, Norton AJ. Extranodal Lymphomas. Edinburgh: Churchill Livingstone, 1994; 285–286
5. Ferry JA, Young RH. Malignant lymphoma of the genitourinary tract. Curr Diagnost Pathol 1997; 4: 145–169
6. Bates AW, Norton AJ, Baithun SI. Malignant lymphoma of the urinary bladder: a clinicopathological study of 11 cases. J Clin Pathol 2000; 53: 458–461
7. Melicow MM. Tumours of the urinary bladder: a clinico-pathological analysis of over 2500 specimens and biopsies. J Urol 1955; 74: 498–521
8. Goldstein AG. Metastatic carcinoma to the bladder. J Urol 1967; 98: 209–215
9. Roberts DI. Secondary neoplasms of the genito-urinary tract. Br J Urol 1978; 50: 68
10. Bates AW, Baithun SI. Secondary neoplasms of the bladder are histological mimics of nontransitional cell primary tumours: clinicopathological and histological features of 282 cases. Histopathology 2000; 36: 32–40
11. Bates AW, Baithun SI. The differential diagnosis of secondary and unusual primary tumours of the bladder. Curr Diagn Pathol 1998; 5: 188–197
12. Saphir O, Parker ML. Metastasis of primary carcinoma of the breast. With special reference to spleen, adrenal glands and ovaries. Arch Surg 1941; 42: 1003–1018
13. Warren S, Witham EM. Studies on tumor metastasis. 2. The distribution of metastases in cancer of the breast. Surg Gynecol Obstet 1933; 57: 81–85
14. Warren S. Studies on tumor metastasis. IV. Metastases of cancer of the stomach. New Engl J Med 1933; 209: 825–827
15. Das Gupta T, Brasfield R. Metastatic melanoma. A clinicopathological study. Cancer 1964; 17: 1323–1339
16. Einhorn LH, Burgess MA, Vallejas C, Bodey Sr GP, Gutterman J, Mavligit G, Hersh EM, Luce JK, Frei 3rd E, Freireich EJ, Gottlieb JA. Prognostic correlations and response to treatment in advanced metastatic malignant melanoma. Cancer Res 1974; 34: 1995–2004
17. Bartone FF. Metastatic melanoma of the bladder. J Urol 1964; 91: 151–155
18. Leddy FF, Peterson NE, Ning TC. Urogenital linitis plastica metastatic from the stomach. Urology 1992; 39: 464–467
19. Silverstein LI, Plaine L, Davis JE, Kabakow B. Breast carcinoma metastatic to bladder. Urology 1987; 29: 544–547
20. Chin JL, Sales JL, Silver MM, Sweeney JP. Melanoma metastatic to the bladder and bowel: an unusual case. J Urol 1982; 127: 541–542
21. Wheeler JD, Hill WT. Adenocarcinoma involving the urinary bladder. Cancer 1954; 7: 119–135
22. Mostofi FK, Thomson RV, Dean AL. Mucous adenocarcinoma of the urinary bladder. Cancer 1955; 8: 741–758
23. Thomas DG, Ward AM, Williams JL. A study of 52 cases of adenocarcinoma of the bladder. Br J Urol 1971; 43: 4–15
24. Haupt HM, Mann RB, Trump DL, Abeloff MD. Metastatic carcinoma involving the testis. Clinical and pathologic distinction from primary testicular neoplasms. Cancer 1984; 10: 592–595
25. Mostofi FK. Pathological aspects and spread of carcinoma of the bladder. J Am Med Assoc 1968; 206: 1764–1769
26. Grignon DG, Ro JY, Ayala AG, Johnson DE, Ordonez NG. Primary adenocarcinoma of the urinary bladder: a clinicopathologic analysis of 72 cases. Cancer 1991; 67: 2165–2172
27. Eble JN. Abnormalities of the urachus. In Young RH (Ed.) Pathology of the Urinary Bladder. New York: Churchill Livingstone, 1989; 213–243
28. Clement PB, Young RH. Endocervicosis of the urinary bladder: a report of six cases of a benign Mullerian lesion that may mimic adenocarcinoma. Am J Surg Pathol 1992; 16: 533–542

29. Seman EI, Stewart CJ. Endocervicosis of the urinary bladder. Aust NZ J Obstet Gyn 1994; 34: 496–497
30. Parivar F, Bolton DM, Stoller ML. Endocervicosis of the bladder. J Urol 1995; 153: 1218–1219
31. Young RH, Clement PB. Mullerianosis of the urinary bladder. Mod Pathol 1996; 9: 731–737
32. Rodriguez R, Alfert H. Endocervicosis of the bladder: a rare mucinous analogue of endometriosis. J Urol 1997; 157: 1355
33. Al-Izzi MS, Horton LWL, Kelleher J, Fawcett D. Malignant transformation in endometriosis of the urinary bladder. Histopathology 1989; 14: 191–198
34. Sakata K, Hareyama M, Yama N, Oouchi A, Shido M, Nagakura H, Morita K, Kudo R. Long survival of patients with unresectable cervical carcinoma after radiotherapy. Jpn J Clin Oncol 1997; 27: 285–287
35. Faysal MH. Squamous cell carcinoma of the bladder. J Urol 1981; 126: 598–599
36. Dimmette RM, Sproat HF, Sayegh ES. The classification of carcinoma of the urinary bladder associated with schistosomiasis and metaplasia. J Urol 1956; 75: 680–686
37. Koss LG. Mapping of the urinary bladder: its impact on the concepts of bladder cancer. Hum Pathol 1979; 10: 533–548
38. Tsutsumi M, Tsai YC, Gonzalgo ML, Nichols PW, Jones PA. Early acquisition of homozygous deletions of p16/p19 during squamous cell carcinogenesis and genetic mosaicism in bladder cancer. Oncogene 1998; 17: 3021–3027
39. Benson RC, Swanson SK, Farrow GM. Relationship of leukoplakia to urothelial malignancy. J Urol 1984; 131: 507–511
40. Braslis KG, Jones A, Murphy D. Clear-cell transitional cell carcinoma. Aust NZ J Surg 1997; 67: 906–908
41. Young RH, Scully RE. Clear cell adenocarcinoma of the bladder and urethra. A report of three cases and review of the literature. Am J Surg Pathol 1985; 9: 816–826
42. Balat O, Kudelka AP, Edwards CL, Silva E, Kavanagh JJ. Malignant transformation in endometriosis of the urinary bladder: case report of clear cell adenocarcinoma. Eur J Gynaecol Oncol 1996; 17: 13–16
43. Novak RN, Raines RB, Sollee AN. Clear cell carcinoma in a Mullerian duct cyst. Am J Clin Pathol 1981; 76: 339–341
44. Bagharan BS, Tiamson EM, Wenk RE, Hamamoto G, Eggleston JC. Nephrogenic adenoma of the urinary bladder and urethra. Hum Pathol 1981; 12: 907–916
45. Alsanjari N, Lynch MJ, Fisher C, Parkinson MC. Vesical clear cell adenocarcinoma v. nephrogenic adenoma: a diagnostic problem. Histopathology 1995; 27: 43–49
46. Sorensen FB, Jacobsen F, Nielsen JB, Mommsen S. Nephroid metaplasia of the urinary tract. A survey of the literature, with the contribution of 5 new immunohistochemically studied cases, including one case examined by electron microscopy. Acta Pathol Microbiol Immunol Scand A 1987; 95: 67–81
47. Bates AW, Baithun SI. Renal cell carcinoma metastatic to the bladder. A report of three cases. J Urol Pathol 1999; 10: 71–76
48. Abeshouse BS. Metastasis to ureters and urinary bladder from renal cell carcinoma; report of 2 cases. J Intern Coll Surg 1956; 25: 117–126
49. Blomjous CEM, Vos W, de Voogt HJ, Van der Valk P, Meijer CJ. Small cell carcinoma of the urinary bladder: a clinicopathologic, morphometric, immunohistochemical, and ultrastructural study of 18 cases. Cancer 1989; 64: 1347–1357
50. Mills SE, Wolfe JT, Weiss MA, Swanson PE, Wick MR, Fowler JE, Young RH. Small cell undifferentiated carcinoma of the urinary bladder. A light-microscopic, immunocytochemical, and ultrastructural study of 12 cases. Am J Surg Pathol 1987; 11: 606–617
51. Stein BS, Kendall AR. Malignant melanoma of the urinary tract. J Urol 1984; 132: 859–868
52. Newbould M, McWilliam LJ. A study of vesical adenocarcinoma, intestinal metaplasia and related lesions using mucin histochemistry. Histopathology 1998; 32: 20–27
53. Okada H, Takehana K, Takahashi K, Matsukawa K. Histochemistry of glandular metaplasia at the trigone of the urinary bladder in cows. J Comp Pathol 1992; 107: 185–194
54. Torenbeek R, Lagendijk JH, Van Diest PJ, Bril H, van der Molengraft FJ, Meijer CJ. Value of a panel of antibodies to identify the primary origin of adenocarcinomas presenting as bladder carcinoma. Histopathology 1998; 32: 20–27

55. Bassily NH, Vallorosi CJ, Akdas G, Montie JE, Rubin MA. Coordinate expression of cytokeratins 7 and 20 in prostate adenocarcinoma and bladder urothelial carcinoma. Am J Clin Pathol 2000; 113: 383–388

56. Ordóñez NG. Value of thyroid transcription factor-1 immunostaining in distinguishing small cell lung carcinomas from other small cell carcinomas. Am J Surg Pathol 2000; 24: 1217–1223

57. Agoff SN, Lamps LW, Philip AT, Amin MB, Schmidt RA, True LD, Folpe AL. Thyroid transcription factor-1 is expressed in extrapulmonary small cell carcinomas but not in other extrapulmonary neuroendocrine tumours. Mod Pathol 2000; 13: 238–242

58. Zein TA, Huben R, Lane W, Pontes JE, Englander LS. Secondary tumours of the prostate. J Urol 1955; 133: 615–616

59. Johnson DE, Chalbaud R, Ayala AG. Secondary tumours of the prostate. J Urol 1974; 112: 507–508

60. Chin Aleong J, Bates AW, Baithun SI. Secondary neoplasms of the kidney: a clinico-pathological review of 443 cases. J Pathol 2000; 190 (suppl.): 42A

61. Bamberger MH, Romas NA. Clinically significant metastatic melanoma to prostate. Urology 1990; 35: 445–447

62. Bates AW, Baithun SI. Secondary solid neoplasms of the prostate: a clinico-pathological series of 51 cases. Virchows Arch 2002; 440: 392–396

63. Ito T, Wada T, Furusato M, Aizawa S. Prostatic involvement of bladder carcinoma. Nippon Hinyokika Gakkai Zasshi 1997; 88: 677–683

64. Pagano F, Bassi P, Ferrante GL, Piazza N, Abatangelo G, Pappagallo GL, Garbeglio A. Is stage pT4a (D1) reliable in assessing transitional cell carcinoma involvement of the prostate in patients with a concurrent bladder cancer? A necessary distinction for contiguous or noncontiguous involvement. J Urol 1996; 155: 244–247

65. Mahadevia PS, Koss LG, Tar IJ. Prostatic involvement in bladder cancer. Prostate mapping in 20 cystoprostatectomy specimens. Cancer 1986; 58: 2096–2102

66. Cheville JC, Dundore PA, Bostwick DG, Lieber MM, Batts KP, Sebo TJ, Farrow GM. Transitional cell carcinoma of the prostate: clinicopathologic study of 50 cases. Cancer 1998; 82: 703–707

67. Oliai BR, Kahane H, Epstein JI. A clinicopathologic analysis of urothelial carcinomas diagnosed on prostate needle biopsy. Am J Surg Pathol 2001; 25: 794–801

68. Madersbacher S, Schatzl G, Susani M, Maier U. Prostatic metastasis of a small cell lung cancer in a young male. Eur Urol 1994; 26: 267–269

69. Helpap B, Köllermann J. Immunohistochemical analysis of the proliferative activity of neuroendocrine tumors from various organs. Are there indications for a neuroendocrine tumor – carcinoma sequence? Virchows Arch 2001; 438: 86–91

70. Grignon DJ, Ro JY, Ayala AG. Malignant melanoma with metastasis to adenocarcinoma of the prostate. Cancer 1989; 63: 196–198

71. Segawa T, Kakehi Y. Primary signet ring cell adenocarcinoma of the prostate: a case report and literature review. Hinyokika Kiyo 1993; 39: 565–568

72. Matsushita Y, Katoh T, Isurugi K, Obara W, Suzuki T, Tamura T, Tanji S, Fujioka T. Metastatic renal tumour originating from oesophageal carcinoma: a case report. Hinyokika Kiyo – Acta Urologica Japonica 1998; 44: 591–594

73. Czader M, Eberhart CG, Bhatti N, Cummings C, Westra WH. Metastasizing mixed tumour of the parotid: initial presentation as a solitary kidney tumour and ultimate carcinomatous transformation at the primary site. Am J Surg Pathol 2000; 24: 1159–1164

74. Ogose A, Morita T, Emura I, Nemoto K, Hirata Y. Osteosarcoma metastatic to the kidneys without lung involvement. Jpn J Clin Oncol 1999; 29: 395–398

75. Parsi B, Beylot J, Turner K, Risch M, Lacoste D, Chomy P, Le Treut A, Grelet P. Diagnostic des tumeurs secondaires bilaterales du rein. Apport de la cytologie. A propos de deux observations. Ann Med Interne (Paris) 1989; 140: 368–371

76. Seifert AL, Pearse HD, Keller FS. Secondary tumors of the kidney: a new diagnostic procedure. J Urol 1979; 122: 542–543

77. Nomura S, Takeda M, Manabe T, Tsukayama C, Tamai H, Ban N, Osawa G, Tsuda T. Case report: intraglomerular metastasis with neoplastic cell interposition. Am J Med Sci 1995; 309: 179–182

78. Sridevi D, Jain D, Vasishta RK, Joshi K. Intraglomerular metastasis: a necropsy study. J Clin Pathol 1999; 52: 307–309

79. Iskandar SS, Jenette JC, Weis LS. Primary cerebral lymphoma with glomerular renal involvement. Arch Pathol Lab Med 1985; 109: 524–528
80. Tolia BM, Newman HR, Fruchtman B, Bekirov H, Freed SZ. Xanthogranulomatous pyelonephritis: segmental or generalized disease? J Urol 1980; 124: 122–124
81. McDonald GS. Xanthogranulomatous pyelonephritis associated with papillary transitional cell carcinoma of the pelvis. J Pathol 1981; 133: 203–213
82. Bates AW, Fegan AW, Baithun SI. Xanthogranulomatous cystitis associated with malignant neoplasms of the bladder. Histopathology 1998; 33: 212–215
83. Hanash KA, Carney JA, Kelalis PP. Metastatic tumours to testicles: routes of metastasis. J Urol 1969; 120: 465–468
84. Price EB, Mostofi FK. Secondary carcinoma of the testis. Cancer 1957; 10: 592–595
85. Pienkos EJ, Jablokow VR. Secondary testicular tumours. Cancer 1972; 30: 481–485
86. Grignon DJ, Shum DT, Hayman WP. Metastatic tumours of the testis. Can J Surg 1986; 29: 359–361
87. Patel SR, Richardson RL, Kvols L. Metastatic cancer to the testis: a report of 20 cases and review of the literature. J Urol 1989; 142: 1003–1005
88. Lowell DM, Lewis EL. Melanospermia: a hitherto undescribed entity. J Urol 1966; 95: 407–411
89. Powell BL, Craig JB, Muss HB. Secondary malignancies of the penis and epididymis: a case report and review of the literature. J Clin Oncol 1985; 3: 110–116
90. Algaba F, Santaularia JM, Villavicencio H. Metastatic tumour of the epididymis and spermatic cord. Eur Urol 1983; 9: 56–59
91. Wachtel TL, Mehan DJ. Metastatic tumours of the epididymis. J Urol 1970; 103: 624–627
92. Gutjahr P, Humpl T. Testicular lymphoblastic leukaemia/lymphoma. World J Urol 1995; 13: 230–232
93. Kushner BH, Vogel R, Hajdu SI, Helson L. Metastatic neuroblastoma and testicular involvement. Cancer 1985; 56: 1730–1732
94. Hayes WT, Young JM. Metastatic carcinoma of the penis. J Chron Dis 1967; 20: 891–895
95. Dutt N, Bates AW, Baithun SI. Secondary neoplasms of the male genital tract with different patterns of involvement in adults and children. Histopathology 2000; 37: 323–331
96. Kay S, Hennigar GR, Hooper JW. Carcinoma of the testis metastatic from carcinoma of the prostate. AMA Arch Pathol 1954; 57: 121–129
97. Ulbright TM, Amin MB, Young RH. Tumors of the Testis, Adnexa, Spermatic Cord, and Scrotum. Bethesda, Armed Forces Institute of Pathology, 1999; 283–284
98. Bhasin SD, Shrikhande SS. Secondary carcinoma of testis – a clinicopathologic study of 10 cases. Ind J Cancer 1990; 27: 83–90
99. Hunter DT, Hutcheson JB. Krukenberg tumor of the testicle, report of a second case. J Urol 1959; 81: 305–308
100. Berdjis CC, Mostofi FK. Carcinoid tumours of the testis. J Urol 1977; 118: 777–782
101. Ballotta MR, Borghi L, Barucchello G. Adenocarcinoma of the rete testis. Report of two cases. Adv Clin Path 2000; 4: 169–173
102. Nochomovitz LE, Orenstein JM. Adenocarcinoma of the rete testis: consolidation and analysis of 31 reported cases with a review of the literature. J Urol Pathol 1994; 2: 1–37
103. Cummings OW, Ulbright TM, Young RH, Del Tos AP, Fletcher CDM, Hull MT. Desmoplastic small round cell tumours of the para-testicular region: a report of six cases. Am J Surg Pathol 1997; 21: 219–225
104. Johnson RE, Scheithauer BW, Dahlin DC. Melanotic neuroectodermal tumor of infancy. A review of seven cases. Cancer 1983; 52: 661–666
105. Young RH, Srigley JR, Amin MB, Ulbright TM, Cubilla AL. Tumors of the Prostate Gland, Seminal Vesicles, Male Urethra, and Penis. Bethesda, Armed Forces Institute of Pathology, 2000
106. Ramani P, Shipley J. Recent advances in the diagnosis, prognosis and classification of childhood solid tumours. Br Med Bull 1996; 52: 724–741
107. Cohn SL. Diagnosis and classification of the small round-cell tumors of childhood. Am J Pathol 1999; 155: 11–15
108. Mills SE, Bova SG, Wick MR, Young RH. Leiomyosarcoma of the urinary bladder. A clinicopathologic and immunohistochemical study of 15 cases. Am J Surg Pathol 1989; 13: 480–489

109. Tzakas K, Ioannidis S, Dimitriadis G, Kotakidou R, Kalinderis A. Primary osteochondrosarcoma of the urinary bladder. Br J Urol 1994; 73: 320–321

110. Ghalayini IF, Bani-Hani IH, Almasri NM. Osteosarcoma of the urinary bladder occurring simultaneously with prostate and bowel carcinomas: report of a case and review of the literature. Arch Pathol Lab Med 2001; 125: 793–795

111. Mentzel T, Flaschka J, Mentzel HJ, Eschholz G, Katenkamp D. Primarer primitiver neuroektodermaler Tumor der Harnblase. Klinisch pathologischer Fallbericht und Differentialdiagnose kleinzelliger Tumoren in dieser Lokalisation. Pathologe 1998; 19: 154–158

112. Desai S. Primary primitive neuroectodermal tumour of the urinary bladder. Histopathology 1998; 32: 477–485

113. Puig Rullan AM, Furio Bacete V, Martin Davila F, Delgado Portela M, Casanueva T, Polanco A, Gijon Rodriguez J. Coriocarcinoma primario de vejiga urinaria. Aportacion de un caso con estudio immunohirtoquimico y ultrastructural. Arch Esp Urol 1993; 46: 415–418

114. Sievert K, Weber EA, Herwig R, Schmid H, Roos S, Eickenberg HU. Pure primary choriocarcinoma of the urinary bladder with long-term survival. Urology 2000; 56: 856

115. Komatsu H, Kinoshita K, Mikata N, Honma Y. Spindle and giant cell carcinoma of the bladder: report of 3 cases. Eur Urol 1985; 11: 141–144

116. Young RH, Eble JN. Lymphoepithelioma-like carcinoma of the urinary bladder. J Urol Pathol 1993; 1: 63–67

117. Amin MB, Ro JY, Lee KM, Ordónez NG, Dinney CP, Gulley ML, Ayala AG. Lymphoepithelioma-like carcinoma of the urinary bladder. Am J Surg Pathol 1994; 18: 466–473

118. Taylor G, Jordan M, Churchill B, Mancer K. Yolk sac tumour of the bladder. J Urol 1983; 129: 591–594

8

Pathology of maternal deaths

G.H. Millward-Sadler

DEFINITIONS

A maternal death in the UK is defined as any death that occurs during pregnancy or within 12 months of parturition. This differs from the international definition, which only includes the first 6 weeks after parturition. For this reason, all maternal deaths occurring later than 6 weeks after parturition are classified as late. The UK definition was revised because of prolonged survival of some patients and the need to review maternal deaths from peripartum mental disease. Maternal deaths are otherwise categorised as follows:

- *Direct*: diseases specifically related to pregnancy.
- *Indirect*: pre-existing disease exacerbated by pregnancy.
- *Coincidental*: deaths not necessarily related to pregnancy.
- *Late*: deaths are also subdivided into the three previous categories.

There are some anomalies and inconsistencies in the use of these definitions. For instance, a puerperal cardiomyopathy is classified with the other cardiac diseases as Indirect and Coincidental suicides are similarly assessed with all suicides due to postnatal depression in the Indirect category.

QUALITY OF THE AUTOPSY

When there has been so much adverse media attention about the autopsy, it is essential that the autopsy is relevant, addresses the clinical issues and carefully excludes unexpected pathology. Achieving these objectives frequently requires histological sampling of several organs. Despite improvements in diagnostic imaging and other techniques, significant clinical discrepancies in approximately 15% of all autopsies can still be identified, indicating that the autopsy is still important in reviewing and confirming clinical diagnoses,[1] and is valuable as an audit and quality control tool. These criteria for the autopsy are even more

G. Harry Millward-Sadler BSc MB ChB FRCPath MHSM, Consultant and Honorary Senior Lecturer, Department of Pathology, Southampton University Hospitals, Southampton, UK

important in maternal deaths. By definition, this group of deaths is occurring in a young population and is usually unexpected. Each has a considerable, devastating impact on the family. Any autopsy in this situation must command a thorough and detailed investigation with careful clinicopathological correlation. A good autopsy should include a review of the circumstances prior to death, should establish the cause of death as well as confirm ancillary diagnoses and identify unexpected pathology, and finally should correlate all these features with the clinical history. This often requires close liaison with clinical staff and every effort should be made to allow them to attend the autopsy itself.

The pathologist also has a significant role in identifying maternal deaths for the Confidential Enquiry, if necessary by notifying the local Director of Public Health (DPH), who has responsibility for initiating the investigation. This is perhaps of greatest value in the group of deaths classified as Indirect and Coincidental – suicides, domestic violence and road traffic accidents. The latest Confidential Enquiry[2] on reviewing maternal suicides found a high incidence of death using violent methods – hangings, jumping from heights, etc. It is difficult to evaluate these fully without knowing the denominator of all suicides occurring in the first year after parturition. Similarly, for road traffic accidents, information on the role of seatbelts in causing injury to the woman in the pregnant state is of value. Frequently, the pathologist is in the prime position to ensure that such information is available.

The autopsy report plays a crucial role for the Confidential Enquiry in the clinical evaluation of maternal deaths, but the quality of the reports is variable and of poor standard in too many instances. Over the years, the Confidential Enquiries have regularly been critical about the quality, consistently commenting on the failure to address the clinical issues and on the failure to perform appropriate histology – or if done, to include the report in the return. For instance, in the Enquiry Report for the years 1979–1981,[3] 172 autopsy reports were analysed: the macroscopic report was considered inadequate in 39 of these and only 87 had satisfactory histology. In the latest Enquiry,[2] analysis of the autopsy report in Direct maternal deaths showed a distinct regional variation (Table 8.1), particularly, in the poor quality of the autopsy report performed for medico-legal purposes in many of the London and Home County areas. Autopsy reports were graded into five categories of excellent, good, adequate, deficient and appalling. From the London and Home Counties area, eight out of the 19 Direct deaths were considered to be appalling reports or to have significant deficiencies. This compared to 10 of 62 Direct maternal deaths in the remainder of the UK.

There, probably, are multifactorial reasons for this difference. However, in the London area, medico-legal deaths and even hospital deaths reported to the Coroner commonly are transferred to a distant public mortuary. Consequently, not only is liaison between clinical staff and the pathologist minimal, but also the pathologist conducting the autopsy may not necessarily be local to the area

Table 8.1 Quality of autopsy reports on Direct maternal deaths – UK 1996–1999[2]

Area	Excellent	Good	Adequate	Deficient	Appalling
London	0	4	7	2	6
Other UK	13	25	14	9	1

or from a nearby hospital. Public mortuaries are not linked to any laboratory service, and consequently, histology of tissues, bacteriological cultures and drug assays are rarely undertaken for non-forensic cases. There have been instances where the autopsy has been delayed for up to 6 days, while awaiting the attendance of the visiting pathologist.

The major reason for the poor quality of the autopsy is simply a failure to observe the criteria laid down by The Royal College of Pathologists.[4] Although there are specific features to be addressed in some maternal deaths, it would be rare for an autopsy performed to the College's criteria to be inadequate. Those recommendations more specific to maternal deaths have been made in the Confidential Enquiries Report (1997–1999)[2] and are reproduced in this chapter (Annex).

DIRECT MATERNAL DEATHS

PULMONARY EMBOLUS

The cause of death from pulmonary embolus is not usually a difficult diagnosis to make at autopsy, but it is surprising, from review of these deaths, how infrequently there is any attempt to provide true clinicopathological correlation. While ultrasound and Doppler studies have shown that the pelvic veins are the most common source of emboli, at autopsy the source of pulmonary emboli is often not sought. Similarly, patients dying with pulmonary embolus frequently have had earlier clinical episodes of breathlessness or chest pain that have been treated as chest infections or dismissed as part of the pregnant state. Only rarely, has there been any attempt at autopsy, either macroscopically or histologically, to confirm the presence or absence of multiple embolic episodes.

Thus, the nature of the emboli should be established: most will be 'standard' histology of laminated thrombus but instances of metastatic choriocarcinoma masquerading as pulmonary thromboembolic disease have been recorded.[5] Recently, a young woman had a lower lobectomy for a pulmonary abscess (clinically attributed to bronchiectasis) that in the resection specimen had complicated a pulmonary artery embolus. Unexpectedly, choriocarcinoma surrounded by laminated thrombus was present on histology (Figs 8.1 and 8.2): blood β-HCG levels were 6,000 i.u. on further investigation (personal observations). Retrospective questioning revealed that she had missed one period approximately 3 months earlier.

As well as identifying the source and nature of the emboli, possible aetiological factors of deep vein thrombosis and embolus should be identified. Morbid obesity (BMI > 30) is strongly associated with increased risk but it is surprising how rarely nutritional status is identified in the pathologist's report. Even if body weight cannot be provided, a simple measure such as thickness of abdominal wall fat could be given. Such factors as family history of deep vein thrombosis should be available in clinical notes but in the last triennial report eight of the 31 embolic deaths occurred in the first trimester and a family history may have to be sought through direct questioning of the Coroner's Officer or General Practitioner (GP). Deep vein thrombosis and pulmonary thromboembolus from the use of antipsychotic drugs have also been recently identified,[6] which again may require specific enquiry.

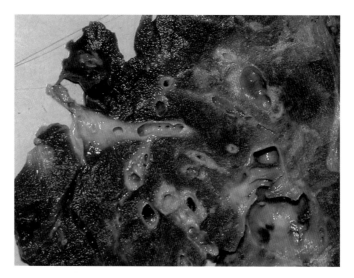

Fig. 8.1 Cut section of lung demonstrating lower right pulmonary abscess. Major pulmonary arteries are patent as can be identified in the centre, but in the lower centre two arteries are occluded by thrombus.

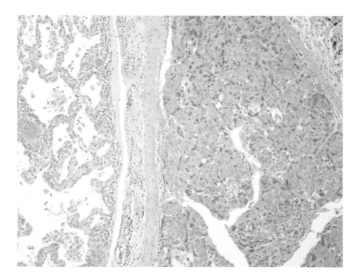

Fig. 8.2 A large tumour embolus fills the pulmonary artery on the right-hand side of the figure. The tumour is composed mostly of the plump cells with prominent nuclei and nucleoli of cytotrophoblast, but small foci of syncytiocytotrophoblast can also be identified (H&E ×20).

PRE-ECLAMPTIC TOXAEMIA

Hypertensive disease in pregnancy is common. Deaths are reducing in number (27 in 1988–1990 and 16 in 1997–1999), but it remains one of the most important causes of maternal deaths. The disease can be fulminant. Four deaths in the last report occurred from sudden clinical deterioration between the decision to

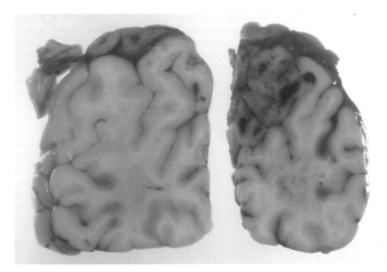

Fig. 8.3 Coronal slice through the occipital lobes of the cerebral cortex shows an area of haemorrhagic infarction in the right lobe. Multiple smaller foci of similar infarction were present elsewhere in the cerebral cortex.

deliver and the actual act of delivery. There is also evidence that fulminating pre-eclampsia can occur in the interval between antenatal appointments and present as sudden death in the community. Deaths have also occurred from eclampsia arising in the immediate post-partum period.

Almost half of the 16 deaths in the period 1996–1999 were due to intracranial haemorrhage (Fig. 8.3), reflecting a failure of effective antihypertensive treatment and five deaths were associated with the HELLP syndrome (haemolysis, elevated liver enzymes, low platelets). It is, therefore, mandatory that evidence of pre-eclamptic toxaemia (PET) at autopsy should be carefully sought, particularly in sudden deaths in the last trimester or in the peripartum period, in cases of cerebral haemorrhage, hepatic rupture or significant liver disease or where there are clinical features of disseminated intravascular coagulation (DIC).

The major pathological features of PET are DIC, which may be present in multiple organs, and the more specific pathology in the placental bed site of the uterus, kidneys and liver. Care must be taken to differentiate the pathological changes of PET in the uterus from the normal physiological adaptation and to differentiate the renal disease of PET from unsuspected pre-existing renal disease.

PLACENTAL BED SITE CHANGES

In normal pregnancy, there are major changes to the spiral arteries in the uterine myometrium and in the decidua underlying the placenta. Within the decidua, trophoblast replaces the endothelium of the spiral arteries and there is fibrinoid necrosis with focal destruction of the arterial wall. In the second trimester, the endovascular trophoblast spreads to involve spiral arteries within the underlying myometrium. This again is associated with fibrinoid disruption of the wall (Fig. 8.4). Basal arteries of the myometrium are not invaded by trophoblast. In pre-existing essential hypertension, myometrial spiral arteries will commonly

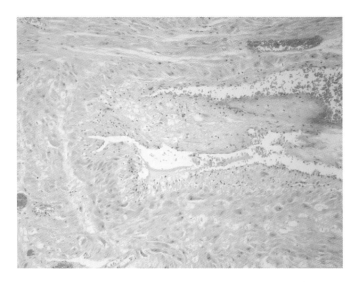

Fig. 8.4 There is marked intimal proliferation in the wall of this superficial uterine vessel and many foamy macrophages and mononuclear cells are present within this zone. In a non-eclamptic uterus, the vessel wall would be infiltrated by trophoblast and shows fibrinoid necrosis without such inflammatory features (H&E ×20).

show arteriolosclerosis: this feature is much more severe than in other organs but the depth and extent of endovascular trophoblastic invasion and fibrinoid disruption of the wall is normal. In contrast, in PET there is failure of the endovascular trophoblast to extend beyond the decidual–myometrial junction. This feature is also associated with foetal growth retardation, where there is no evidence of pre-eclampsia. The fibrinoid necrosis in the wall of the arteries is associated with large numbers of foamy macrophages and mononuclear cells and is usually found in both myometrial and decidual spiral arteries. This infiltrate is considered to be more specific for PET. There is both increased mitotic activity and apoptosis in the endovascular trophoblast in PET and the trophoblast also shows evidence of immaturity, failing to express human placental lactogen.[7]

RENAL CHANGES

In approximately 20% of women with hypertension in pregnancy, there is evidence of pre-existing underlying renal disease and such patients are more likely to have gestational proteinuria or pre-eclampsia prior to 30-week gestation.[8] In PET, the characteristic lesion in the kidney is glomerular endothelial proliferation with reduplication of capillary walls (Fig. 8.5). There are subendothelial fibrinoid deposits and the glomerular capillary lumen is reduced. This activation of glomerular endothelial cells (glomerular capillary endotheliosis) has been associated with the deposition of complement 4D and cofactor C4B-binding protein in the glomerular capillary walls.[10] Mesangial deposition occurs and there are electron dense droplets in glomerular epithelial cells. The subendothelial fibrinoid deposits quickly resolve after parturition, disappearing progressively in the first week after delivery. As these deposits disappear, foam cells become progressively more prominent.[9]

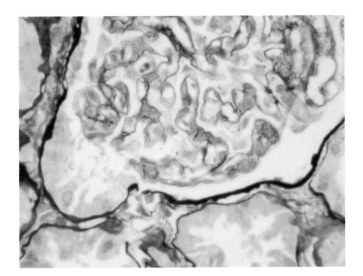

Fig. 8.5 Glomerulus showing the reduplication of the basement membrane, which is sometimes referred to as tramlines. This can be particularly well seen on the lower edge of the glomerular tuft in the centre. Glomerular endothelial cells are also prominent as can be identified from the very large nuclei in this section. Sometimes, this is so florid that the lumen is apparently occluded (Jones ×40, courtesy of Dr Danielle Peat).

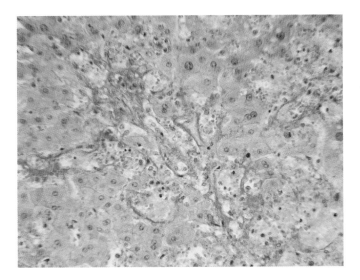

Fig. 8.6 Liver in PET: not only are periportal sinusoids dilated and filled with red cells (yellow), but there are numerous fibrin strands layered along the sinusoidal walls (red). Lesions of this severity can quickly progress to frank periportal necrosis (MSB ×40).

LIVER DISEASE

While periportal sinusoidal ectasia is a common feature in the third trimester of a normal pregnancy, in PET and eclampsia the ectasia is more marked and sometimes there is evident periportal hepatic necrosis. Fibrin is deposited in the dilated sinusoids and can be visualised with trichrome stains (Fig. 8.6).

Sometimes, these lesions lead to haematoma and rupture of a subcapsular haematoma can present as a massive haemoperitoneum. Two deaths from a ruptured liver were recorded in the last triennial report and a third was only just avoided by emergency hepatic resection and massive (>100 units) blood transfusion (personal observation).

In the HELLP syndrome, the liver changes are very similar, but frequently there is also microvesicular fatty change. There seems to be overlap between the liver changes in PET and the acute fatty liver of pregnancy (*vide infra*).

DISSEMINATED INTRAVASCULAR COAGULATION

DIC is a feature of pre-eclampsia (as well as other major obstetric emergencies). Tissues, therefore, should be carefully examined for evidence of microthrombi. Their absence of course does not exclude the condition, as there is also con-comitant fibrinolysis. This extensive DIC has been attributed to alterations in endothelial function.[11] Certainly, endothelial activation is demonstrable in women with pre-eclampsia; these markers precede clinically evident disease and disappear with resolution of the disease. Mechanisms promoting this endothelial activation are poorly understood. Reduced placental perfusion alone is not sufficient to produce the syndrome as foetal growth retardation is not automatically associated with pre-eclampsia and it has been suggested that it is a combination of reduced perfusion with inherent maternal factors.

OBSTETRIC HAEMORRHAGE

Deaths from obstetric haemorrhages can occur due to ante-partum haemorrhage (APH), abruption, placenta praevia or post-partum haemorrhage (PPH).

ABRUPTION

Deaths from placental abruption have fallen dramatically from 44 in the 3-year period 1985–1987 to only three in the last CEMD (Confidential Enquiries into Maternal Deaths in the United Kingdom) report.[2] Of these three deaths, one was associated with amniotic fluid embolus. A second occurred in a woman with pulmonary hypertension and the blood loss precipitated cardiogenic shock from which she could not be resuscitated. In the third case, the woman was admitted to a unit several miles distant from the laboratory and blood bank, so that shock and DIC were not adequately treated for several hours. Thus, death from abruption is usually associated with compounding factors, which may only be revealed during a careful autopsy.

PLACENTA PRAEVIA

There were four deaths from placenta praevia in the last triennial report, which represents no significant change compared with previous reports. Usually, the cause of death is massive haemorrhage with shock and DIC supervening. The massive haemorrhage is usually due to the presence of placenta accreta or occasionally a placenta percreta. In placenta accreta, the placental villi extend directly into the myometrium or cervix; in placenta percreta, chorionic villi penetrate the full thickness of the uterine or cervical wall. It is obviously mandatory in such situations for histology of the placental implantation site to be taken; should hysterectomy have been done prior to death, then the histology of the surgical specimen should be reviewed.

POST-PARTUM HAEMORRHAGE (PPH)

There were six deaths associated with PPH in the last report with two being associated with PET, one with genital tract sepsis and one with vaginal trauma during delivery. In each of these cases, the DIC associated with the primary condition precipitated the PPH. However, PPH can also occur from placenta accreta, when placenta praevia is not present and this condition should be particularly suspected if there is a history of previous uterine surgery. Again, it is mandatory that histology of the placental bed site should be examined for these causes or the resected specimens retrieved and reviewed.

AMNIOTIC FLUID EMBOLISM

There were eight deaths from amniotic fluid embolism (AFE) from 1997 to 1999[2] and this rate, apart from a sudden unexplained increase in the 3 years 1994–1996, has not changed significantly over the years. The majority of women are over the age of 25. The condition, classically, has a precipitous onset during or immediately after labour with cyanosis, shock and fulminating DIC, but the diagnosis has very occasionally been made when these features have appeared prior to the onset of contractions. It has also been described as a complication of termination of pregnancy. In these more dubious circumstances, it is essential that the diagnosis be corroborated by meticulous autopsy examination. As DIC also complicates other obstetric emergencies (such as PET, abruption and PPH), it is also important that AFE is carefully excluded in all cases where DIC is a dominant clinical feature.

The interval between collapse and death can be less than one hour and in the last report only one case survived more than 24 hours. Although the diagnosis has previously been made on pathological criteria, the Confidential Enquiry now accepts the diagnosis on clinical criteria because of the poor quality of the pathology in some suspected cases. Clinical criteria are also used because we have no information on how long foetal squames survive in the pulmonary capillary bed and it is conceivable that modern intensive care can prolong survival to the point at which this evidence may not be demonstrable.

Identification of foetal squames in catheter samples of pulmonary arterial blood have been used to establish the diagnosis but squames have also been found in similar samples of non-maternal blood and have been attributed to unavoidable contamination.[12] Occasionally, the diagnosis can be made ante-mortem from identification of meconium, vernix or lanugo hairs in the pulmonary arteries but after death histological examination of the lungs is essential.

The pathology is well documented. Macroscopically, the lungs can show oedema with intrapulmonary haemorrhages and pleural petechiae but may be almost normal. On histology, all of the components of AFE may be identified in routine hematoxylin and eosin (H&E) sections, particularly in florid cases but in many instances, they may be easily overlooked. While the mucin in meconium can be demonstrated with mucin stains, such as alcian blue, foetal squames are the most commonly identified component (Fig. 8.7). A search for the squames can be simplified using immunocytochemistry (Fig. 8.8). In this respect, the antibody LP34 is superior to CAM 5.2, AE1 or AE3. These three latter antibodies also stain the alveolar epithelial cells.

In all cases of AFE, a careful search for a tear as the source of the embolus should be made. This requires careful examination of the placenta and uterus. The portal of entry may be minute, so that careful examination is mandatory.

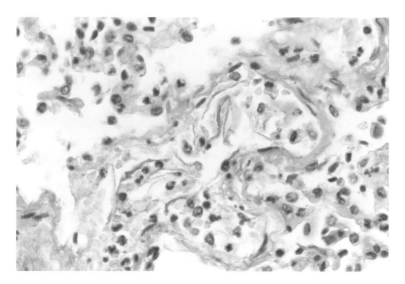

Fig. 8.7 Slender foetal squames (stained red) are present in the lumen of this pulmonary capillary. Differentiation from fibrin can be difficult even at high magnification (MSB ×40).

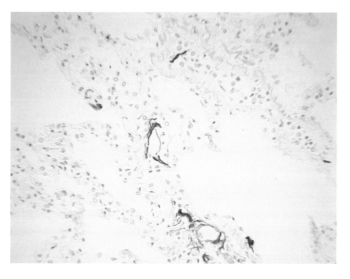

Fig. 8.8 Numerous foetal squames are easily identified even on low power by immunocytochemical techniques (LP 34 × 20).

EARLY PREGNANCY DEATHS

There are three main categories contributing to early pregnancy death. These are ectopic pregnancies, miscarriages and termination of pregnancies. Seventeen deaths from complications of early pregnancy were identified in the triennial report in 1997–1999. Of these, there were 13 deaths from ectopic pregnancy (12 tubal and one cervical, two deaths after miscarriage and two deaths after termination of pregnancy). In five other cases, sepsis causing death complicated a miscarriage.

ECTOPIC PREGNANCY

The death rate from ectopic pregnancy does not seem to have altered despite more accurate means of diagnosis. There were 13 deaths in the period from 1997 to 1999[2] compared with 16 from 1985 to 1987 and 15 from 1988 to 1990. The major problem identified in this last triennium was a failure clinically to suspect ectopic pregnancy: the majority of women who died had treatment directed at symptoms suggestive of gastrointestinal or urinary tract disease. Such women, even when referred for secondary care, usually presented in an Accident and Emergency Department, were treated with antibiotics and were found dead with haemoperitoneum from ruptured ectopic a few hours or days later.

While the majority of ectopic pregnancies are tubal, implantation in the cervix and onto the ovary as well as other organs can occur (Fig. 8.9). It is important in all cases that the amount of blood loss and location of the ectopic pregnancy and if possible an estimation of its gestational age should be made. Any resected tissues referred to the laboratory prior to death should be retrieved and reviewed and the findings incorporated in the autopsy report.

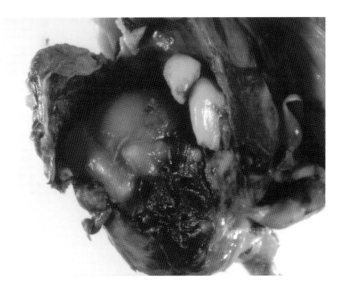

Fig. 8.9 Ectopic pregnancy of ovary. The thorax and foetal limbs including a bent knee can just be identified through the gestational sac in this 16-week gestational pregnancy. The pregnancy and associated haemorrhage has completely destroyed the ovary, but fallopian tube could be separately identified. The uterine fundus is to the right.

MISCARRIAGES

Sepsis is the most common cause of death after miscarriage and will be considered in that section. Some of the other deaths have had to be classified under this heading because of poor autopsy assessment. In the recent CEMD report,[2] we document the history of a known alcoholic with a history of fits following alcohol withdrawal. She had a grand mal seizure the day before a spontaneous abortion. Evacuation of retained products was performed and she was discharged. She was found dead at home the next morning. The autopsy report attributed death to uterine haemorrhage from her miscarriage but there were clear contraindications within the autopsy itself and between the autopsy and the clinical events. The autopsy demonstrated an enlarged heart, heavy oedematous lungs and an enlarged uterus weighing 220 g. The liver was enlarged to twice normal and showed fatty change and there was pancreatic fibrosis. Histology showed early bronchopneumonia in the lungs with fibrosis, ischaemic changes in the heart, severe fatty change in the liver, interstitial nephritis in the kidneys and a congested spleen. No toxicology or microbiology were undertaken. It seems difficult to claim significant blood loss from a uterus weighing only 220 g with a congested spleen and with no identifiable blood loss elsewhere. The fatty liver was proposed to have contributed to death by causing abnormal clotting and electrolyte disturbance; but at the time of evacuation, the patient had normal electrolytes and clotting profile. The possibilities of acute alcohol poisoning or drug overdose were not excluded and the role of the interstitial nephritis and the fibrotic pancreas were not explored.

Some of the deaths from sepsis were associated with medical interventions; others complicated retained intrauterine death. In such deaths, careful search for uterine and bowel perforations and careful microbiological investigations must be performed. One parous patient was admitted at 12-week gestation with a short history of vomiting and abdominal pain after she had been treated for urinary tract infection by her GP. Ultrasound quickly established the intrauterine death and evacuation was done but cardiac arrest occurred at the end of the procedure. Initial successful resuscitation was soon followed by further cardiac arrest. There was evidence of a fulminating streptococcal infection at autopsy.

TERMINATION OF PREGNANCY

The major complications from termination of pregnancy relate to sepsis or to accidental perforation of the uterus and abdominal organs. The termination, though legally performed, may have been concealed from parents or next of kin so that there is no clinical history to direct investigations. It follows that very careful inspection of the uterus and intestines for damage, supported by microbiology and histology, is required, and the evacuated products should be traced and re-examined in detail for myometrium and non-uterine tissues.

OTHER DIRECT CAUSES

SEPSIS

In the last triennial report, there were 14 deaths from genital tract sepsis of which five followed miscarriage. There were six deaths due to streptococcal septicaemia and in five of these there was no clinical evidence that the primary route of infection was through the genital tract. Most frequently, there is a history of sore throat, diarrhoea and vomiting or a 'flu'-like illness. The illness progresses with dramatic speed and such patients from being mildly unwell can be dead within 24–36 hours. For instance, in the last report, a 30-week pregnant woman had a history of sore throat, diarrhoea and vomiting with abdominal pain of a few hours. She collapsed on arrival in hospital and foetal heart rate dropped to 40 beats per minute. A live baby was delivered by emergency caesarean section; there was no evidence of abruption, which was the clinical diagnosis. Septic shock rapidly supervened and despite multiple antibiotics and intensive care, she died the next day. Group A streptococci were cultured from the placenta.

At autopsy, a characteristic feature is the presence of a blotchy lividity and marbling of the skin that becomes quickly evident after death (Fig. 8.10). This is associated with intense haemolytic staining of the intimal surfaces of veins and arteries. In such deaths, an attempt should always be made to identify the portal of entry using microbiological sampling, but frequently the beta haemolytic streptococci are present as a heavy growth from all sampled sites.

ACUTE FATTY LIVER

The aetiology of acute fatty liver of pregnancy is unknown but, recently, cases have been identified with a deficiency of a long chain hydroxyacyl-CoA dehydrogenase (LCHAD) mitochondrial enzyme. This enzyme plays a role in the β-oxidation of fatty acids. A high proportion of mothers, heterozygous for this deficiency and bearing children who also have the trait, develop acute fatty liver.[13] The strong links of acute fatty liver with toxaemia of pregnancy have also suggested that the two entities are related.

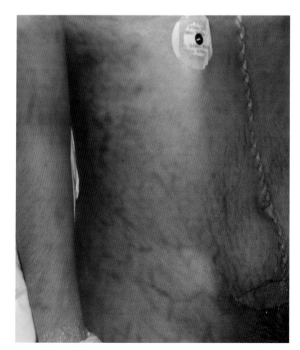

Fig. 8.10 The marbling of the skin by haemolytic staining of the veins and venules is an early and prominent post-mortem feature in streptococcal septicaemia. Post-mortem was conducted less than 6 h after death. Also noticeable is a blotchy erythema with poorly defined margins that after death quickly acquires a purple cyanotic hue.

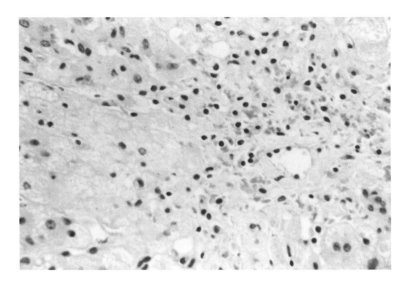

Fig. 8.11 Fatty liver of pregnancy. The hepatocytes have finely vacuolated cytoplasm and pale staining due to the presence of microvesicular fat. Hepatocytes are separated from the hepatic vein (centre right) by mononuclear macrophages and lymphocytes that are within a zone of perivenular necrosis and collapse immediately around the wall (H&E ×40).

Acute fatty liver occurs mostly in primigravida in the third trimester but rare cases have been reported at less than 28 weeks with the earliest being in the 22nd week. The incidence is not accurately known as mild forms of the disease may go undiagnosed but the fulminating clinical presentation occurs in about one in 6000–7000 births. Clinically, as well as the signs and symptoms of mild pre-eclampsia, nausea and vomiting with abdominal pain are commonly present. This can progress very rapidly to jaundice and encephalopathy with oliguria and uraemia. Hypoglycaemia may also be a significant problem. All patients have evidence of DIC and a severe metabolic lactic acidosis can develop.[14]

Macroscopically, the liver is both pale from fatty change and wrinkled from loss of liver cell mass. The liver histologically shows microvesicular fatty change with canalicular and intrahepatic cholestasis. Although liver cell death is not always obvious, considerable cell death can be identified on careful examination of reticulin and diastase PAS stains (Fig. 8.11). Evidence of DIC is seen in other organs and there may be cerebral oedema and acute haemorrhagic pancreatitis.

INDIRECT DEATHS

CARDIOVASCULAR DISEASES

A full spectrum of cardiac pathology is seen in the maternal deaths that have been reported to the Confidential Enquiry ranging from congenital heart disease and ischaemic heart disease to cardiomyopathies and aneurysms.

CONGENITAL HEART DISEASE

Congenital heart disease is a major cause of maternal death: most deaths are related to pulmonary hypertension, either primary or secondary to Eisenmenger's syndrome. In the 6 years from 1994 to 1999, there had been 13 deaths from pulmonary hypertension. These include seven cases of primary pulmonary hypertension and five secondary to Eisenmenger's. In one case, the clinical history identified that the proband's mother had died of possible pulmonary hypertension. Both autopsies were reviewed and death from primary pulmonary hypertension confirmed. A genetic abnormality has been identified in cases of familial pulmonary hypertension[15,16] and was retrospectively identified in these cases using polymerase chain reaction (PCR) on autopsy samples.

Obviously, the differentiation of primary from secondary pulmonary hypertension is by exclusion of other causes: histologically, the pulmonary arterial lesions are identical. The lesion is a necrotising fibrinoid arteriopathy that focally destroys the media. It then resolves with obliterative intimal fibrosis and the formation of a plexus of fine capillary channels. These channels can dilate and mimic a small haemangioma.

The differential diagnosis of either type of pulmonary hypertension is from recurrent pulmonary emboli and requires careful exclusion of sources of emboli as well as histological confirmation of the plexogenic pulmonary arterial changes, which at this stage should be advanced. Secondary thrombotic changes in the arteries can make differentiation of non-embolic pulmonary hypertension from organising thromboemboli very difficult but destruction of the media is rarely found with an organised embolus.

CARDIOMYOPATHIES

There have been 20 maternal deaths from cardiomyopathies between 1994 and 1999 and 11 of these have been categorised as puerperal cardiomyopathy. The differentiation of the puerperal cardiomyopathy from hypertrophic and particularly from congestive cardiomyopathies is difficult and sometimes impossible. The last CEMD report recorded the death of a young multiparous woman, who suddenly collapsed a few days after an uneventful pregnancy and normal full-term vaginal delivery. She died 4 days later after an echocardiogram had demonstrated an enlarged heart consistent with hypertrophic cardiomyopathy. The cardiomegaly was confirmed at autopsy but the characteristic myocardial fibre disarray of hypertrophic cardiomyopathy was not present on histology. Expert cardiac pathological opinion was sought and it was confirmed that the findings were atypical and could not be characterised as puerperal, dilated or hypertrophic cardiomyopathy. A category of pseudohypertrophic cardiomyopathy was suggested because this did not have the same familial implications as hypertrophic cardiomyopathy.

The familial and genetic basis for hypertrophic cardiomyopathies is now well established, and in the past 10 years, genetic abnormalities in some of the dilated cardiomyopathies have also been identified.[17] Accurate diagnosis obviously has implications for counselling of the family.

A puerperal (or peripartum) cardiomyopathy occurs during the last trimester or within 6 months of delivery and most cases are dilated cardiomyopathies. Morphologically, there are no differences from a non-puerperal dilated cardiomyopathy and there is the same spectrum of histological changes. The heart is increased in mass with a dilated left ventricular cavity though the wall is thinned. Histologically, there is interstitial fibrosis with a pericellular pattern. Myocytes show increased nuclear size but there is also loss of cytoplasmic myofibrils that give the cells a moth-eaten appearance. There may be an increase in chronic inflammatory cells in the interstitial tissues, which when prominent is sometimes labelled as a myocarditis.

Despite the similarities, peripartum cardiomyopathy has a worse prognosis compared with dilated cardiomyopathy. This may simply reflect the cardiovascular strain of pregnancy but nonetheless suggests that more work separating and defining these conditions is required.[18] The problems now experienced with organ retention indicate that, in many cases, there will be great difficulty in getting the necessary expert cardiac opinion on the macroscopic appearances. Therefore adequate histological sampling of the chambers of the heart including the interventricular septum is required to establish a diagnosis of cardiomyopathy.

ANEURYSMS

There were 10 deaths from dissecting aortic aneurysms and six deaths from ruptured aneurysms of coronary, splenic or renal/adrenal arteries from 1994 to 1999. When histologically sampled, the aortic aneurysms showed cystic medial necrosis but a fully developed Marfan's syndrome was present in only three patients. The pathogenesis of the other aneurysms is unknown but these particular arteries seem most susceptible to rupture during pregnancy (Fig. 8.12), although any artery is potentially at risk from this rare complication.

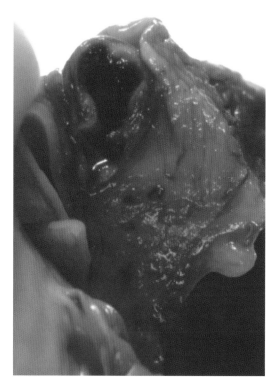

Fig. 8.12 Coronary artery aneurysm. The aorta is to the left. This aneurysm of the left coronary artery arose immediately proximal to its division into anterior descending and circumflex branches and had ruptured giving rise to haemoperitoneum. Myxoid degeneration of the media was evident on histology.

SUICIDE

In the last triennial report,[2] it was identified that psychiatric disorders caused or contributed to 12% of maternal deaths. Twenty-eight of the 42 maternal deaths linked with psychiatric illness were due to suicide. These have been classified as 13 Indirect and 15 Late Indirect deaths. Other studies also suggest that a large number of late deaths associated with psychiatric causes are not included in the CEMD reports. It is likely that, if these were reported, then psychiatric illnesses would be a leading cause of maternal death. It is worth commenting that of the 28 suicides in the last report, 24 were committed by violent methods. Ten died by hanging, five by jumping from height, four from cutting their throats or self stabbing, two from gunshot wounds and one each from self immolation, drowning and an intentional road traffic accident. Only three women died by taking a drug overdose. The Central Assessors wish to investigate this group of deaths in more detail, which will require better ascertainment and sufficient clinical detail. The pathologist is in a prime position to

1. identify such deaths to the Enquiry,
2. provide a detailed comprehensive account of the known circumstances surrounding the death,
3. produce an autopsy report of high quality.

EPILEPSY

The overall effect of pregnancy on epilepsy is unknown. In some instances, epilepsy improves during pregnancy, whereas in others there is increased risk of fitting. Various reasons for the increased risk have been proposed, including haemodilution in the last trimester, failure to adjust drug levels and even non-compliance with drug therapy because of its potential teratogenic effects. Given that deaths have occurred in all three trimesters of pregnancy, it is prob-able that there is no single explanation. In known epilepsy, treatment is controlled by the clinical response to the drug therapy, but it is still valuable at autopsy to have drug levels estimated. In such circumstances, non-compliance with therapy or a rapid change in drug levels can be documented and will significantly contribute to an appropriate analysis of the death.

Unexpected deaths that are attributed to epileptiform seizures have also been recorded in pregnant women with no history of fits for over 2 years and, occasionally, with no history of fits at all. Such diagnoses obviously require a careful and detailed autopsy to exclude other causes of fits, such as eclampsia.

In many instances in these reports, death from epilepsy has been associated with drowning in the bath. Therefore, although the risks are low, the recommendations made in the report are that the woman should only bathe in shallow water or take a shower. This should be undertaken preferably when another adult is in the house.

Therefore, before a maternal death is attributed to epilepsy, careful exclusion of other causes particularly eclampsia should be made. This will usually require histology. Blood for post-mortem levels of anticonvulsant drugs should also be taken.

OTHER INDIRECT DEATHS

In the last report, there were 52 deaths from malignancy and 75 other Indirect deaths: as might be expected, the latter were from many different causes.

MALIGNANCY

Twenty-eight of the deaths from malignancy were classified as Indirect and the remainder as Coincidental. Apart from melanoma, where there is a slight increase, there is no evidence that the frequency of cancer is increased in pregnancy, apart from, of course, placental malignancies, and the range and types of cancer are as expected in an equivalent non-pregnant population. It is often thought that the immunosuppressive effects of pregnancy accelerate the growth and spread of cancer and there are anecdotal examples to support this view. However, the numbers are too small for reliable epidemiological studies. For melanoma[19] and for carcinoma of colon and rectum,[20] the prognosis, stage for stage, seems unaffected by pregnancy.

What is apparent from the Confidential Enquiry Reports is that diagnosis, investigation and/or treatment may have been delayed because of the pregnancy. Most common among these is failure to request imaging investigations because of the theoretical risks to the foetus. For instance, one young patient had severe lower back pain throughout pregnancy with scarring of her legs from repeated hot water bottle burns. Only pain-relieving drugs were given and it was not until she became incontinent and confined to a wheelchair that a magnetic resonance (MR) scan was performed. This revealed an extensive paraspinal tumour and she died a few months after delivery.

CENTRAL NERVOUS SYSTEM DISORDERS

Among the other Indirect causes, almost half the deaths were due to the diseases of the central nervous system, subarachnoid and intracerebral haemorrhages, cerebral thrombosis and epilepsy forming the bulk of these. Obviously, it is important in examples of cerebral haemorrhage to exclude pregnancy-related causes, such as eclampsia.

INFECTIONS

Deaths from a variety of infections including tuberculosis, varicella, influenza, HIV and toxoplasmosis also constitute another large group. There is always the risk that the immunosuppressive effects of pregnancy will enhance the virulence of any infection. A maternal death from acute phlegmonous gastritis was recorded in the last report: only one other such maternal death has been recorded.[21] Regardless of the infection, careful identification/exclusion of a genital tract portal of entry is always necessary.

RESPIRATORY DISEASES

Acute asthma is the most common cause of death among the diseases of the respiratory system. Deaths are not always in severe asthmatics with an acute attack in the last trimester as might be expected: several deaths reviewed in the last two CEMD reports occurred unexpectedly in mild asthmatics though severe mucus plugging was found at autopsy. In some instances, this was associated with stopping steroids because of the potential risk to the foetus and the risks to the mother from this course of action seem to have been underestimated.

Patients with cystic fibrosis are becoming pregnant following improved treatment and maintenance therapy and the adverse effects of the gravid uterus on respiratory function in these patients resulted in two deaths in the last report.

OTHER SYSTEM GROUPS

There are also, as might be expected, deaths in all system groups from metabolic to gastrointestinal and some of these are exotic. One patient developed pancreatitis secondary to hypertriglyceridemia during pregnancy. On further investigation, she was shown to have complete lipoprotein lipase deficiency, a rare autosomal recessive disorder associated with elevated triglyceride levels from birth. Deterioration in pregnancy with pancreatitis is a recognised complication of this condition.

COINCIDENTAL DEATHS

Obviously, any cause of death may occur coincidentally during pregnancy or in the post-partum period and it is impossible to consider all of these in this chapter. It has often been argued that there is no need to report these deaths to the Confidential Enquiry. However, without ascertainment of all deaths occurring within the definitions of maternal mortality, it is impossible to gain information that could reclassify a particular cause as Indirect or even Direct. The importance of assessing all maternal deaths due to suicide has already been alluded to, even when there is no apparent connection: the circumstantial evidence suggests that suicide may be one of the most important causes of an Indirect and even Direct death.

Additional information of social or socioeconomic importance can also be derived. For instance, information about the type of injuries sustained in road traffic accidents can influence the advice to pregnant mothers on wearing and how to wear seatbelts. In addition, 12% of all deaths reviewed in the last CEMD Report had reported or had autopsy evidence of domestic violence. Information about these deaths is now influencing policy.[2]

SUMMARY

Maternal deaths are defined as deaths during pregnancy or within 1 year of delivery. The major categories are Direct, Indirect and Coincidental with further subclassification as Late, if death occurs more than 42 days after delivery.

The causes of death are many and varied and the pathologist has a key role in verifying or establishing the cause of death as well as providing a report that forms the basis of clinical audit.

It is important that autopsy examinations in cases of maternal death are conducted in time and place so that the clinicians involved can attend.

The Royal College Guidelines provide the basis for a high quality autopsy and report.[4] Points more specific to a maternal death are identified in the Annex.

ANNEX

RECOMMENDATIONS FOR PATHOLOGISTS

The following abbreviated guide to the requirements for a maternal death autopsy should be regarded as supplementing, and not replacing, the guidelines issued by the Royal College of Pathologists. If in doubt, advice and help should be sought from the local CEMD Regional Pathology Assessor.

IN GENERAL

Maternal deaths are still under-reported and pathologists performing autopsies on women who are pregnant or are known have been pregnant within a year of their death should contact their local Director of Public Health (DPH) to check the case has been reported.

Clinical information for the enquiry is sometimes incomplete and pathologists should provide review of the clinical history in autopsy reports including height and weight of the woman.

SPECIFIC DISORDERS

Hypertensive diseases
- Check and note existence of local guidelines for the management of hypertensive disorders of pregnancy.
- Identify fluid balance; minimum histology of lungs, liver, kidney, brain, placental site; exclude previous hypertension.

Thromboembolus
- Identify any local risk factors protocol, note family history, tests for thrombophilia, where appropriate, significance of chest symptoms, heparin prophylaxis.
- Describe the nature and distribution of emboli, site of origin, evidence of previous episodes, histology.

Haemorrhage: APH and PPH
- Macroscopic: identify the site and severity of bleeding, location of placenta, detail genital tract trauma.
- Histology: placental histology, search for DIC, exclude AFE, review other tissues resected.

Early pregnancy
- Ectopics: diagnostic awareness, ultrasound monitoring and diagnosis, location and size of ectopic, estimate blood loss, review other tissues resected.
- Abortions: sites and locations of bowel perforations, culture of tissues.

Amniotic fluid embolism
- Macroscopic: detailed examination of genital tract for trauma.
- Histology: detailed histology of both lungs, immunocytochemistry for cytokeratins using LP34 or AE1/2 rather than CAM5.2, if in doubt.
- Women dying after labour of causes other than suspected AFE should have their lungs examined for amniotic squames to check whether amniotic fluid can enter the circulation without a fatal outcome.

Hyperemesis
- Exclude acute Wernicke's encephalopathy.

Epilepsy
- Macroscopic: exclude specific brain pathology, establish anticonvulsant drug levels.
- Histology: exclude eclampsia as cause of fits.

Cardiac deaths
- Macroscopic: full description of heart, weigh/measure ventricles separately.
- Histology: both ventricles, assess conducting system, seek cardiac pathology opinion if in doubt.

Aneurysms
- Macroscopic: nature and site of aneurysm.
- Histology: distribution of arterial pathology.

REFERENCES

1. Sonderegger-Iseli K, Burger S, Muntwyler J, Salomon F. Diagnostic errors in three medical eras: a necropsy study. Lancet 2000; 355: 2027–2031
2. Drife J, Lewis G (Eds). Why Mothers Die 1997–1999. The Confidential Enquiries into Maternal Deaths in the United Kingdom. London: RCOG Press, 2001
3. Report on Confidential Enquiries into Maternal Deaths in England and Wales 1979–81. The Maternal Autopsy – The Role of the Pathologist. London: HMSO, 1986; 111–116
4. Royal College of Pathologists. Guidelines for Post Mortem Reports. London: RCPath, 1993
5. Rubery E, Bourdillon P, Hibbard B (Eds). Report on Confidential Enquiries into Maternal Deaths in the United Kingdom 1991–1993. London: HMSO, 1996
6. Zornberg GL, Jick H. Antipsychotic drug use and risk of first-time idiopathic venous thromboembolism: a case–control study. Lancet 2000; 356: 1219–1223
7. Redline RW, Patterson P. Pre-eclampsia is associated with an excess of proliferative immature intermediate trophoblast. Human Pathol 1995; 26: 594–600
8. Murakami S, Saitoh M, Kubo T, Koyama T, Kobayashi M. Renal disease in women with severe eclampsia or gestational proteinuria. Obstet Gynaecol 2000; 96: 945–949
9. Kincaid Smith P. The renal lesion of pre-eclampsia revisited. Am J Kidney Dis 1991; 17: 144–148
10. Joyama S, Yoshida T, Koshikawa M, Sawai K, Yokoi H, Tanaka A, Gotoh M, Ueda S, Sugawara A, Kuwahara T. C4d and C4BT deposition along the glomerular capillary walls in a patient with pre-eclampsia. Am J Kidney Dis 2001; 37: E6
11. Robert JM. Endothelial dysfunction in pre-eclampsia. Sem Reprod Endocrinol 1998; 16: 5–15
12. Clark SL, Pavlova Z, Greenspoon J, Horenstein J, Phelan JP. Squamous cells in the maternal pulmonary circulation. Am J Obstet Gynecol 1986; 154: 104–106
13. Ibdah JA, Bennett MJ, Rinaldo P, Zhao Y, Gibson B, Sims HF, Straus AW. A fetal fatty-acid oxidation disorder as a cause of liver disease in pregnant women. N Engl J Med 1999; 340: 1723–1731

14. Castro MA, Fassett MJ, Reynolds TB, Shaw KJ, Goodwin TM. Reversible peripartum liver failure: a new perspective on the diagnosis, treatment, and cause of acute fatty liver of pregnancy, based on 28 consecutive cases. Am J Obstet Gynecol 1999; 181: 389–395

15. Thomson JR, Trembath RC. Primary pulmonary hypertension: the pressure rises for a gene. J Clin Pathol 2000; 53: 899–903

16. De Caestecker M, Meyrick B. Bone morphogenetic proteins, genetics and the pathophysiology of primary pulmonary hypertension. Resp Res 2001; 2: 193–197

17. Suomalainen A, Paetau A, Leinonen H, Majander A, Peltonen L, Somer H. Inherited idiopathic dilated cardiomyopathy with multiple deletions of mitochondrial DNA. Lancet 1992; 340: 1319–1320

18. Bernstein PS, Magriples U. Cardiomyopathy in pregnancy: a retrospective study. Am J Perinatol 2001; 18: 163–168

19. Drife JO. The contribution of cancer to maternal mortality. In O'Brien PMS, McLean AB (Eds) Hormones and Cancer. London: RCOG Press, 2000; 299–310

20. Bernstein MA, Madoff RD, Caushaj PF. Colon and rectal cancer in pregnancy. Dis Colon Rectum 1993; 36: 172–178

21. Anaes S, Pedersen SN, Theilade P. Phlegmonous gastritis in pregnancy: a case with fatal outcome. Ugeskr Laeger 1993; 155: 1806–1807

9

Sudden adult death and the heart

M.N. Sheppard

INTRODUCTION

Pathologists are faced with many complex cardiac diseases that cause sudden natural death in the absence of coronary artery disease. There may be a familial and genetic basis for these diseases, which is of major importance for the families. In order that the causes can be readily identified, detailed case history, meticulous post-mortem examination and complete toxicological screening are essential to arrive at the underlying cause of death. In this context, sudden means death within minutes of symptoms occurring and is usually due to the onset of a ventricular arrhythmia. Such sudden arrhythmic deaths can be invoked by both solvent abuse and cocaine, so toxicological investigation is essential in all such cases.

EPIDEMIOLOGY OF SUDDEN DEATH

Ischaemic heart disease is the commonest cause of death in the western world today. A substantial proportion of persons experience sudden death as the first clinical expression of underlying coronary artery disease. In the US, it is estimated that 2/1000 population die from sudden cardiac death (SCD), making up 500 000 per year.[1] The Framingham study found that 13% of all deaths in its prospectively followed cohort were sudden, with 90% of these attributed to cardiac disease.[2] Sudden death can occur in up to 23% of cases as a first episode as reported from the UK. As the first clinical presentation of ischaemic heart disease, angina represents 30–34%, other ischaemic episodes, e.g. cardiac failure 10%, acute myocardial infarction 33% and sudden death 23% of cases. In a British Regional Heart Study of males between the ages of 40 and 59 years, 217 died

Mary N. Sheppard FRCPath, Consultant Histopathologist, Royal Brompton and Harefield Trust, London, UK

of ischaemic heart disease. Among those 217, 117 (54%) died suddenly. In that study, the risk factors associated with sudden adult death were the usual ones linked to atherosclerosis, but heavy drinking and a previous history of arrhythmias was also important.[3] Extensive coronary atheroma is found in most victims of sudden death. One autopsy study of 168 sudden death victims demonstrated three vessel disease in 47%, two vessel disease in 27% and single vessel disease in 15%.[4]

Many of the above studies suffer from the fact that they are retrospective with all the limitations that implies. In order to overcome these arguments, we carried out a prospective study sponsored by the British Heart Foundation of the English population aged from 16 to 64 years with no history of ischaemic heart disease, who were last seen alive within 12 h of being found dead and in whom a Coroner's post-mortem examination found either a cardiac or no identifiable cause of death. The median time from symptom onset to death was 40 min. Sixty-seven per cent were taken ill at home, 12% at work, 12% in a public place and 10% elsewhere. The certified cause of death was ischaemic heart disease in 86% and non-ischaemic heart disease in 7%. 2.7% had a history of alcohol abuse and epilepsy with no abnormality in the myocardium and finally, in 4.7% of cases after detailed pathological examination of the whole heart, no cause of death could be established. These were termed sudden adult death cases to highlight that death can occur in apparently fit individuals in whom toxicology and detailed examination of the heart for structural abnormalities were negative.[5]

More recently we have completed a study with the British Heart Foundation, which has focused on these sudden adult deaths. One hundred and fifteen Coroners' cases were reported and 56 (49%) were reported as sudden unexplained cardiac deaths, mean age 32 (male 31, female 34), with range 7–64 years and 5 (9%) <16 years. Thirty-five (63%) were male with a male to female ratio of 1.7:1. Informants for 39 (70%) cases reported one or more cardiac symptoms in 27 (69%) and a family history of sudden deaths in 7 (18%), unexplained accidents in 2 (5%) and childhood or cot death in 5 (13%). The estimated incidence rate of these unexplained cardiac deaths is 0.16 per 100 000 per annum for males and 0.13 for females. Combined with the Office of National Statistics information on all 'unascertained causes of death', the rate is 1.34 per 100 000 per annum, a potential of over 500 sudden arrhythmic deaths in England per annum. This study recommends the term sudden arrhythmic death syndrome (SADS) as the officially certified cause of death to emphasise the arrhythmic cardiac nature of the death and to facilitate systematic population-based research, through a national register, into the environmental and genetic causes of these unexplained deaths.

In the Veneto region of Italy, 200 cases of sudden death in the young (≤35 years) were reported.[6] Sudden death was cerebral in 15 cases (7.5%), respiratory in 10 (5%) and cardiovascular in 163 (81.5%), whereas it remained unexplained in 12 cases (6%). Among cardiovascular sudden death, obstructive coronary atherosclerosis accounted for 23%, arrhythmogenic right ventricular cardiomyopathy (ARVC) for 12.5%, mitral valve prolapse for 10%, conduction-system abnormalities for 10%, congenital coronary artery anomalies for 8.5%, myocarditis for 7.5%, hypertrophic cardiomyopathy (HCM) for 5.5%, aortic rupture for 5.5%, dilated cardiomyopathy (DCM) for 5%, nonatherosclerotic-acquired coronary artery disease for 3.5%, post-operative congenital heart disease for 3%, aortic stenosis for 2%, pulmonary embolism for 2% and other causes for 2%. Cardiac arrest remained unexplained in 6% of the cases. Thus, a large spectrum of cardiovascular disorders, both congenital and acquired, may represent the organic substrate of sudden death in the young. The underlying abnormality is frequently only discovered at post-mortem examination.[6]

Other studies on sudden unexplained death are limited to case reports, but a small retrospective study from Ireland found a large proportion of sudden deaths in young adults were secondary to epilepsy and chemical/drug poisoning accounting for 34% and 31.8%, respectively. Sudden adult death syndrome accounted for 9% of the study population.[7]

AUTOPSY

In a study of sudden death in Ireland, only 18 (13%) underwent Coroner's autopsy and 16 were found to have extensive coronary disease.[8] This study illustrates that not all sudden deaths have autopsies, especially in situations where the patient has had a history of previous illness, particularly cardiac disease. How does the pathologist investigate a sudden unexpected death in young subjects without any prior known medical history? A full autopsy with toxicology is essential. Giving the cause of a sudden death for purposes of death certification is an exercise in probabilities rather than certainties. Pathologists, therefore, need to consider the cause of death carefully. In our study,[5] 7% of cardiac sudden death were not related to coronary artery disease. Individuals dying suddenly from other causes form a complex group. These causes include:

ANOMALIES OF CORONARY ARTERIES

In subjects over the age of 30, coronary atherosclerosis increasingly becomes a major cause of death. There are, however, other vascular causes of sudden death, particularly in younger subjects. Any examination of the heart in sudden death must specify the coronary artery orifices. Always check the ostia and probe the proximal coronary arteries to check their position and patency. Normally, one orifice is present in each of the two forward facing aortic sinuses (right and left). Anomalies in the coronary artery anatomy may be safe or lethal. Lethal anomalies fall into two clear groups. In the first group, one artery arises in the aorta while the other ostium is in the pulmonary artery. Sudden death often occurs in early adult life without prior symptoms. Thus, always check the coronary orifices and, if one is not identified, always check the pulmonary artery. The second dangerous group of anomalies occurs when two coronary ostia arise in one aortic sinus. In such cases, an arterial branch has to cross from right to left or left to right, depending in which sinus the ostia are present. If the crossing artery lies between the pulmonary and aortic trunk, the subject is at risk of sudden death on exercise. If the crossing artery lies in front of the pulmonary trunk, there is no danger.[9] Another dangerous anomaly in children is where the proximal portion of the left coronary artery or the ostium is atretic (Fig. 9.1) as we have previously reported.[10]

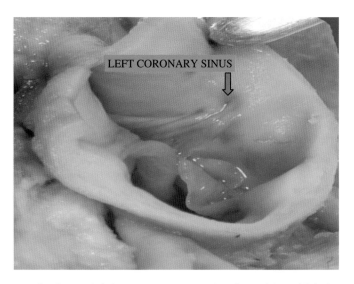

LEFT CORONARY SINUS

Fig. 9.1 A completely atretic left coronary artery ostium (arrow) in a child who died suddenly, aged one year.

Coronary ostia, which arise from the aorta above their usual site at the sinu-tubular junction and have to run through the media at an acute downward angle, which have a shelf-like fold of aortic wall at their upper border, have been described as causing death, but these appearances can be found in control hearts. We did a study of the origin of coronary arteries in 23 normal hearts from autopsied adults. The left coronary artery arose within the left aortic sinus in 16 (69%) subjects, above the sinutubular junction in five (22%) and at the level of the junction in two (9%). The right coronary artery arose within the right aortic sinus in 18 (78%) subjects, above the junction in three (13%) and at the level of the junction in two (9%). An accessory coronary orifice was found in the right aortic sinus in 17 (74%) subjects, whereas a third orifice in this sinus was found in five hearts.[11] If a large probe can be passed easily into the coronary artery, the lesion cannot be regarded as a cause of death. However, the role of spasm with an intramural course of a coronary artery needs to be considered, especially if there are ischaemic changes in the myocardium supplied by that vessel.

Kawasaki disease is recognisable as aneurysmally dilated arteries containing thrombus. Spontaneous dissection of a coronary artery is seen as a focal mass of red thrombus in an artery with minimal atherosclerosis, which by histology is a subadventitial haematoma rather than intraluminal thrombus (Fig. 9.2). Bridging, where a layer of myocardium covers the epicardial surface of a major coronary artery (Fig. 9.3), is a contentious cause of sudden death. Many normal hearts (from 5 to 25%) have 10 to 20 mm of a bridged epicardial coronary artery covered by a layer of cardiac muscle, but it is usually superficial with little muscle covering the vessel. Therefore, most of these must be functionally of no consequence. The bridge of muscle must be 20 mm long and 5 mm in depth in order to be of significance and capable of causing compression of a coronary artery with myocardial ischaemia. To ascribe a bridged or tunnelled section of coronary artery as

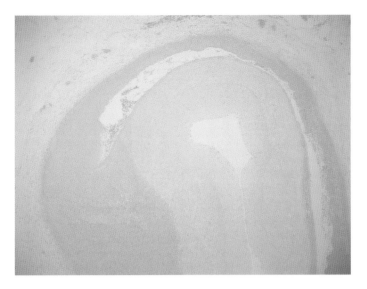

Fig. 9.2 A transverse section of a coronary artery with spontaneous dissection in a 35-year-old female. Note the intramural haematoma (H&E ×100).

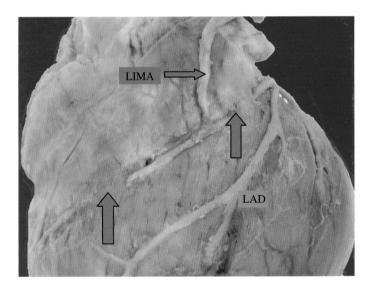

Fig. 9.3 A diagonal branch of the left anterior descending (LAD) coronary artery with two muscular bridges (arrows) in a child, who died with myocardial infarction aged 3 years. Note the left internal mammary artery (LIMA) bypass graft.

a cause of death requires additional evidence. This may take the form of a history of episodic anginal-type pain prior to death or histological evidence of ischaemia in the myocardium, particularly contraction bands in large numbers, acute infarction or fibrosis confined to the segment of myocardium supplied by the artery. However, it has been argued that, while superficial bridging may not be clinically significant, deep bridging greater than 5 mm in depth may lead to sudden death without ischaemic changes at autopsy.[12]

CARDIOMYOPATHIES

A significant proportion of natural sudden deaths are due to heart muscle disease (cardiomyopathy). Hypertrophic, dilated and restrictive cardiomyopathy can lead to sudden death. Hypertrophic cardiomyopathy (HCM) is one of the most common causes of sudden death in young people and athletes,[13] especially in the 12–35 years bracket. In the Italian study, HCM accounted for 5.5% of the 200 cases.[6] The risk declines with increasing age. The heart pathology is usually obvious at autopsy with increase in heart size, hypertrophy (either eccentric or concentric in the left ventricle (LV) with outflow tract obstruction and an impact lesion on the interventricular septum) an area of endocardial thickening on the septum, which has a very discrete lower border and is the exact mirror image of the anterior cusp of the mitral valve. Such a lesion is pathognomonic of HCM, but is only found in about 40% of cases (Fig. 9.4). Diffuse endocardial thickening over the left side of the interventricular septum is non-specific. Myocardial bridging is associated with HCM. Myocardial bridging of the left anterior descending coronary artery in children with HCM showed a 67% survival among patients with bridging and 94% among those without bridging. Myocardial bridging is, thus, associated with a poor outcome in children with HCM.[14]

Fifty per cent of HCM cases are familial with an autosomal dominant pattern of inheritance. In HCM, nine genetic loci and more than 130 mutations in 10 different sarcomeric genes and in the γ2 subunit of AMP-activated protein kinase (AMPK) have been identified, indicating impaired force production associated with inefficient use of ATP as the crucial disease mechanism. Certain mutations are more associated with sudden death. The Gly256Glu, Val606Met and Leu908Val mutations in the β-MyHC are associated with a benign prognosis. In contrast, Arg403Gln, Arg719Trp and Arg453Cys mutations are associated with a

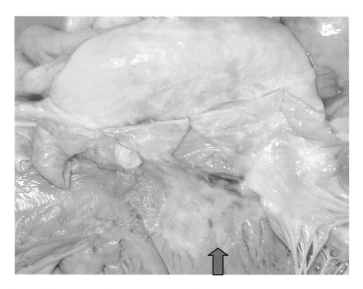

Fig. 9.4 The outflow tract of the LV in a case of HCM with sudden death in male aged 23. Note the thickened ridge present on the endocardium, which matches the lower edge of the anterior leaflet of the mitral valve (arrow).

high incidence of SCD. Mutations in troponin are associated with a mild degree of hypertrophy, but a high incidence of sudden death.[15]

The macroscopic appearances produced by the myofibrillary gene mutations now are so wide that it is impossible to exclude HCM by naked-eye examination. Widespread disarray and a risk of sudden death can be present in hearts in which the weight is not increased and the LV is close to normal which occurs with mutations in troponin T.[15] With time, HCM can progress to dilatation of the LV.[16] Thus, the phenotypic characteristics of HCM are much wider than previously thought. Detailed histology of the myocardium is, therefore, essential. For the pathologist, this means the LV has to be studied with at least 8–10 histological blocks to exclude a myofibrillary gene defect cardiomyopathy. The histological marker of HCM is disarray of myocytes in which the cells run in circular whorls around a small focus of connective tissue (Fig. 9.5). Disarray is associated with marked nuclear enlargement in myocytes. Disarray is, however, very rarely present throughout the LV and is patchy, meaning that a single random histology block cannot exclude the diagnosis. Many cases of HCM have segments of myocardium which are totally normal.

A family history of sudden death, recurrent syncope, non-sustained ventricular tachycardia and an abnormal response of blood pressure to exercise, all have prognostic value in families in predicting the risk of sudden death.[17]

Cases are also encountered in which the LV mass is increased considerably with some fibrosis but no disarray is present on histology. The pathogenesis of such cases is widely debated. The phenomenon is often encountered in subjects of Afro-Caribbean origin and a LV, which can be described as 'Hocoid' (that is like 'Hocum', an alternative abbreviation for HCM) but without disarray. Some may be associated with hypertension but a history is often lacking. Similar hearts are seen in athletes and there is the inevitable question of anabolic steroid use in their causation. What seems likely is that a number of genes control LV hypertrophy and that mutations or polymorphisms can allow a disproportionate

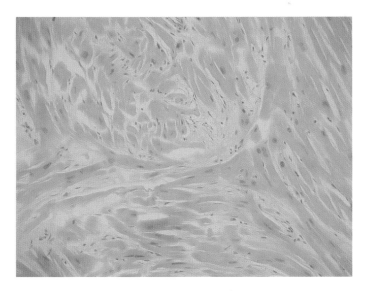

Fig. 9.5 Myocyte disarray in a case of HCM (H&E ×500).

increase in LV mass in response to exercise or mild hypertension, and there is a risk of sudden death. Infants of diabetic mothers develop a large thick-walled LV, probably, as a response to insulin-like growth factors. The relation of LV hypertrophy to sudden death means that pathologists must record heart weight. Total heart weight is an excellent surrogate for isolated LV mass and avoids the accurate but time consuming Fulton dissection method. Total heart weight must be equated to body size and a number of tables and equations allow adjustments to be made. Heart weight must be at least outside the 95% confidence limits for body size to be credible as a cause of death alone. Many pathologists adopt an arbitrary upper limit of 450–500 g for total heart weight, but this depends on ideal body weight of 70 kg. Today the average adult is taller and heavier than his/her predecessor, so these heart weights need reassessing also. Thickness of the LV or RV wall may also be useful but dilatation can occur with time, and ischaemic damage and fibrosis may also alter the thickness of the ventricles.

Dilated cardiomyopathy (DCM) is not a common cause of SCD. The majority of patients present with evidence of cardiac disease prior to death. However, these patients can die suddenly and this risk progressively increases during long-term follow-up, especially in those with persistent severe LV dilation and dysfunction, who are not on β-blockers.[18] Familial cause has been shown in 35% of patients with DCM. Sixteen chromosomal loci with defects of several proteins also involved in the development of skeletal myopathies have been detected. Myotonic dystrophy is associated with marked cardiac involvement, LV fibrosis and high risk of sudden death. Families with myotonic dystrophy may have sudden deaths without skeletal muscle expression of the abnormal gene. A lamin gene defect is responsible for autosomal dominant DCM and conduction system disease. This gene defect is on chromosome 1p1-q21, where the gene for nuclear envelope proteins lamin A and lamin C are located. Mutations in the head or tail domain of this gene cause Emery–Dreifuss muscular dystrophy, a childhood-onset disease characterised by joint contractures and in some cases by abnormalities of cardiac conduction during adulthood. Five novel missense mutations in the lamin A/C gene and one in the lamin C tail domain cause heritable, progressive conduction system disease (sinus bradycardia, atrioventricular (AV) conduction block or atrial arrhythmias) and DCM. Heart failure and sudden death occur frequently within these families and no family members with mutations have either joint contractures or skeletal myopathy.[19]

These mutated cytoskeletal and nuclear transporter proteins may alter force transmission or disrupt nuclear function, resulting in cell death. Further, DCM mutations have also been identified in sarcomeric genes, which indicate that different defects of the same protein can result in either HCM or DCM.[20]

Restrictive cardiomyopathy is the rarest form of cardiomyopathy but can present as sudden death in sarcoidosis and amyloid infiltration.[21] Sudden death in subjects can occur when the heart looks macroscopically normal with no hypertrophy but widespread myocardial fibrosis is present on histology with normal coronary arteries. Fibrosis may take the form of discrete linear scars or be diffuse and perimyocyte in distribution.[22] The genetic basis is not known but the cases can be designated as idiopathic fibrosis (IF). Connective tissue disease, such as systemic lupus erythematosus, can be associated with ventricular fibrosis with or without inflammation and cause sudden death.[23]

ARRHYTHMOGENIC RIGHT VENTRICULAR CARDIOMYOPATHY

RV cardiomyopathy is a heart muscle disease that is often familial and is anatomically characterised by adipose or fibroadipose infiltration of the RV myocardium. It is the most recently recognised of the cardiomyopathies and differs from the others by predominantly involving the RV. In Italy, RV cardiomyopathy may be more frequent and represents an important cause of sudden death among young people, especially with exertion.[24]

This is another genetic cardiomyopathy with a high risk of sudden death in gene carriers. There is a familial incidence in 30% with ARVC. In ARVC, six genetic loci and mutations in the cardiac ryanodine receptor (which controls electro-mechanical coupling) and in plakoglobin and desmoglobin (molecules involved in desmosomal cell junction integrity), have been identified.[20] Studies of large families with the disease have shown that, like HCM, the heart phenotype can be wide. In established cases, the right side of the heart appears yellowish or whitish as to suggest a fatty or fibrofatty infiltration of the underlying myocardium (Fig. 9.6); the myocardial loss frequently accounts for a parchment-like, translucent look of the RV free wall. Aneurysms of the RV free wall, whether single or multiple, are reported in about 50% of cases and are considered a pathognomonic feature of ARVC; they are typically located in the inferior, diaphragmatic wall, underneath the posterior leaflet of the tricuspid valve as well as in the infundibulum and at the apex. RV enlargement, whether mild, moderate or severe, is a feature. At histology, the pathological process generally starts from the subepicardium and extends to the endocardium in a wave-front phenomenon. The residual, spared myocytes are located within the subendocardial trabeculas and few myocardial fascicles are scattered throughout the fibrofatty tissue. All stages of myocardial injury and repair are recognisable: acute cell death with myocytolysis and inflammatory infiltrates, active fibrosis with lymphocytes and macrophages, mature adipocytes replacing vanished myocytes and, eventually,

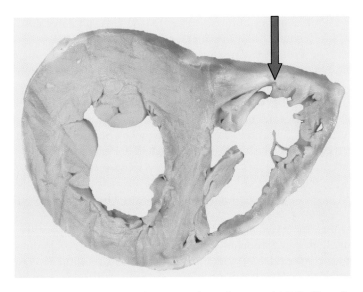

Fig. 9.6 The transverse section of the LV and RV of a case of ARVD. Note the thinning and fatty replacement of the RV (arrow).

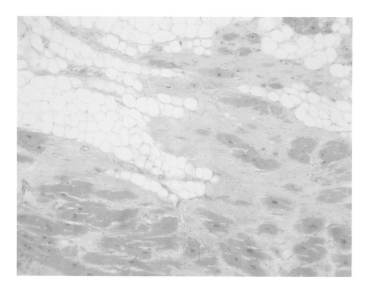

Fig. 9.7 Fatty infiltration fibrosis and residual myocytes in a case of ARVD (H&E ×400).

a chronic stage with fibrous tissue and adipocytes surrounding residual surviving myocytes (Fig. 9.7).

The areas of thinning may be focal and small (10–20 mm^2) and one has to look at the RV in some detail to find them. The extremes of the phenotype are even more difficult with some cases looking macroscopically normal. Thus, microscopic findings are diagnostic and may be present in the absence of gross findings.[25] About 30% of cases of ARVD have some LV involvement and patients may present with biventricular involvement with thin-walled ventricles with foci of fibrofatty replacement of myocytes, often in a band-like distribution on the posterior wall. Cases are seen in which the LV is involved by this change in isolation. Whether this is part of the spectrum of ARVD is still debatable.

Marked fat replacement is not essential for the diagnosis of RV dysplasia; it is the fibrosis with or without the inflammation, which is necessary for diagnosis. The RV should be extensively sampled histologically in all cases of sudden unexpected death, especially those that are exercise-related.[25] It can be difficult to distinguish simple adipose tissue infiltration of the RV muscle without fibrosis. This is a common change in normal subjects, particularly obese middle aged and elderly women, and is believed to be of no consequence. Studies of large families with known ARVD, however, suggest that occasional cases of sudden death occur with this picture of fatty infiltration in the RV in isolation.

THE CONDUCTION SYSTEM AND SUDDEN DEATH

As already mentioned, mutations in the lamin gene cause Emery–Dreifuss muscular dystrophy, characterised by abnormalities of cardiac conduction and progressive conduction system disease (sinus bradycardia, AV conduction block or atrial arrhythmias). Sudden death can occur indicating that this lamin intermediate filament protein has an important role in cardiac conduction.[19]

Patients with complete AV block or with pre-excitation (Wolff–Parkinson–White syndrome) have a risk of sudden death, yet the number of cases who die in their very first syncopal attack is uncertain. The 116 452 consecutive 12-lead electro-cardiograms (ECG), belonging to the entire cohort of 18-year-old young boys in Italy, identified 173 cases of overt WPW pattern (short PR interval, delta wave, anomalous configuration of QRS complex) with a calculated incidence of 1.48/1000. Accessory pathway location was: left free wall (70 patients), right free wall (39 patients), postero-septal (37 patients), antero-septal (15 patients) and unde-termined (12 patients). Mitral valve prolapse was diagnosed in eight patients.[26]

It is impossible to make a diagnosis of Wolff–Parkinson–White syndrome in true SCD, unless there is previous ECG evidence. Serial sectioning of the entire AV ring to detect abnormal pathways would be totally impractical.

Unless there is again clear evidence of AV block on ECG, histological exam-ination of the conduction system is not rewarding. Study of 177 cases of permanent AV block showed idiopathic bilateral bundle branch fibrosis to be the commonest single cause (33%). There is locaised loss of conduction fibres in the proximal left bundle branch and bifurcating main bundle (Lev's disease) to more periphery loss of conduction fibres in the bundle branches alone (Lenegre's disease). The aetiological factors in idiopathic bundle branch fibrosis are still obscure. Ischaemic damage is responsible for 17% of cases and is usually in patients who have sur-vived destruction of the bundle branches in septal infarction. Calcific AV block is the term applied to destruction of the main bundle by large masses of calcifi-cation in the mitral or aortic valve rings and is responsible for 10% of cases of chronic AV block.

Cardiomyopathies of all types (except hypertrophic obstructive cardiomy-opathy) involve the conduction system and produce 14% of cases of AV block. The remaining numerous causes of chronic AV block are individually very rare, ranging through tumour involvement, congenital defects, collagen vascular dis-eases and surgical or traumatic damage.[27] Detailed serial sectioning is necessary with hundreds of sections to examine. The difficulty of such examinations is that normal hearts often contain minor anatomical abnormalities of the conduc-tion system, such as nodo-ventricular connections or small accessory masses of AV nodal tissue. The presence of these abnormalities, therefore, cannot be taken to be a cause of sudden death, although many case reports in the literature do so. The changes consist of abnormalities in His bundle position (branching bun-dle in membranous septum or left-sided bundle), AV node fibrosis and inter-atrial lipoma. Other age-related minor abnormalities are mild fibrosis, fatty change or fibrointimal hyperplasia of AV nodal arteries, downward displace-ment of the tricuspid valve with AV node elongation, His compression by HCM, Mannheim fibres, focal ischaemia of bundle, AV node division, AV node dissec-tion by oedema and intramural left bundle branch.[28]

Dysplasia of the AV node artery with intimal thickening and mucopolysac-charide deposition has been described in a substantial portion of patients with unexplained sudden death.[29] However, the conduction system is a complex structure and all these changes described are difficult to assess because there is such wide variation in the adult and knowledge of these variations and ageing effects are not familiar to most pathologists. It is, however, always worth look-ing at the AV nodal area with the naked eye to exclude the small benign tumour (AV nodal mesothelioma) that arises in the node. This is seen as a cystic nodule

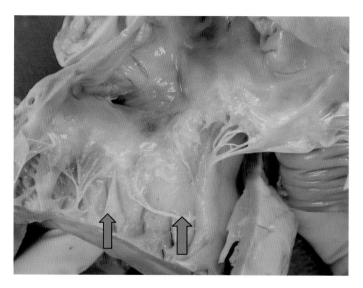

Fig. 9.8 View of the triangle of Koch containing the AV node outlined by the mouth of the coronary sinus and the septal leaflet of the tricuspid valve. Note the thickening (arrows) involving this area in a case of sudden death due to cardiac sarcoidosis.

just anterior to the coronary sinus in the right atrium.[30] Sarcoidosis can also involve the conduction system (Fig. 9.8).

MYOCARDITIS

Myocarditis is a rare disease in adults and an ever rarer cause of sudden adult death.[31] Myocarditis as a cause of acute or sudden death in infancy has been given little emphasis in the literature. However, in a 40-year autopsy review in Canada (3086 cases), 20 cases of isolated myocarditis were found, of which 17 occurred in infants less than 12 months of age, often with no antecedent clinical signs and who presented with sudden death or had a clinical history of less than 24 h.[32] Myocarditis can occur as an acute lethal illness in early life. The presentation in the paediatric age group may vary from an asymptomatic incidental finding to a well-defined illness lasting several weeks to sudden death cases.[33] The histological sections of 35 autopsies of infants diagnosed as sudden infant death syndrome (SIDS) victims revealed myocarditis in seven cases. Therefore, in SIDS-suspected cases, a meticulous post-mortem microscopic examination of the heart should be carried out.[34]

SUDDEN INFANT DEATH

Other causes should be ruled out before diagnosing SIDS. Cardiac causes for sudden infant death include viral myocarditis (see above), congenital heart disease, particularly congenital aortic stenosis, endocardial fibroelastosis and anomalous origin of the left coronary artery from the pulmonary artery. Other cardiac conditions that may result in sudden death include rhabdomyomas of the heart

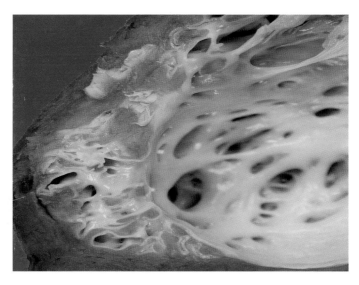

Fig. 9.9 Section of right ventricle apex from a case of sudden death with thickening and irregular spongy pattern of trabeculae (non-compaction of ventricle).

in tuberous sclerosis and fibromas. The most frequent conduction system disorders include involvement by histiocytoid cardiomyopathy and congenital heart block that may be associated with maternal lupus erythematosus. Cardiomyopathies include arrhythmogenic RV dysplasia, non-compaction of the LV (Fig. 9.9) and long QT syndrome (LQTS).[35] There is a history of sudden infant death in LQTS[36] and our study confirms this. Thus, in medicolegal cases it is important to consider this possibility.

SUDDEN DEATH AND A MORPHOLOGICALLY NORMAL HEART

Sudden deaths do occur in which, despite taking adequate histology of the heart, no structural abnormality is found and toxicology is negative. It is being increasingly recognised that gene defects in ion channels in the myocyte can lead to rhythm disturbances, ECG abnormalities and a risk of sudden death, but no morphological abnormality in the heart. Examples are the LQT and Brugada syndromes. The only way these conditions can be confirmed are ECGs taken earlier in the subject's life or by discovering other family members whose ECGs show the characteristic appearances. The frequency of the LQTS as a cause of sudden death can only be guessed at; in our survey of families of sudden death cases, 25% had evidence of LQTS (in press).

ARRHYTHMIAS

The pathogenesis of familial inherited arrhythmias is being progressively clarified, thanks to the insights provided by molecular biology and by functional studies. Transmembrane or intracellular ion channel mutations have been identified in genetically determined forms of polymorphic ventricular tachycardia and sudden death, such as catecholaminergic ventricular tachycardia, LQT and Brugada syndromes. The role of molecular abnormalities in the genesis of monomorphic idiopathic ventricular tachycardias is less well defined, mainly because of the lack of a Mendelian pattern of inheritance. Interestingly, the presence of somatic mutations has been suggested as the mechanism for monomorphic ventricular tachycardia originating from the RV outflow tract.[37]

The LQTS is a familial disease characterised by prolonged ventricular repolarisation and a high incidence of malignant ventricular tachyarrhythmias, often occurring in conditions of adrenergic activation.

The genes for the LQTS have been identified as SCN5A, the cardiac sodium channel gene, and as HERG and KvLQT1 potassium channel genes.[38] It is becoming clear that mutations in the KVLQT1, cardiac voltage-dependent sodium channel gene, minK and MiRP1 genes, respectively, are responsible for the LQT1, LQT2, LQT3, LQT5 and LQT6 variants of the LQTS or Romano–Ward syndrome, characterised by autosomal dominant transmission and no deafness. The much rarer Jervell–Lange–Nielsen syndrome (with marked QT prolongation and sensorineural deafness) arises when a child inherits mutant KVLQT1 or minK alleles from both parents. In addition, some families are not linked to the known genetic loci. Cardiac voltage-dependent sodium channel gene encoding the cardiac sodium channel and LQTS mutations prolong action potentials by increasing inward plateau sodium current. The other mutations cause a decrease in net repolarising current by reducing potassium currents through 'dominant negative' or 'loss of function' mechanisms. Clinical presentations vary with the specific gene affected and the specific mutation.[39]

The incidence of cardiac events is highest in LQT1 and LQT2, but sudden death is highest in LQT3. These episodes are characteristically associated with sudden increases in sympathetic activity, such as during violent emotions (particularly fright, but also anger) or physical activity (notably swimming). Sudden awakening (alarm clock, telephone ring and thunder) seems to be a trigger for some patients. Based on LQT registry, 427 patients were classified as arousal, 345 as non-arousal and the remaining 553 were unknown. The age at first cardiac event was significantly younger in the arousal than the non-arousal group (11.7 versus 15.5 years, respectively; $P < 0.001$). Arousal-related cardiac events occurred in 85% of LQT1, 67% of LQT2 and 33% of LQT3 patients. This study provides evidence that the genotype is an important determinant of the LQTS phenotype in terms of arousal and non-arousal-related cardiac events.

In another study, LQT1 patients experienced the majority of their events (62%) during exercise and only 3% occurred during rest/sleep. These percentages are almost reversed among LQT2 and LQT3 patients, who were less likely to have events during exercise (13%) and more likely to have events during rest/sleep (29% and 39%). Life-threatening arrhythmias in LQTS patients tend to occur under specific circumstances in a gene-specific manner.[40] The identification of LQTS genes has provided tremendous new insights for our understanding of normal cardiac electrophysiology and its perturbation in a wide range of conditions associated with sudden death. It seems likely that the approach of applying information from the genetics of uncommon congenital syndromes to the study of common acquired diseases will be an increasingly important one in this millennium.

Jervell–Lange–Nielsen syndrome is a rare form of profound congenital deafness combined with syncopal attacks and sudden death due to prolonged QTc; it is inherited as an autosomal recessive trait. First described in Norway in 1957, it has a prevalence of at least 1:200 000. Later reports from many other countries have confirmed its occurrence. The KCNQ1 and KCNE1 proteins co-assemble in a potassium channel and mutations in either the KCNQ1 gene or the KCNE1 gene disrupt endolymph production in the stria vascularis in the cochlea, causing deafness. Some heterozygous carriers of JLNS mutations in either gene may suffer from prolonged QTc.

SUDDEN DEATH IN EPILEPSY

It has also become apparent that sudden deaths occur in epileptic subjects without a clear cardiac morphological abnormality and in whom the final event was not related to a grand mal seizure. The mechanisms are not clear but may be related to sympathetic over-activity in the prodomal phase of an epileptic attack to alterations in the QT interval and due to electrical instability of the heart related to therapeutic drugs or to cerebral neuronal activity arrest leading to respiratory arrest, hypoxia and then ventricular fibrillation (VF). About 612 deaths were associated with epilepsy in 1997. Forty-four deaths were certified as being attributable to sudden death in epilepsy (SUDEP) and a further 292 deaths were considered to be probable SUDEP cases. It is estimated that between 350 and 400 cases of SUDEP occurred in England and Wales, in 1997, in those aged 16–50 years. SUDEP is the commonest category of epilepsy-related death.[41] Among patients between 20 and 45, sudden unexpected death is the most frequently occurring epilepsy-related cause of death. In patients with refractory epilepsy, sudden unexpected death comprises about 10% of deaths; the incidence is about 1:200–300 per year. Risk factors are symptomatic epilepsy, tonic-clonic seizures, early onset of the epilepsy, polytherapy and non-compliance.[42]

ALCOHOL AND SUDDEN DEATH

Alcohol with toxic effect resulting in DCM may be responsible for SCD. However, there are cases of sudden death in people with a history of alcohol abuse with a normal heart found at autopsy with marked fatty change in the liver.[43] The mechanisms are unclear but heavy use and alcohol withdrawal may play a role.[44,45]

In our survey, alcohol abuse or epilepsy was recorded in 2.7% of cases with a morphologically normal heart.

TRAUMA

Blunt trauma to the anterior chest wall, such as being hit by a cricket or hockey ball, can invoke sudden VF without either acute structural damage to the sternum, pericardium and myocardium or prior heart disease. This is known as commotio cordis. Seventy cases, including 34 occurring during organised competitive athletics and 36 others that occurred during informal recreational sports at home, school or the playground, or during non-sporting activities have been described. Ages were 2–38 (mean age, 12) with 70% <16-year old. Most common sports involved were youth baseball ($n = 40$), softball ($n = 7$) and ice hockey ($n = 7$). Seven (10%) of the 70 commotio cordis victims, including six with documented VF, have survived the consequences of their chest blow. Eleven of the events (16%) occurred despite the presence of chest padding believed to be potentially protective. An experimental model of low-energy chest wall impact demonstrates that commotio cordis events are largely due to the exquisite timing of blows during a narrow window within the repolarisation phase of the cardiac cycle, 15–30 ms prior to the peak of the T-wave.[46]

RESPONSIBILITIES OF THE PATHOLOGIST

The pathologist has a responsibility to accurately record data that will allow the cause of death to be identified. This cannot be done without histological examination of the myocardium. It is still unclear as to the responsibility on the medicolegal authority requesting the autopsy or the pathologist to inform the deceased person's family practitioner of the possibility of a familial cause being present or to explain the possible causes of death. Medicolegal authorities vary in their approach to cases where no morphological cause of death was found. In England and Wales, some Coroners will order an inquest while others record causes, such as spontaneous cardiac arrhythmia or even sudden adult death syndrome. The public has increasing awareness of their right to know and will ask questions about risk to other family members. Advice can only be based on knowledge of what the true cause of death is. If the death is due to a familial condition, such as cardiomyopathies or the LQTS, more than 90% of these families will have others carrying the abnormal gene. There has been a view that to identify asymptomatic gene carriers is unethical because anxiety is created without benefit. There now is benefit: gene carriers of the LQT, Brugada syndrome, HCM, DCM and ARVD are at risk of sudden death and this can be reduced by drug therapy or implantable defibrillators. No one would suggest forcing family investigations in sudden unexplained cardiac death, but at the very least the deceased person's general practitioner should be informed of the details of the post-mortem report to allow a discussion on whether to seek further investigation.

We are entering the molecular age in pathology but it is still reassuring to us jobbing non-molecular pathologists that often the cornerstone of the diagnosis rests with a thorough, professionally done autopsy in sudden death cases. We owe it to the deceased and their family to do our jobs properly and retain tissue for diagnosis.

REFERENCES

1. Kannel W, Schatzkin A. Sudden death: lessons from subsets in population studies. J Am Coll Cardiol 1985; 5: 141–149
2. Kannel W, Thomas H. Sudden death: the Framingham study. Ann NY Acad Sci 1982; 382: 3–21
3. Wannamethee G, Shaper AG, Macfarlane PW, Walker M. Risk factors for sudden cardiac death in middle-aged British men. Circulation 1995; 91: 1749–1756

4. Warnes C, Roberts W. Sudden coronary death: relation of amount and distribution of coronary narrowing at necropsy to previous symptoms of myocardial ischaemia, left ventricular scarring and heart weight. Am J Cardiol 1984; 54: 65–73

5. Bowker TJ, Wood DA, Davies MJ. Sudden unexpected cardiac death: methods and results of a national pilot survey. Int J Cardiol 1995; 52: 241–250

6. Basso C, Corrado D, Thiene G. Cardiovascular causes of sudden death in young individuals including athletes. Cardiol Rev 1999; 7: 127–135

7. Bennani FK, Connolly CE. Sudden unexpected death in young adults including four cases of SADS: a 10-year review from the west of Ireland (1985–1994). Med Sci Law 1997; 37: 242–247

8. Kearney P, Vaughan C, Fennell F, McKiernan S, Fennell W. Sudden death in Cork and Kerry – results of a one year survey and a review of the literature. Irish J Med Sci 1994; 163: 16–24

9. Taylor AJ, Rogan KM, Virmani R. Sudden cardiac death associated with isolated congenital coronary artery anomalies. J Am Coll Cardiol 1992; 20: 640–647

10. Gerlis LM, Magee AG, Sheppard MN. Congenital atresia of the orifice of the left coronary artery. Cardiol Young 2002; 12: 57–62

11. Muriago M, Sheppard MN, Ho SY, Anderson RH. Location of the coronary arterial orifices in the normal heart. Clin Anat 1997; 10: 297–302

12. Ferreira Jr AG, Trotter SE, Konig Jr B, Decourt LV, Fox K, Olsen EG. Myocardial bridges: morphological and functional aspects. Br Heart J 1991; 66: 364–367

13. Maron BJ, Shirani J, Poliac LC, Mathenge R, Roberts WC, Mueller FO. Sudden death in young competitive athletes. Clinical, demographic, and pathological profiles. JAMA 1996; 276: 199–204

14. Yetman AT, McCrindle BW, MacDonald C, Freedom RM, Gow R. Myocardial bridging in children with hypertrophic cardiomyopathy – a risk factor for sudden death. N Engl J Med 1998; 339: 1201–1209

15. Marian AJ, Roberts R. Molecular genetic basis of hypertrophic cardiomyopathy: genetic markers for sudden cardiac death. J Cardiovasc Electrophysiol 1998; 9: 88–99

16. Fujino N, Shimizu M, Ino H, Okeie K, Yamaguchi M, Yasuda T et al. Cardiac troponin T Arg92Trp mutation and progression from hypertrophic to dilated cardiomyopathy. Clin Cardiol 2001; 24: 397–402

17. Maron BJ, Casey SA, Poliac LC, Gohman TE, Almquist AK, Aeppli DM. Clinical course of hypertrophic cardiomyopathy in a regional United States cohort. JAMA 1999; 281: 650–655

18. Zecchin M, Lenarda AD, Bonin M, Mazzone C, Zanchi C, Di Chiara C et al. Incidence and predictors of sudden cardiac death during long-term follow-up in patients with dilated cardiomyopathy on optimal medical therapy. Ital Heart J 2001; 2: 213–221

19. Fatkin D, MacRae C, Sasaki T, Wolff MR, Porcu M, Frenneaux M et al. Missense mutations in the rod domain of the lamin A/C gene as causes of dilated cardiomyopathy and conduction-system disease. N Engl J Med 1999; 341: 1715–1724

20. Franz WM, Muller OJ, Katus HA. Cardiomyopathies: from genetics to the prospect of treatment. Lancet 2001; 358: 1627–1637

21. Veinot JP, Johnston B. Cardiac sarcoidosis – an occult cause of sudden death: a case report and literature review. J Forensic Sci 1998; 43: 715–717

22. Katritsis D, Wilmshurst PT, Wendon JA, Davies MJ, Webb-Peploe MM. Primary restrictive cardiomyopathy: clinical and pathologic characteristics. J Am Coll Cardiol 1991; 18: 1230–1235

23. Takahashi T, Suzuki T, Suzuki A, Yamada T, Koido N, Akizuki S et al. A case of systemic lupus erythematosus with interstitial myocarditis leading to sudden death. Ryumachi 1999; 39: 573–579

24. Thiene G, Nava A, Corrado D, Rossi L, Pennelli N. Right ventricular cardiomyopathy and sudden death in young people. New Engl J Med 1988; 318: 129–133

25. Burke AP, Robinson S, Radentz S, Smialek J, Virmani R. Sudden death in right ventricular dysplasia with minimal gross abnormalities. J Forensic Sci 1999; 44: 438–443

26. Sorbo MD, Buja GF, Miorelli M, Nistri S, Perrone C, Manca S et al. The prevalence of the Wolff–Parkinson–White syndrome in a population of 116 542 young males. G Ital Cardiol 1995; 25: 681–687

27. Davies MJ. Pathology of chronic A-V Block. Acta Cardiol 1976; suppl. 21: 19–30

28. Suarez-Mier MP, Fernandez-Simon L, Gawallo C. Pathologic changes of the cardiac conduction tissue in sudden cardiac death. Am J Forensic Med Pathol 1995; 16: 193–202

29. Burke AP, Subramanian R, Smialek J, Virmani R. Nonatherosclerotic narrowing of the atrioventricular node artery and sudden death. J Am Coll Cardiol 1993; 21: 117–122

30. Burke AP, Anderson PG, Virmani R, James TN, Herrera GA, Ceballos R. Tumor of the atrioventricular nodal region. A clinical and immunohistochemical study. Arch Pathol Lab Med 1990; 114: 1057–1062

31. Phillips M, Robinowitz M, Higgins JR, Boran KJ, Reed T, Virmani R. Sudden cardiac death in Air Force recruits. A 20-year review. JAMA 1986; 256: 2696–2699

32. DeSa DJ. Isolated myocarditis in the first year. Arch Dis Child 1985; 60: 484–485

33. Smith NM, Bourne AJ, Clapton WK, Byard RW. The spectrum of presentation at autopsy of myocarditis in infancy and childhood. Pathology 1992; 24: 129–131

34. Cote A, Russo P, Michaud J. Sudden unexpected deaths in infancy: what are the causes? J Pediatr 1999; 135: 437–443

35. Valdes-Dapena M, Gilbert-Barness E. Cardiovascular causes for sudden infant death. Pediatr Pathol Mol Med 2002; 21: 195–211

36. Bajanowski T, Rossi L, Biondo B, Ortmann C, Haverkamp W, Wedekind H et al. Prolonged QT interval and sudden infant death – report of two cases. Forensic Sci Int 2001; 115: 147–153

37. Napolitano C, Priori SG. Genetics of ventricular tachycardia. Curr Opin Cardiol 2002; 17 (3): 222–228

38. Priori SG, Napolitano C, Paganini V, Cantu F, Schwartz PJ. Molecular biology of the long QT syndrome: impact on management. Pacing Clin Electrophysiol 1997; 20: 2052–2057

39. Chiang CE, Roden DM. The long QT syndromes: genetic basis and clinical implications. J Am Coll Cardiol 2000; 36: 1–12

40. Schwartz PJ, Priori SG, Spazzolini C, Moss AJ, Vincent GM, Napolitano C et al. Genotype-phenotype correlation in the long-QT syndrome: gene-specific triggers for life-threatening arrhythmias. Circulation 2001; 103: 89–95

41. Langan Y, Nashef L, Sander JW. Certification of deaths attributable to epilepsy. J Neurol Neurosurg Psychiat 2002; 73: 751–752

42. Lossius R, Nakken KO. Epilepsy and death. Tidsskr Nor Laegeforen 2002; 122: 1114–1117

43. Randall B. Fatty liver and sudden death. A review. Hum Pathol 1980; 11: 147–153

44. Wannamethee G, Shaper AG. Alcohol and sudden cardiac death. Br Heart J 1992; 68: 443–448

45. Yoshida K, Funahashi M, Masui M, Ogura Y, Wakasugi C. Sudden death of alcohol withdrawal syndrome – report of a case. Nippon Hoigaku Zasshi 1990; 44: 243–247

46. Maron BJ, Link MS, Wang PJ, Estes NA, 3rd. Clinical profile of commotio cordis: an under appreciated cause of sudden death in the young during sports and other activities. J Cardiovasc Electrophysiol 1999; 10: 114–120

10

A new stem cell biology for pathologists

N.C. Direkze   S.L. Preston   R. Poulsom   M.R. Alison   N.A. Wright

ABSTRACT

There has recently been a significant change in the way we think about organ regeneration. In the adult, organ formation and regeneration was thought to occur through the action of organ or tissue restricted stem cells (e.g. haematopoietic stem cells making blood, gut stem cells making gut). However, there is a large body of recent work that has extended this model. Thanks to lineage-tracking techniques, we now believe that stem cells from one organ system, for example the haematopoietic compartment, can develop into the differentiated cells within another organ system, such as the liver, brain or kidney. This cellular *plasticity* occurs not just in experimental conditions but has been shown to take place in humans following bone marrow and organ transplants. This trafficking is potentially bi-directional, and even differentiated cells from different organ systems can interchange, with pancreatic cells able to form hepatocytes, for example. In this review we will detail some of these findings, attempt to explain the biological significance and suggest some possible therapeutic options that are now available.

INTRODUCTION

Stem cells are very much in the scientific – and public – attention at the present time. We have followed the saga of reproductive cloning, observing cloned sheep,

Natalie C. Direkze MA MB BS MRCP, Clinical Research Fellow, Cancer Research UK, London, UK and Department of Histopathology, Imperial College, London, UK

Sean L. Preston BSc MB BS MRCP, Histopathology Unit, Cancer Research UK, London, UK, and Department of Histopathology, Barts and the London Queen Mary's School of Medicine and Dentistry, London, UK

Richard Poulsom BSc PhD MRCPath, Histopathology Unit, Cancer Research UK, London, UK

Malcolm R. Alison BSc PhD DSc FRCPath, Department of Histopathology, Imperial College, London, UK

Nicholas A. Wright MS DSc MD PhD FRCP FRCS FRCPath FMedSci, Histopathology Unit, Cancer Research UK, London, UK and Department of Histopathology, Barts and the London Queen Mary's School of Medicine and Dentistry, London, UK

pigs and mice. We have also marvelled at the possibilities of 'therapeutic cloning' and wondered when such technology would come up with the goods, in the form of custom-made islets of Langerhans or kidneys for transplantation. And we have heard, with some consternation, apparently validated claims that cell populations, such as those in the bone marrow, long regarded as a tissue wholly committed to maintaining the blood vascular system, can colonise other tissues, giving rise to neurones, hepatocytes and renal tubular cells. Such tenets assault the bastions of the biology we were taught as students and trainee pathologists and naturally have distinct repercussions when we consider tumour histogenesis.

Previous work has explored the therapeutic potential of embryonic stem (ES) cells in an attempt to exploit the pluripotent nature of these cells. This has stimulated heated debate and raised huge ethical dilemmas. However, there is now evidence that certain adult, differentiated organ-specific stem cells have the ability to jump lineage boundaries and generate completely new types of cells. The evidence for this adult stem cell plasticity usually depends on the appearance of Y-chromosome-positive cells in a female recipient of a bone marrow transplant from a male donor. Alternatively, other markers, such as *LacZ* or green fluorescent protein (GFP), have been used (Fig. 10.1) and these techniques are usually combined with immunohistochemically defined lineage markers in an attempt to show a switch in the fate (transdifferentiation) of the transplanted cells.

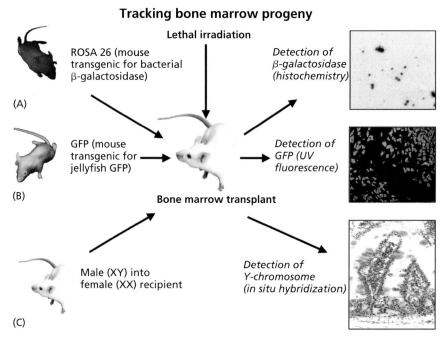

Tracking bone marrow progeny

Fig. 10.1 The techniques used to demonstrate transdifferentiation of transplanted cells. Donor-derived cells are detected via (A) detection of β-galactosidase activity (blue stain). ROSA26 transgenic mice express the enzyme *Escherichia coli* β-galactosidase, encoded by the *LacZ* gene. Following ROSA26 bone marrow transplantation into wild-type mice, donor cells can be detected by X-gal histochemistry. (B) Detection of GFP. GFP transgenic mice express green fluorescent protein. Following bone marrow transplantation into wild-type mice, this protein can be detected by its fluorescence in UV light. (C) Detection of the Y-chromosome following transplantation of male donor bone marrow into female recipients. Reproduced with permission from Ref. [190]. © The Biochemical Society and the Medical Research Society.

These phenomena focus our attention on stem cells and, thus, research in stem cell biology is indeed very topical. This was not always so and workers in this field over the last 30 years have felt isolated, tilling a hard and often barren pasture. But pathologists, an enlightened and far-seeing species, in their contributions to tumour histogenesis, and to the growth phenomena that accompany repair and regeneration, have always acknowledged the important role of stem cells in these processes.

In this chapter, we propose to discuss how the new stem cell biology has impacted on how pathologists view tissue and organ regeneration and repair, and how such advances might alter the way we treat some of these conditions in the future.

WHAT ARE STEM CELLS?

The time-honoured definition is that stem cells are cells with considerable proliferative potential and capable of giving rise to a large family of descendants. In normal circumstances, for example, the human small intestinal epithelium renews itself every 7 days or so; thus, intestinal stem cells have to keep providing the precursors of these epithelial cells every week for many years. Yet a situation in experimental pathology really brings this message home. Mice who have lost both alleles of the gene encoding for fumaryl acetoacetate hydrolase (FAH) develop a condition similar to Type I tyrosinaemia in humans. The ensuing liver damage kills them within about 3 months (mark this model well, since we will return to it, importantly, later). However, if syngeneic normal liver cells – wild-type hepatocytes – are transplanted into these diseased animals, they rescue the mice from a grisly end in liver failure.[1,2] Moreover, if the transplanted wild-type cells express a marker gene, such as *LacZ* (which makes the cells express β-galactosidase, which can be made to turn blue), the blue cells can be seen colonising the diseased liver. This procedure can be carried out a number of times, with the progeny of the original wild-type cells colonising the livers and rescuing successive animals (Fig. 10.2). This underlines the tremendous proliferative potential of this hepatocyte stem cell population.

A second property of stem cells is usually held to be their capacity to produce several different cell lineages – *multilineage differentiation*. This property may not be a prerequisite as illustrated by our friend, the hepatocyte. While undoubtedly capable of sustained proliferation, as we have seen above, it apparently produces only one lineage. Thirdly, mindful that in experimental or indeed therapeutic circumstances, stem cells might find themselves in different anatomical sites, others have added the property of *engraftment*. This might be thought, at first sight, a bit artificial but need not be so if we adopt the somewhat heretical concept that there is a circulating pool of uncommitted stem cells, which engraft any damaged organ and differentiate into lineages specific for that organ. More of this will be discussed later.

Stem cells are a small fraction of the total population, for example the four to five stem cells at the bottom of an intestinal crypt,[3] and are relatively undifferentiated. They are self-maintaining, dividing to replenish the stem cell pool as well as contributing to the transit-amplifying population, which in turn contributes to the resident tissue. Moreover, they slowly cycle compared to the transit-amplifying

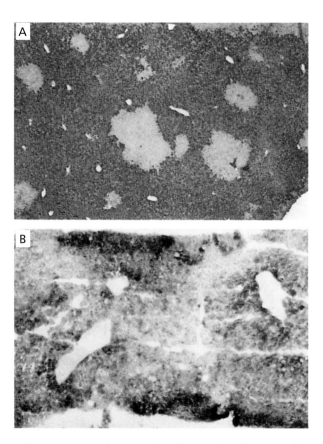

Fig. 10.2 Donor hepatocytes can be transplanted a number of times and have the ability to rescue successive animals. Figure 10.2 illustrates donor-derived cells: (A) after transplantation of FAH-positive donor hepatocytes into FAH-deficient recipients, approximately 80% of hepatocytes were found to express FAH by histochemistry. This sample was taken after the sixth round of serial transplantation. (B) β-galactosidase staining of a frozen section of mutant FAH$^{-/-}$ mice during the fourth round of serial transplantation. The blue staining is indicative of β-galactosidase activity and thus repopulation by transplanted, not revertant, endogenous hepatocytes. From Ref. [1] with permission of the American Society for Investigative Pathology.

cells, avoiding rapid rounds of cell division, which in turn can increase the risk of incorporating errors into the stem cell population.

There are different sorts of stem cells, and we should really try to classify them. A reasonable way forward, in the mammalian situation, might be:

- pluripotent stem cells, such as ES cells and embryonic germ (EG) cells;
- organ-specific stem cells, such as bone marrow or intestinal stem cells;
- mesenchymal stem cells (MSCs).

We should consider all three.

PLURIPOTENT STEM CELLS

ES cells are pluripotent stem cells derived from the inner cell mass of the blastocyst,[4] while EG cells are derived from presumptive gonadal tissue in early embryos. These cells have more or less unlimited self-renewal potential and theoretically, at any rate, are capable of differentiation into any tissue in the body. These cells were initially derived from mouse embryos, but now primate and even human cell lines are available,[5,6] although your access to these obviously depends on where in the world you live. The simple way of demonstrating the pluripotency of ES cells is to introduce them into a mouse blastocyst, where the ES cell line can be seen to contribute to all the tissues of the resulting chimaera, if the embryo is allowed to develop.[7] Moreover, post-natal animals transplanted with ES and EG cells develop teratomas, again emphasising their ability to contribute to all three germ layers.[8]

ES and EG cells, unless transplanted as described above, can be kept in culture as cell lines in an undifferentiated state. This state appears to be maintained by expression of a number of transcription factors, which are probably important in determining cell fate in early embryos. Practically speaking, ES and EG cell lines are grown on feeder layers of fibroblasts themselves derived from foetal tissues, which contribute factors (such as leukaemia inhibitory factor (LIF)) to the medium. If these factors are removed, or growth factors (such as retinoic acid) are added, then the cells differentiate into derivatives of all three germ layers, such as neuroectodermal or cardiomyocyte lineages.[9,10] Indeed, it is through the understanding and manipulation of such differentiation switches that we hope to exploit this property, growing lung lobes, pancreatic islets and other tissues for transplantation.

ORGAN-SPECIFIC STEM CELLS

When analysed closely, most tissues contain a stem cell population. It is now clear that not only do the constantly renewing tissues (such as the bone marrow, the epidermis and the gastrointestinal mucosa) contain stem cells, but solid, parenchymal organs (such as the liver) also contain stem cell systems. These are often complex. In tissues such as the bone marrow and intestine, stem cells are thought to be housed in a *niche*. A niche is a conceptual or indeed anatomical microenvironment, which is thought to help maintain the stem cell(s) in the undifferentiated state[11] (Fig. 10.3). If the progeny of stem cells leave the niche, then they become committed to differentiation – for example, they would become myeloid or erythroid precursors in the marrow or goblet cell precursors in the intestine.[3] As well as providing these precursors, the stem cells must maintain their numbers, so that, on average at any rate, each stem cell division is asymmetric, providing one cell for differentiation and one for the stem cell pool, which remains in the niche. It is possible that the niche, towards the bottom of the intestinal crypt or on the endosteal surface of the medullary cavity, in some way modulates the symmetry of stem cell divisions.

Figure 10.3 shows a conceptual diagram of the niche in the intestinal crypt. The crypt is very closely encased in a dense but fenestrated meshwork of myofibroblasts, the so-called *pericryptal myofibroblast sheath,* which is thought to help form the niche. There is evidence that a good deal of cross-talk goes on between the pericryptal fibroblasts and the epithelial cells; the myofibroblasts express growth factors, such as keratinocyte growth factor (KGF) and hepatocyte growth factor (HGF), the receptors for which are found on the epithelial cells. It has recently been proposed that other growth factors, such as glucagon-like peptide 2 (GLP-2),

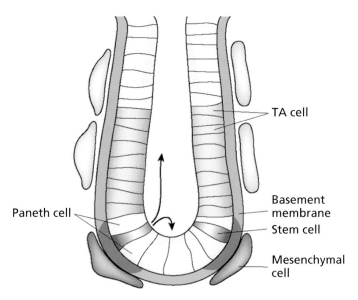

Fig. 10.3 The intestinal stem cell niche. TA cell: transit-amplifying cell. Reprinted by permission from Ref. [11]: Nature; © 2001 Macmillan Publishers Ltd.

a potent mitogen for intestinal epithelial cells, is secreted by enteroendocrine cells and through its interaction with enteric neurones promotes differentiation down the enterocyte rather than the secretory (Paneth, endocrine, goblet) lineages.[12]

As well as self-renewal, multilineage differentiation is also a property of many organ-specific stem cells and there is now abundant emerging evidence that some stem cells are indeed pluripotent (see below). In a now classic experiment, when bone marrow was used to re-constitute lethally irradiated mice, colonies of cells appeared in the spleen which contain all blood cell lineages.[13] These colonies came from one cell clearly demonstrating the multipotentiality of some marrow stem cells. The haematopoietic stem cell (HSC) has now been characterised on the basis of its cell surface markers,[14] its operational behaviour, as seen above and in everyday clinical practice. Human bone marrow transplantation results in donor colonisation of the host tissues with new erythroid, granulocyte, macrophage, megakaryocyte and lymphoid lineages in immune compromised mice, again illustrating the multipotential nature of bone marrow.[15] HSCs also form multiple lineages *in vitro*.[16]

In the intestine, crypts and gastric glands have been shown to be a clonal population (i.e. derived from one cell during histogenesis) in animals and man, and in adult life are maintained as clonal populations.[17] Single colorectal carcinoma cells also show trilineage differentiation – into goblet, endocrine and colonocyte lineages.[18] Thus, gut stem cells are multipotent and, as in the bone marrow, give rise to differentiated progeny, via committed precursor cells[3] (see Wright[19] and Brittan and Wright,[20] for reviews).

In the epidermis, things are quite complex. It was previously thought that the epidermal stem cells were found in the papillae of the interfollicular epidermis, where the so-called 'integrin-bright cells' are housed and which give rise to

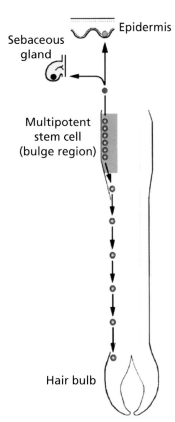

Sebaceous gland

Epidermis

Multipotent stem cell (bulge region)

Hair bulb

Fig. 10.4 The stem cell niche in the mouse skin. Multipotent stem cells are located in the upper region of the vibrissal (whisker) follicle. They may migrate to the upper part of the follicle to generate sebaceous glands and epidermis and to the hair bulb to generate the hair lineages. Reprinted from Ref. [22]; © 2001 with permission from Elsevier Science.

colonies with extended growth *in vitro*.[21] However recent work has concentrated on the hair follicle as a source of skin stem cells. It is now realised that the hair bulge is an important stem cell niche and from here cells migrate in quite a convoluted manner to populate the hair follicle and indeed the adjacent epidermis[22] (see Fig. 10.4). Conceptually, at any rate, there could be considerable lateral migration into the interfollicular epidermis, as seen in the cornea, where the stem cells are found in the limbus, and from here, there is lateral cell migration to populate the whole of the corneal epithelial sheet.[23]

There are two main epithelial cell populations in the liver, the hepatocytes and the cholangiocytes, the cells lining the bile ducts (Fig. 10.5). It is a matter of everyday observation that the resting liver shows few if any mitoses and few cells are in cycle. After we induce damage, however, for example by a partial hepatectomy, all hepatocytes enter the cell cycle and complete several rounds of cell division, making good the deficit. The bile duct epithelial cells also divide, slightly later than the hepatocytes. There is a further stem cell system, which is seen particularly in circumstances where the hepatocytes are prevented from entering the cell cycle, for example after carcinogen treatment. 'Oval cells', so called because of their shape, emerge from the region of the terminal bile ducts and begin to proliferate in the periportal areas (Fig. 10.6). In this situation, the oval cells are bi-potential, and can differentiate into hepatocytes and bile duct epithelial cells.[24] The liver then has two indiginous systems and, while it is commonplace to see hepatocytes proliferating in numbers after acute liver damage

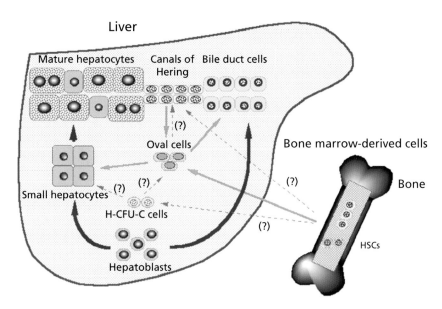

Fig. 10.5 The stem cell compartments in the mouse liver and the interaction between hepatic stem cells. Thick blue arrows show the major stream of hepatic development and the red arrows represent emergent routes. Dotted arrows are other routes for which convincing results are not yet available. Hepatocyte-colony forming units in culture (H-CFU-C) (c-Kit⁻/CD45⁻/TER119⁻) cells were isolated from murine foetal liver cells and express hepatic and bile ductular markers, and have been proposed as hepatic stem cells.[185] Reprinted from Ref. [186]; © 2001 with permission from Elsevier Science.

in man, oval cell reactions are rare in human pathology but are now being described.[25]

It seems natural indeed that the foetal and neonatal brain should contain stem cells that become active at the time of neurogenesis and at this time neural stem cells (NSCs) are concentrated in the subventricular zone (SVZ).[26] However, it is surprising that such stem cells continue to be present in the *adult* human brain, where they can be seen to be proliferating and to produce neurones and glia *in vitro*.[27,28] Moreover, when foetal and indeed adult neural cells are transplanted into the adult brain, they can give rise to both neurones and glia.[29]

MESENCHYMAL STEM CELLS

There has been considerable recent interest in these cells, and particularly in those found in the bone marrow. Our attention was first drawn to these interesting cells by the work of Fridenshtein,[30] who first demonstrated that aspirates of bone marrow contain adherent fibroblast-like cells which can, in culture, form adipocytes and bone-forming cells. These marrow-derived mesenchymal cells have now been purified, starting with the adherent population, and differentiation into chondrocytes, osteoblasts, adipocytes and even skeletal muscle cells has been noted.[31–33] It is possible to expand these cells many times *in vitro*, and when they are transplanted into animals appear to form cartilage and bone;[32] similar results have also been reported in humans.[34]

Of course, there are mesenchymal cell populations in most tissues of the body and not just the bone marrow. We have discussed above the pericryptal

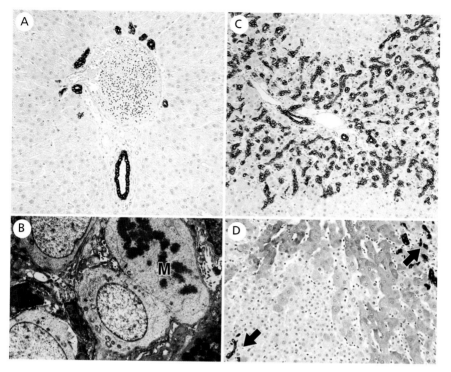

Fig. 10.6 Hepatic stem cell activation in the rat liver. (A) Normal rat liver immunostained for CK19 to highlight biliary epithelia. Note that all positive cells are within or very close to the portal tract. (B) After hepatocyte loss in a liver where hepatocyte regeneration is compromised, oval cells increase in number – an electron micrograph of oval cells with one in mitosis (M). (C) Oval cell reaction in which the biliary cells form branching ducts radiating from the portal tract (CK 19 immunostain). (D) The biliary cells observed in (C) eventually differentiate into hepatocytes that have not yet acquired the cytochrome P450 immunoreactivity of the older and larger hepatocytes; residual ductular structures are still apparent (arrows). Reproduced from Ref. [187]; © John Wiley & Sons with permission.

myofibroblasts in the intestine and there are other examples of important populations of similar cells, such as the stellate cells of the liver and the pancreas, which are critical in the pathogenesis of fibrosis in these organs. Are there separate MSCs for each of these organs, or is it possible that such populations are fed by, and are in equilibrium with, MSCs in the bone marrow? We shall return to this fascinating possibility later on.

The fact that adult MSCs can be expanded *in vitro* and stimulated to form bone, cartilage, tendon, muscle or fat cells makes them attractive for tissue engineering and gene therapy strategies.[32] However, study of MSC plasticity may be hampered by bias introduced when these cells are acquired and/or cultured.[35,36] Despite these problems, techniques used *in vivo* to study these cells have involved intravenous injection of MSCs into the circulation. These studies have supported the plasticity of these cells showing engraftment into many tissue types, for example the brain,[37] where, following the transplantation of labelled MSCs, donor-derived cells in the brain show morphological differentiation and neurone-specific markers. Importantly, these injected MSCs are incorporated into the bone marrow and it is here that they may act as a reservoir of stem cells, which may ultimately engraft into multiple organs.

BONE MARROW

Adult bone marrow is special; it contains HSCs and MSCs. HSCs are a rare but well-characterised subset of the bone marrow stem cell compartment. They are predominantly immature cells that lack the markers of differentiated haemato-poietic cells and are recognised by the presence of various cell surface markers, such as the sialomucin CD34, a highly conserved cell surface marker which has been shown to be downregulated as the HSC matures.[38,39] These cell surface markers have been utilised to extract/obtain enriched samples using techniques such as fluorescence-activated cell sorting (FACS).

HSCs are found in niches within the bone marrow. These niches provide all the factors required to maintain their viability and function.[40–43] Their survival and proliferation *in vivo* is dependent on an intimate association with bone marrow stroma. Bone marrow stroma contains MSCs and their derivatives which provide signals (soluble and adhesive) to support HSCs[40,44–46] including cytokines (e.g. IL-4), chemokines and growth factors (e.g. G-CSF).[47,48]

What factors promote the homing and migration of HSCs? Following bone marrow transplantation, the initial fate of donor HSCs is to home to the bone mar-row niche, which is able to support them and allow their survival. This process of homing and engraftment is incompletely understood but is thought to be a highly complex mechanism involving adhesion molecules and their receptors (e.g. c-Kit). c-Kit allows HSCs to adhere to the stroma via membrane-associated stem cell factor (SCF). Another important factor is the integrin family;[49] recent studies have shown that β-1 integrin is fundamental to the migration of HSCs to the foetal liver.[50] Chemokines are also implicated in the homing of HSCs – for example, transgenic mice without the chemokine SDF1 or its receptor are unable to transfer haematopoiesis from the embryonal liver to bone marrow.[51] There is also evidence to suggest that the bone marrow engraftment after transplantation is not a random process.[52]

Other signals are also thought to be important. G-CSF is an agent capable of mobilising HSCs and is used in a clinical setting to mobilise HSCs prior to their harvesting for transplantation.[43] The *selectins* are also implicated in HSC function and there is interesting evidence that recruitment of HSCs to areas of damage may be facilitated by these molecules. This cell signal may be part of the drive behind the directionality of stem cell trafficking.[40,43]

The proposed plasticity of bone marrow-derived cells is very exciting. Various studies have looked at this using both whole bone marrow and with efforts to separate the various bone marrow constituents. Isolated HSCs have been shown to have potential to transdifferentiate. Importantly, Krause *et al.*[53] showed that a single HSC could engraft into epithelial cells of the liver, lung, gastrointestinal tract and skin and, in addition, observations in humans have also supported this possibility[54,55] (Fig. 10.7), although other studies have suggested that these events are rare.[56]

Bone marrow transplantation is a technique already extensively used in clini-cal practice. It is a well-proven technique and it is exciting to speculate that stem

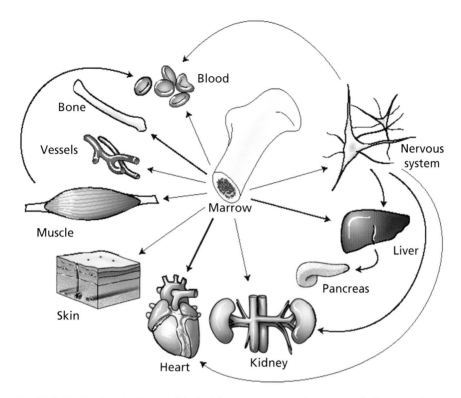

Fig. 10.7 Studies in mice have yielded evidence to suggest that stem cells from a variety of tissues can produce progeny in different organs. Reprinted with permission from Ref. [188]; © 2002 American Association for the Advancement of Science. Illustration by G. Slayden.

cell transplantation could ultimately be used to introduce cells that then migrate to areas of damage and proliferate resulting in functional healing/organ regeneration or, alternatively, to act as vectors for drugs or gene therapy.

SIDE-POPULATION CELLS

Apart from characterising whole bone marrow by separating its constituents using cell surface markers, FACS has revealed a smaller population of cells within the bone marrow on the basis of its ability to exclude fluorescent dyes.[14] This small population is now known as the side population (SP) and characterisation by virtue of cell surface markers has now revealed that these cells in the mouse have a largely similar phenotype to c-Kit$^+$, lin$^-$, Sca1$^+$ (KLS) cells. These cells have now been demonstrated in other species including humans.[57,58]

The SP are interesting as in some circumstances they appear to lack the HSC marker CD34.[59] This suggests that these cells may be uncommitted to haematopoeitic lineages, may be more primitive and, therefore, be able to differentiate into both MSC and HSC lineages.[60] SP cells appear to be able to exclude xenobiotic molecules by virtue of a number of drug efflux membrane transporter proteins and this property may confer a valuable survival advantage.[61]

THE CARDIOVASCULAR SYSTEM

There has been much debate as to the capacity of the heart to regenerate following injury. Although there is now evidence to suggest that the heart is not a terminally differentiated organ and that cardiac stem cells exist,[62] their capacity for regeneration appears to be limited. Nevertheless, cardiac disease is a massive problem and even now the treatment of myocardial infarction and end-stage cardiac failure is limited. There is now evidence emerging to suggest that there is an alternative route by which damaged cardiomyocytes and cardiac endothelium can be repaired. This work is exploring the role of adult stem cells in the heart and vascular system and may ultimately have considerable implications for the treatment of disorders in these organs.

In the vascular system, circulating endothelial progenitor cells have a key role in the repair of damaged endothelium and contribute to neovascularisation. There is *in vitro* evidence to show that circulating cells with cell surface markers also common to HSC can have the capacity to differentiate into endothelial cells.[63] These circulating progenitor cells have also in turn shown to be bone marrow derived.[64] In animal models, circulating endothelial progenitor cells appear to be mobilised by ischaemic injury or cytokine therapy[65] and integrate into new vessels, for example in the heart and skeletal muscle.[66] These cells may be harvested from peripheral blood[67] and can facilitate the repair of injured tissue.[68]

The evidence for recipient-derived cells with a degree of plasticity is not only restricted to animal models. There are also observations in humans following sex-mismatched transplants that support incorporation of recipient-derived/circulating precursors into the donor endothelium. As early as 1969, recipient arterial endothelial cells were reported to engraft into renal transplants.[69] This engraftment of small renal vessels appears to be a sporadic occurrence that is enhanced by graft damage.[70] The degree of engraftment appears to be related to the severity of the vascular rejection.[71] Poulsom *et al.*[72] have reported the occasional recipient-derived endothelial cell in sex-mismatched human renal transplants, but the evidence is mixed and other studies have failed to show endothelial engraftment even in the face of organ failure.[73] The glomerular endothelium appears to be different and to date recipient-derived endothelium has not been reported in engrafted donor kidneys.[70,71,73]

In the larger vessels (e.g. the aorta) there are further reports of host endothelium engrafting into donor tissue,[69,74] although this engraftment is less pronounced when the recipient is immunosuppressed. Similarly, in human liver transplantation, portal and hepatic veins show recipient-derived cells and following bone marrow transplantation in mice similar endothelial engraftment is seen[75] again suggesting that there are cells with endothelial plasticity residing in the bone marrow.

Following myocardial infarction necrotic cardiomyocytes are removed, granulation tissue forms and neovascularisation occurs. There is now some evidence to suggest that a population of cardiac myocytes then divide within the heart.[62] The natural history of the infarct is then for a process of remodelling to occur with subsequent scarring. The scarring and its sequelae can result in deteriorating cardiac function and heart failure. In considering stem cells and the heart, it is important to consider both cardiomyocytes and the vasculature, since the neo-vascularisation and cardiomyocyte regeneration are both required to improve cardiac function in this setting.

There is some evidence to suggest that it is possible to improve revascularisation in injured myocardium. There is animal model evidence to suggest injection of bone marrow cells can promote angiogenesis in damaged heart muscle and improved cardiac function.[76] The improved cardiac function appears to be due in part to revascularisation of the heart. Following left anterior descending artery ligation and transplantation of adult human bone marrow-derived cells into rats, new human capillaries are found within the infarct that improved the survival of rat myocytes.[77] This is supported by work in patients with chronic myeloid leukaemia; in these patients endothelial cells with the leukaemic translocation (i.e. bone marrow derived) were found. In addition, following bone marrow transplantation some endothelial cells were found that appeared to originate from the therapeutic graft.[78]

Cardiomyocytes themselves have a limited capacity for self-renewal but this appears to be maximal in areas adjacent to infarcted myocardium.[62] Improved cardiac function has been achieved by transplanting cells directly into the damaged myocardium. The main question that arises from this is which are the best cells to implant and can they have a similar effect if transplanted peripherally? There is some work involving ES cells,[79] but more excitingly there is evidence that adult bone marrow-derived stem cells can contribute to the regeneration of cardiomyocytes. Adult mouse MSC can generate spontaneously beating cardiomyocytes in culture.[80] Orlic et al. have shown that bone marrow can generate endothelial cells, smooth muscle cells and cardiomyocytes.[81–83] In vivo, bone marrow-derived MSCs have been shown to stably engraft into myocardial scar tissue in the rat when treated with 5-azacytidine after cryoprobe-induced infarction.[76] In addition, haematopoietic SP stem cells can differentiate into cardiomyocytes and endothelial cells in the context of ischaemic injury in mice.[84] Other supportive evidence for cardiomyocyte engraftment comes from other mouse studies where host and recipient tissues can be differentiated. For example, in dystrophic female mice following wild-type male donor bone marrow transplantation not only were Y-chromosome-positive muscle fibres found in the heart but these fibres were seen to express myogenic proteins.[85] It is not only bone marrow that appears to have the capacity to differentiate into cardiomyocytes, but labelled cultured liver cells have also been shown to develop cardiomyocyte phenotype after intracardiac injection.[86] Nevertheless, the evidence is mixed and some other groups have been unable to detect bone marrow-derived cardiomyocytes,[77,87] although even in these groups bone marrow transplantation has reduced ventricular remodelling by improving angiogenesis as described above.

There is now more work emerging suggesting these processes are relevant to humans. In sex-mismatched cardiac transplants a number of cardiomyocytes, coronary arterioles and capillaries have been identified as being of recipient origin.[88] Strauer et al. treated a patient with acute myocardial infarction with primary angioplasty and autologous bone marrow transplantation into the coronary arteries. A functional benefit was documented following this but the histological correlate of engraftment and transdifferentation is yet to be described.[89] Will we one day see the acute myocardial infarct treated with thrombolytic therapy in conjunction with stem cell transplantation to promote cardiac angiogenesis and replenish cardiomyocytes? This question remains unanswered as do the potential problems with stem cell transplantation in this setting. Do the cells engraft in the appropriate place? Do they integrate with functioning host cardiomyocytes? What is the longevity of the transplant? Fascinating questions for the future!

LUNG

There are stem cells within the lung with the capacity to proliferate and produce functional progeny after injury. These stem cells appear to be partially committed and in the lung the proliferative populations differ according to anatomical site; the trachea and bronchus are thought to be repopulated by basal and tracheal ductal cells, while the Clara cell is the proliferative cell of the bronchiole[90] and the Type II pneumocyte is the proliferative cell of the alveolus that can give rise to Type I pneumocytes. The evidence for this comes from a variety of studies, mainly in mice and has recently been reviewed.[91]

But what about lung stem cells originating from outside the lung? There is evidence to suggest that bone marrow-derived cells can engraft into the lung. Janes *et al.* found that following sex-mismatched whole bone marrow transplant donor-derived Y-chromosome-positive cells were found in the lung parenchyma.[92] Krause *et al.*'s study, in which single HSCs were successfully engrafted into lethally irradiated mice, demonstrated donor-derived epithelial cells in the lung[53] (Fig. 10.8), an observation that cannot be explained by trapping of transplanted

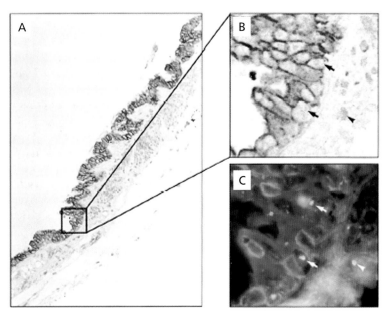

Fig. 10.8 Donor-derived epithelial cells found in the lung following transplantation of a single male donor cell.[53] (A,B) Brochus stained with CAM 5.2 (specific for cytokeratins 8, 18 and 19). Epithelial cells are positive with dim cytoplasmic and dark membranous staining. In (B) the arrows indicate Y-chromosome-positive epithelial cells. On the right a Y-chromosome-positive cell not stained with CAM 5.2 is probably a stromal cell or a cell of haemopoietic lineage. (C) FISH for Y-chromosome (pseudocoloured pale yellow green) with DAPI (blue) nuclear counterstain. Y-chromosomes are marked with white arrows. Reprinted from Ref. [53]; © 2001 with permission from Elsevier Science.

cells alone. Importantly, this study showed differentiation to Type II pneumo-cytes – the apparent stem cell of the alveolus. Kotton et al.[93] reported somewhat different findings following the intravenous injection of bone marrow-derived cells into mice treated with intra-tracheal bleomycin. The lung was the only organ with significant engraftment and only Type I pneumocytes of donor origin were seen. This could have been because the Type I pneumocytes were the cells that were maximally damaged at the time of bone marrow transplantation or could be due to a different population of bone marrow being transplanted, but such findings are difficult to explain if the Type II pneumocyte is indeed the stem cell for the alveolar epithelium, unless the HSC takes its place.

There is as yet little evidence that bone marrow stem cell transdifferentiation occurs in human lung and a number of questions remain to be answered; is the engraftment seen in animals related to stem cell trapping in the lung in any way? Is this process seen as the lung is damaged by the lethal irradiation required prior to bone marrow transplantation? Are there other models of acute lung damage that can promote engraftment?

GASTROINTESTINAL TRACT

The gastrointestinal tract is subject to continual chemical and mechanical stress and, to maintain gut structure and function, there is a continual turnover of cells: the epithelium is replaced every 2–7 days. This repopulation is in turn dependent on the presence of gastrointestinal stem cells – multipotential cells capable of giving rise to all gut cell lineages.[19] These cells are difficult to identify as there are no specific stem cell markers, but histologically undifferentiated cells with the capacity to repopulate the epithelium are found at defined sites in the gut. In the gastric epithelium these cells are found just below the neck/isthmus of the gland, and in the intestine these cells are found close to the crypt base.[94]

The stem cells within the gut have remarkable regenerative capacity and indeed, following radiation injury, a single surviving gut stem cell can regenerate a whole crypt as is shown by its clonality. However, there also appears to be a bone marrow/gut axis that could contribute to the repopulation of gut stem cells and, therefore, gut structure in the face of injury. Krause et al.[53] reported that 0.19–1.81% of cells within the gastrointestinal tract were HSC derived and strongly resembled, for example, absorptive villus epithelial cells, columnar oesophageal epithelium and gastric pit cells. However, it must be remembered that the mice in this study required lethal irradiation prior to bone marrow transplantation and, therefore, a significant degree of gut injury was inflicted. Gastrointestinal epithelial engraftment has also been noted in humans after sex-mismatched peripheral blood stem cell transplantation;[95] in addition, significant epithelial engraftment has been noted by Okamoto et al. in cases of graft versus disease (GVHD) after male bone marrow transplantation into female recipients.[96] Rather than epithelial engraftment, Brittan et al.[97] found that, following whole bone marrow transplantation in mice and humans, pericryptal myofibroblasts in the small intestine and colon were bone marrow-derived. Myofibroblasts are ubiquitous cells with some of the properties of fibroblasts and smooth muscle cells. They have a key role in development and healing and can produce collagens and other matrix proteins. In the intestine they form a fenestrated sheath around the crypt and also have a barrier function. When over-activated they can contribute to scarring and fibrosis in the gut and other organs.[98,99]

There is also evidence that stem cells derived from other organs can be coaxed toward gastrointestinal lineages. Foetal liver stem cells can be encouraged not only to maintain their population and differentiate into hepatocytes, but in addition if transplanted into the duodenal wall can form villus and crypt epithelial cells.[100] Studies involving mouse–chick aggregation chimeras have shown that even adult NSCs can apparently form gut. When mouse–chick aggregation chimeras are created by injecting adult mouse NSCs into chick embryos 12% of embryos contained cells derived from the mouse. These mouse cells were found in the heart, lung, liver and intestine of the progeny[101] illustrating the capacity for adult cells to become part of all three germ layers in the correct environment.

This work illustrates the role of stem cells in the gut and also suggests how, in the face of damage, there is potentially an extra reserve in the form of the bone marrow and other stem cells which have the capacity to assist in gastrointestinal repair. How might stem cell transplantation have a role in the treatment of disorders of the gut? Bone marrow-derived myofibroblasts are deeply engrafted into the intestinal wall and have a role in fibrosis. Their over-activation may be implicated in the fibrosis of Crohn's disease. Stem cell transplantation may allow targeting of therapy (e.g. cells carrying an anti-fibrotic cytokine gene) to areas of disease in this setting. The role of stem cell transplantation in this and other diseases of the gastrointestinal tract (e.g. colitis and cancer) remain to be investigated but may provide exciting possibilities.

LIVER

The liver is an organ with massive proliferative capacity; following partial hepatectomy liver mass is rapidly restored by cell proliferation – only one to two cycles are required to restore liver mass after a two-thirds partial hepatectomy. This proliferative capacity is essential if the liver is to survive the constant chemical insult it may be subjected to, in the form of alcohol, hepatitis virus infection and other hepatotoxic agents. To combat these there are three major sources of stem cells that could contribute to this regeneration – hepatocytes, cholangiocytes and bone marrow-derived cells.[102]

Hepatocytes are cells with a great proliferative capacity. Although it appears that simple cell division of hepatocytes can result in restoration of liver mass after injury, some hepatocytes may be deserving of being labelled as stem cells, being capable of producing a large family of descendants. In mice, transplanted hepatocytes are capable of significant clonal expansion[1] illustrating the potential of transplanted hepatocytes for treatment of intractable liver disease. Cholangiocytes form a potential stem cell compartment that is available in the face of massive liver damage. These *potential stem cells* are in the form of a population of 'oval cells' in the terminal branches of the intrahepatic biliary tree. In the face of massive injury these cells proliferate and then differentiate into hepatocytes.[103–106] Oval cells proliferate forming arborising ducts prior to differentiating into hepatocytes (Fig. 10.6) and this process is also documented in humans where the response is proportional to the injury sustained.[25] Interestingly, oval cells have cell surface markers, such as c-Kit, Thy-1, flt-3 and CD34, in common with HSCs.[107–110]

This brings us to the third and most recently considered source of hepatocytes – the bone marrow. In addition to all the tissues already mentioned, bone marrow-derived cells have been seen to differentiate into hepatocytes. The initial evidence for bone marrow stem cells differentiating into hepatocytes came from Petersen et al.,[111] who treated female rats with lethal irradiation followed by male bone marrow transplantation. These animals were administered a regime of hepatotoxic agent designed to promote hepatic necrosis and inhibit hepatic regeneration. Following this, Y-chromosome-positive oval cells were seen at day 9 and hepatocytes at day 13 consistent with the natural history of liver repair following an insult. Sex-mismatched transplantation has also been used by other groups to show the bone marrow derivation of hepatocytes in mice[112] and observations in humans support these findings.[54,55] Krause et al.[53] also found donor-derived cholangiocytes when they transplanted a single male HSC into female recipients. Engraftment appears to be a continuous process, which is upregulated in the face of liver damage. This upregulation is seen in samples taken from patients following sex-mismatched liver transplantation with ongoing liver injury.[55] Increased hepatocyte chimerism is noted in those with recurrent hepatitis after liver transplantation.[113] There have also been proposals as to how the homing of HSC might be achieved, but the mechanisms involved await confirmation.[114]

Importantly, as already mentioned, the engrafted bone marrow-derived cells appear to have significant functional capacity at least in the FAH$^{-/-}$ mouse[2] (Fig. 10.9). As hepatocytes differentiate and replicate, they become polyploid. Following sex-mismatched bone marrow transplantation with male HSCs, polyploid Y-chromosome-positive hepatocytes are found – consistent with normal function.[115]

There is currently a shortage of transplantable livers with an ongoing demand to support/cure patients with end-stage liver disease due to toxins, infections, metabolic disorders and inflammatory conditions, to name but a few. This ongoing

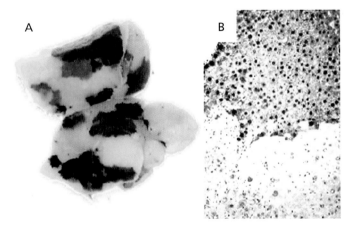

Fig. 10.9 Repopulating liver nodules following bone marrow transplantation into FAH$^{-/-}$ mice. Liver of the FAH$^{-/-}$ mice 7 months after bone marrow transplantation from ROSA26/129SvJ mice. (A) Repopulating nodules are stained blue. (B) FAH staining of the nodule. The dark red areas are FAH-positive hepatocytes and are adjacent to FAH-negative areas. Reproduced from Ref. [2] with permission.

pressure is driving the search for alternative methods to help those individuals. The demonstrated proliferative capacity of hepatic stem cells and bone marrow-derived cells offers a potential route to support hepatic function.

Thus, stem cell transplantation offers a number of exciting avenues for exploration. Metabolic disorders, such as hereditary tyrosinaemia, may benefit from stem cell transplantation, and other metabolic disorders, such as the Crigler–Najjar syndrome, in which there is failure of bilirubin conjugation also have their own animal models. Hepatocyte transplantation experiments have already shown an improvement in conjugation capacity[116] in rats and this has been replicated in humans with some success.[117] Transplantation techniques may also be developed with a view to manipulating HSCs to supplement whole organ/partial organ transplant. They may be used to expedite organ regeneration in the face of a single toxic insult or may be used in conjunction with extra-corporeal liver-replacement therapies (such as the molecular-adsorbent recycling system (MARS) or bioartificial liver (BAL)[118]) as holding measures, while the liver regenerates or in those unfit for surgery.

Stem cell transplantation may be used as a vehicle to target drugs and therapeutic genes to the liver, such as interferons in hepatitis B and anti-inflammatory cytokines in autoimmune disease. Functional repopulation may offer cures for haemophilia. These exciting areas await exploration.

PANCREAS

The pancreas is composed of two components, the exocrine portion organised into acini and secretory ducts and the endocrine portion organised into islets of Langerhans. The islets contain the pancreatic β-cells and are responsible for plasma glucose homeostasis via the production of insulin. In diabetes mellitus, there is inadequate insulin production due to destruction or poor function of these pancreatic islets. Diabetes is a massive health problem, affecting 1% of the UK population. Stem cell transplantation could provide a possible solution. However, there are ongoing questions standing in the way of these developments. The exact nature of pancreatic stem cells is yet to be defined but there are several possible candidates.

Nestin (an intermediate filament) has been identified as a marker for NSCs.[119] Nestin-positive cells have been found in the islets and pancreatic ducts of adult rats which have the capacity to differentiate into pancreatic exocrine and endocrine cell types *ex vivo*.[120] These nestin-positive cells can even produce hepatocytes. Although these cells do not spontaneously produce the pancreatic islet hormones, they can be persuaded to do so by altering their growth factor exposure. Nestin-positive cells are widely distributed and they are considered a likely candidate for the pancreatic stem cell but their exact role awaits confirmation.

A second candidate pancreatic stem cell was reported by Guz *et al.*,[121] who treated mice with streptozotocin to destroy pancreatic islets. If the animals were supported by administration of exogenous insulin, they noted a proportion of regenerating islets and concluded this was secondary to β-cell neogenesis via precursor cell types, although this work cannot be considered conclusive.

Pancreatic oval cells have also been postulated as stem cells; hepatic oval cells are selectively stained by the antibody MAb 374.3, which also stains certain cells in the pancreatic duct, islets and acini.[122] These pancreatic oval cells have been documented in copper-deficient rats; however, copper supplementation results in their differentiation into hepatocytes and it is not clear if these represent true pancreatic stem cells.

Although the nature of true pancreatic stem cells is unclear, what is clear is that there is ongoing β-cell replication in adulthood[123] albeit at very low levels. It is now thought that the pancreatic duct cells act as functional stem cells. Pancreatic ducts appear to be the site of multipotential stem cells with the potential to generate endocrine and ductular cells phenotypes[124] when presented with a functional demand. Following partial pancreatectomy there is pancreatic regeneration, probably via two pathways: (1) replication of differentiated cells and (2) proliferation of ductules which then differentiate into both acini and islets.[125] Pancreatic ductal cells have a higher capacity to proliferate and differentiate than previously thought and, given the correct environment, they can be made to proliferate and, in some circumstances to form, functional islet β-cells.[126]

Thus, there are various candidates for pancreatic stem cells but functionally pancreatic ductules appear to be the most promising source of islet cells. There is evidence to support transdifferentiation of pancreatic cells into hepatocytes,[125] although this is perhaps unsurprising due to the close embryological derivation of the pancreas and liver. However, it is as yet unclear how this axis may be exploited to therapeutic effect. It is hoped that stem cell transplantation may result in the repopulation with functioning islets in Type II diabetics.

KIDNEY

Exploration and exploitation of stem cells in the kidney is also at an early stage. Similar to the pancreas, renal stem cells have not as yet been clearly identified. However, a degree of plasticity has already been noted; tubular cells have been shown to have the capacity to regenerate after injury and various studies have demonstrated both the plasticity of renal cells themselves as well as other stem cells in the body which may transdifferentiate into renal tissue.

In mice adult NSCs have been shown to transdifferentiate into renal cells when transplanted into early embryos.[101] Not only do adult cells have the ability to transdifferentiate into renal cells but there is considerable evidence to suggest that renal cells can transdifferentiate within the kidney. Strutz and Müller[127] have reviewed the evidence that transdifferentiation occurs between epithelial cells and fibroblasts; this phenomenon is most marked in damaged areas where there is disruption of cell contacts with the basement membrane[128] and is dependent on the cytokines and growth factors that are expressed locally. It is possible that, when injured, epithelial cells transdifferentiate into myofibroblasts and contribute to the interstitial fibrosis that marks terminal renal disease. Alternatively, myofibroblasts are recruited from an extra-renal circulating source, such as the bone marrow. These myofibroblasts may act to repair the basement membrane and may then be involved in a further transdifferentiation into epithelial cells or continue to function as myofibroblasts and begin the process of fibrosis and scarring. Evidence to support this hypothesis includes the observation that in the repair of renal tubules a population of vimentin-positive cells with myofibroblast morphology are seen to line the damaged tubules.[129] In addition to this, epithelial tubular cells and glomerular podocytes have already been shown to be bone marrow derived in mice.[72]

Work in humans has also demonstrated extra-renal involvement in kidney turnover. In adult male patients, who have been transplanted with female kidneys, male tubular epithelial cells have been seen[72] but others have not found similar engraftment.[73] In addition, myofibroblasts of recipient origin are also frequently found in the renal allografts of patients undergoing chronic rejection suggesting that a circulating population of cells have the capacity to migrate to and engraft in areas of inflammation.[130] Indeed, there is evidence to suggest that the bone marrow contributes to a circulating population of cells that are recruited to areas of damage in any site in the body where they begin to contribute to the process of healing and repair (unpublished work).

There are conditions, such as congenital nephropathy of Finnish type and Alport's syndrome, where progressive renal failure occurs. In nephropathy of the Finnish type there is an abnormality of podocyte structure and function. In Alport's syndrome there is an absence of Type IV collagen. Exploiting the bone marrow–renal axis could result in a functional repopulation of such kidneys. If exploited effectively, other conditions (such as obstructive uropathy, drug-induced nephropathy or acute tubular necrosis) could be aided.

NERVOUS SYSTEM

The adult central nervous system has a limited capacity to recover following injury. Despite this, there is evidence indicating ongoing neurogenesis in the adult and two areas where this is occurring have been identified: firstly, cells in the adult SVZ and secondly cells in the adult hippocampus. It has previously been shown that cells from the SVZ had trilineage potential and were capable of differentiating into astrocytes, oligodendrocytes or neurones.[26,131–133] In addition to this, an area in the dentate gyrus of the hippocampus in rats was identified where active neural cell proliferation and neurogenesis was thought to be occurring.[134,135] Even after death in humans, cells can be isolated which retain the capacity to form astrocytes and neurones.[136]

Further studies have shown there is also evidence that neural-derived stem cells have the capacity to transdifferentiate. Single NSCs are clonogenic and can form neurospheres that when injected into sublethally irradiated mice transdifferentiate into several haematopoetic lineages[137] but this has not been confirmed by others.[138] NSCs can also be manipulated to show features of myogenic differentiation.[101,139] However, this is not thought to be a common occurrence and appears only to apply in specific circumstances.

Non-neural tissues have cells that have the capacity to differentiate into neural cells. Sex-mismatched bone marrow transplantation studies have shown evidence of bone marrow-derived cells differentiating into neurones and glial cells.[140,141] Stromal cells may also show this capacity *in vitro*[142] and, thus, marrow stromal cells may ultimately have a role in transplantation to treat neurodegenerative diseases.

Despite the now apparent regenerative capacity of NSCs and the observed plasticity in other tissues, recovery from brain injury is a slow and often incomplete process and degenerative brain disorders are often treated supportively. There has been considerable effort into the use of stem cell transplantation to treat these conditions. To date the most successful approach has involved the use of foetal NSCs; patients with Parkinson's disease have already been treated with these cells, although success has been limited by the occurrence of dyskinesias in 15%.[143] Further work is ongoing looking into the use of immortalised and ES cells. Despite this, the work into the use of embryo/foetal-derived cells is beset with ethical and moral dilemmas and so work into the use of adult NSCs for this purpose is to be encouraged. Studies to date suggest that newly formed adult neurones have the ability to integrate and function in the mature brain[144] but problems to be overcome include the fact that adult NSC plasticity appears to reduce with age and the days when adult NSCs are used to treat stroke patients and those with degenerative brain disorders, such as Parkinson's disease, are not yet in sight.

SKIN

The skin is the barrier to the environment. Thus epidermal and hair cells are constantly being damaged and repaired and the rate of turnover of the epidermis is estimated to be 7 days in mice[145,146] and approximately 60 days in humans.[147] This rapid turnover requires the existence of a population of stem cells that can maintain this turnover for life. In addition, these stem cells have to be able to proliferate and differentiate above a background level to meet the demands of injury, such as trauma and burns.

The proliferating cells of the skin are found in the basal layer. Epidermal stem cells divide on average asymmetrically, yielding a daughter stem cell to maintain the stem cell population and a cell with a more limited proliferative capacity known as a *transit-amplifying cell*. This strategy allows the stem cell population to remain relatively quiescent, possibly reducing its mutation risk.[21,145]

Epidermal stem cells are difficult to identify but various possible molecular markers have been identified. The β-1 integrin is downregulated as keratinocytes leave the basal layer[148,149] (Fig. 10.10). β-1 integrin is seemingly required in the maintenance of the keratinocytes in an undifferentiated state.[150] Other markers include other integrins, p63 (a homologue of the tumour suppressor p53) and P-glycoprotein (a multidrug resistance pump). Since stem cells are thought to be relatively slowly cycling, their ability to retain a marker (such as BrdU or tritiated

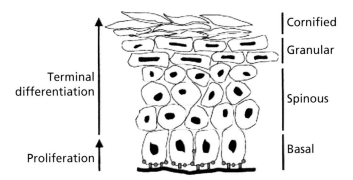

Fig.10.10 The layers of the human epidermis and some of the markers of keratinocyte differentiation. β1 integrins (indicated in red), hemidesmosomes by β4 integrins (indicated in blue). Reproduced from Ref. [189]; © John Wiley & Sons with permission.

thymidine) which is normally diluted with successive cell divisions, is thought to be a good indicator of stem cells, the so-called label-retaining cells.[145,151]

The epidermal stem cells of the basal layer of the interfollicular epidermis are continuous with those of the hair follicle. In the hair follicle a region adjacent to the insertion of the arrector pili muscle is known as the bulge region and is an area with a cluster of what appear to be stem cells. Cells from this region in the mouse have the capacity to differentiate into follicular, sebaceous and epidermal lineages[22] (Fig. 10.4), but it is not clear if there are also other stem cell compartments found in different areas of the follicle. This is seen in clinical situations, where following a burn, regenerating epithelium grows out from the hair follicle and interfollicular keratinocytes can contribute to hair formation.[152]

There is also evidence of plasticity involving skin; Krause *et al.*[53] found that 2% of epidermal cells were Y-chromosome- and cytokeratin-positive 11 months after sex-mismatched bone marrow transplantation of a single male HSC. Bone marrow-derived cells may also assist with skin repair; human MSCs injected into sheep at the time of skin injury become fibroblast-type cells in the dermis.[153] Skin-derived cells in rodents and humans have been shown to have considerable plasticity.[23,154] This plasticity may yet be used to promote healing in wounds and burns.

MUSCLE

Within skeletal muscle there is a cell with a significant proliferative capacity known as the *satellite cell.*[155] This cell is involved in the maintenance, repair and regeneration of muscle tissue throughout life and may either represent a skeletal muscle stem cell[156] or be derived from an as yet unidentified precursor cell. There is now accumulating evidence that the muscle stem cell population is not homogeneous,[157] but to date much of the work on the regenerative capacity of skeletal muscle has involved satellite cells. There is now evidence that these cells are not only derived from within the muscle but in certain circumstances appear to be derived from other sources by transdifferentiation. This alternative source of satellite cells may be capable of repairing damaged or diseased tissue.

There are several studies demonstrating bone marrow-derived cells with the capacity to differentiate into muscle fibres. Whole bone marrow can migrate to and repair damaged skeletal muscle[158] and this ability may be manipulated therapeutically. In primary muscle disease, introduction of genetically normal cells with the capacity to replicate and integrate into the abnormal muscle and function normally may result in clinical improvement. Thus, in humans, muscle myoblasts injected directly into the muscle of patients with Duchenne muscular dystrophy (DMD) can engraft and express normally absent transcripts.[159] When bone marrow-derived MSCs,[160] HSCs or SP cells[161] are transplanted into mice with muscular dystrophy, a proportion of muscle fibres with dystrophin (the protein absent in this condition) are found, supporting a potential role for stem cell transplantation for primary muscle disorders, although the possibility of fusion of engrafted cells is a potential explanation for these observations (*vide infra*).

As already discussed, there are cells in the nervous system[101,139] and skin[162–165] capable of differentiating into cells with a muscle phenotype. In addition, cells from adipose tissue derived from liposuction can also be induced to show a muscle phenotype.[166]

There are, therefore, various sources of cells that appear to be able to contribute to skeletal muscle repair and regeneration. Although some (such as neural tissue) seem unlikely candidates to be of significant therapeutic use, there may be possibilities for others to be used to help heal injury or use in primary muscle disorders.

BONE

The plasticity of adult bone marrow-derived cells also extends to the skeletal system and appears to be able to contribute to bone metabolism and turnover. Stem cells from both muscle[167] and bone marrow have been shown to engraft into bony tissue and produce bone. In mice, in studies using sex-mismatched transplantation, whole bone marrow has been shown to engraft into long bones[31] to function as osteoblasts, producing bone before terminally differentiating into osteocytes. Muscle stem cells have been induced to produce bone *in vitro* and these cells have been shown to make bone after injection into ectopic sites.[167]

This ability has been investigated in disease, osteogenesis imperfecta, a condition where mutation in the Type I collagen gene results in abnormal mesenchymal function, osteopaenia and, therefore, bony fragility and multiple fractures. In a mouse model of this condition, sex-mismatched bone marrow transplantation showed that transplantation of male marrow stromal cells resulted in an increase in concentration in bone collagen and mineral content in female-recipient mice.[87] Male cells comprised 7% of long bone and 15% of calvaria cells. This was repeated in humans with a similar increase in bone mineral content as well as improved growth and fewer fractures despite only a small degree of engraftment (1.5%).[34] Work is ongoing to investigate whether further transplants may increase this effect and result in improved benefit.[168] The balance between osteoclast and osteoblast activity may also be a potential target for work in this area.

CARTILAGE

There is some evidence that bone marrow-derived cells can contribute to the turnover of cartilage. *In vitro* studies suggest that expanded MSCs can be induced to secrete an extracellular matrix.[169] This is echoed *in vivo*, and following sex-mismatched transplantation of MSC into osteogenesis imperfecta mice, 8% of cartilage cells are donor-derived.[87] Following transplant of labelled MSC into arthritic mice, labelled cells are found in the joint cavities and synovial tissues.[170] Human chondrocytes are also found in the joints of sheep following human MSC transplantation.[153]

This evidence again demonstrates the plasticity of bone marrow-derived cells, although it is too early to say that there may be a potential role for stem cell transplant in degenerative joint disease.

MECHANISMS OF STEM CELL PLASTICITY

There are three postulated mechanisms of stem cell plasticity:

- incorporation of early pluripotential stem cells
- transdifferentiation
- cell fusion

INCORPORATION OF EARLY PLURIPOTENTIAL STEM CELLS

It is naturally impossible to exclude the possibility that, intermingled with organ-specific stem cells (such as HSCs), there may be residual primitive cells capable of multilineage differentiation when engrafted in an appropriate environment.

TRANSDIFFERENTIATION

To date, studies looking at the plasticity of adult bone marrow have concentrated on tracking donor-derived bone marrow cells in the recipient. This has been by virtue of tracking the Y-chromosome in sex-mismatched transplantation or some other label, such as GFP or *LacZ*. The fact that these cells are clearly found documented in a variety of tissues has been taken as evidence of transdifferentiation of bone marrow cells. It is acknowledged that, at least in the liver, these events are rare but clonal expansion allows these events to result in significant volumes of donor-derived tissue.[171]

CELL FUSION

It has more recently been argued that Y-chromosome-tracking techniques cannot distinguish between donor-derived cells differentiating and proliferating in the recipient as opposed to donor cells fusing with recipient cells and taking on their phenotype. Studies have shown that on occasion adult murine bone marrow/neural cells can fuse with ES cells *in vitro* and subsequently behave as the latter.[172,173]

To date, cell fusion as an explanation for stem cell plasticity has not gained credence except for in the FAM knockout mouse. Indeed, there are a growing number of observations that would be difficult to explain by fusion. For example, polyploidy is rarely seen outside the liver (where it is a common phenomenon even in the non-transplanted state). Moreover, in a study of postpartum women with male children who developed thyroid disorders (such as Hashimoto's thyroiditis and thyroid cancer), male cells and in one case male thyroid follicular cells were found. These cells contained one X- and one Y-chromosome but no polyploid (XXXY) cells were reported.[174] Likewise, Korbling *et al.*[95] observed only hepatocytes and gut mucosal cells with no more than one X- and one Y-chromosome in female recipients of male peripheral blood stem cells. In a similar vein, the *in vitro* studies of Verfaillie and colleagues[175] on the differentiation of multipotent adult progenitor cells (MAPCs) into cells from the three germ layers are testimony to the enormous plasticity of these cells and, of course, cannot be ascribed to cell fusion. Further evidence for transdifferentiation comes from a study by Campbell *et al.*[176] They investigated mice who have had foreign bodies (devoid of stem cells) implanted into the abdominal cavity after bone marrow transplantation. These free-floating bodies become coated with donor-derived cells which firstly express and then loose haematopoietic markers. These cells then go on to change phenotype, become embedded in a collagen matrix and become α-smooth muscle actin positive over a course of 2 weeks.

STEM CELLS IN CARCINOGENESIS AND IN TUMOURS

This is scarcely the place for an exhaustive discussion of this topic which has been reviewed recently elsewhere.[177,178] There is now increasing evidence that stem cells are intimately concerned in the development of tumours and that even established tumours, such as colorectal adenomas, retain a stem cell architecture, with stem cells forming a minority population, feeding a transit-amplifying population.[179] Moreover, we have known for many years that tumours are heterogeneous, with sub-populations differing in their replicative and indeed tumourigenic capacity.[180]

However, there are now interesting observations which point to the fact that cell plasticity is important in the histogenesis of tumours as well; to give one example, juvenile polyps are usually described histologically as hamartomas of the lamina propria, and when these lesions are multiple, as in the juvenile polyposis syndrome (JPS), there is an increased risk of the development of colorectal and other cancers. A percentage of these cases are due to a mutation in the SMAD4 gene, a molecule in the TGFβ pathway of signal transduction. The usual explanation of such malignant progression is that it is the stromal cells which bear the mutation, and cross-talk between these cells and the epithelial cells results in the development of the tumour – the so-called 'landscaper hypothesis' of Vogelstein.[181] However, recent work has shown that the SMAD4 mutation is present in the stroma and the epithelial cells in the JPS polyps without neoplastic change.[182] This demonstration of a clonal lesion present on both lineages dispenses with the need to incriminate any 'landscaper' hypothesis, since here SMAD4 is behaving as any other tumour suppressor gene. Moreover, the presence of this clonal lesion is strongly suggestive that the stroma and the epithelium is of the same derivation – either the lesion has been present very early in intestinal histogenesis or else there has been transdifferentiation between the lineages during the development of the lesion in post-natal life. Similar observations are now being made amongst the several cell lineages seen in breast carcinomas and other tumours. Thus, such considerations of stem cell plasticity will indeed have far-reaching effects on our ideas of the origins and development of even the commonest tumours.

CONCLUSION

There has recently been a radical change in the way the scientific community thinks about the biology of stem cells. It is now considered that the adult stem cell is far less committed than previously thought and that there are some populations of stem cells that can contribute to tissues from all three germ layers. Thus, stem cells appear to home to sites of damaged tissue and occupy a new local environment or niche which then defines the new characteristics of the engrafted cells.[11] This is well illustrated in bone where bone marrow-derived MSCs differentiate according to the environment they become resident in.[35,183] This is exciting, since the use of adult stem cells is far less controversial and emotive than the use of foetal or ES cells.

Stem cells from organs previously thought to have a very limited capacity for regeneration, such as the brain, are proving to have a far greater regenerative capacity and can even appear to be able to change lineages.[137] This, although exciting in itself since it may help in the development of strategies to encourage healing of damaged brain by already resident stem cells, is unlikely to be useful for stem cell transplantation. Some of the more exciting possibilities are areas where stem cells are easily accessible or plentiful such as the bone marrow and skin. This accessibility allows more scope for investigation and may more easily be utilised in a therapeutic setting.

There is now evidence to suggest that stem cell transplantation may be helpful in the repair of almost every organ. Transplanted bone marrow has been demonstrated to become incorporated in injured tissue or those with metabolic and degenerative disorders. Although early days, there is already evidence in humans that these techniques may be of clinical benefit.

However, there are problems. The doubts about observations demonstrating fusion rather than transdifferentiation await clarification, although if the transplantation results in lasting clinical benefit it is still a reasonable strategy, whatever the underlying mechanism. The side effects and risks of bone marrow transplantation are also a potential problem with the application of the technique. The irradiation and the immunosuppression required in addition to the risks of GVHD would minimise the use of stem cell allografts for life-threatening conditions. This problem can be overcome by the use of autografts, such as those used in the studies of patients' post-myocardial infarction.[89] Moreover, extending the use of autografts by using the patient's own marrow and genetically modifying it using it as a vector for gene therapy, avoids these other risks.

The number of bone marrow cells in a single individual capable of being appropriate for bone marrow transplantation may not be sufficient for transplantation. Cell culture techniques may allow amplification of the appropriate cells prior to transplantation, but do cells expanded *ex vivo* behave normally when returned to the body? Are they as controllable? Will their progress through the cell cycle be difficult to control and will they form tumours?

The possibilities of the plasticity of adult stem cells have been illustrated; adult bone marrow-derived cells have been found engrafted into other tissues in a number of circumstances. However, the functionality, longevity and robustness of these cells is yet to be demonstrated.[184] A higher standard of evidence has been called for, particularly on the functional side, and work is now progressing to investigate this aspect of stem cell biology. Nevertheless, the next few years should prove exciting for all involved in stem cells, particularly pathologists.

GLOSSARY

BAL	Bioartificial liver
DMD	Duchenne muscular dystrophy
EG	Embryonic germ
ES	Embryonic stem
FACS	Fluorescence-activated cell sorting
FAH	Fumaryl acetoacetate hydrolase
GFP	Green fluorescent protein
GLP-2	Glucagon-like peptide 2

GVHD	Graft versus host disease
H-CFU-C	Hepatocyte-colony forming units in culture
HGF	Hepatocyte growth factor
HSC	Haematopoietic stem cell
JPS	Juvenile polyposis syndrome
KGF	Keratinocyte growth factor
LIF	Leukaemia inhibitory factor
MAPCs	Multipotent adult progenitor cells
MARS	Molecular-adsorbent recycling system
MSCs	Mesenchymal stem cells
NSCs	Neural stem cells
SCF	Stem cell factor
SP	Side population
SVZ	Subventricular zone

REFERENCES

1. Overturf K, Al-Dhalimy M, Ou CN, Finegold M, Grompe M. Serial transplantation reveals the stem-cell-like regenerative potential of adult mouse hepatocytes. Am J Pathol 1997; 151: 1273–1280
2. Lagasse E, Connors H, Al-Dhalimy M, Reitsma M, Dohse M, Osborne L et al. Purified hematopoietic stem cells can differentiate into hepatocytes in vivo. Nat Med 2000; 6: 1229–1234
3. Bjerknes M, Cheng H. Clonal analysis of mouse intestinal epithelial progenitors. Gastroenterology 1999; 116: 7–14
4. Martin GR. Isolation of a pluripotent cell line from early mouse embryos cultured in medium conditioned by teratocarcinoma stem cells. Proc Natl Acad Sci USA 1981; 78: 7634–7638
5. Thomson JA, Itskovitz-Eldor J, Shapiro SS, Waknitz MA, Swiergiel JJ, Marshall VS et al. Embryonic stem cell lines derived from human blastocysts. Science 1998; 282: 1145–1147
6. Shamblott MJ, Axelman J, Wang S, Bugg EM, Littlefield JW, Donovan PJ et al. Derivation of pluripotent stem cells from cultured human primordial germ cells. Proc Natl Acad Sci USA 1998; 95: 13726–13731
7. Orkin SH. Embryonic stem cells and transgenic mice in the study of hematopoiesis. Int J Dev Biol 1998; 42: 927–934
8. Wobus AM, Holzhausen H, Jakel P, Schoneich J. Characterization of a pluripotent stem cell line derived from a mouse embryo. Exp Cell Res 1984; 152: 212–219
9. Wobus AM, Wallukat G, Hescheler J. Pluripotent mouse embryonic stem cells are able to differentiate into cardiomyocytes expressing chronotropic responses to adrenergic and cholinergic agents and Ca^{2+} channel blockers. Differentiation 1991; 48: 173–182
10. Itskovitz-Eldor J, Schuldiner M, Karsenti D, Eden A, Yanuka O, Amit M et al. Differentiation of human embryonic stem cells into embryoid bodies compromising the three embryonic germ layers. Mol Med 2000; 6: 88–95
11. Spradling A, Drummond-Barbosa D, Kai T. Stem cells find their niche. Nature 2001; 414: 98–104
12. Bjerknes M, Cheng H. Modulation of specific intestinal epithelial progenitors by enteric neurons. Proc Natl Acad Sci USA 2001; 98: 12497–12502
13. Till JE, McCulloch EA. A direct measurement of the radiation sensitivity of normal mouse bone marrow cells. Radiat Res 1961; 14: 213–222
14. Goodell MA, Brose K, Paradis G, Conner AS, Mulligan RC. Isolation and functional properties of murine hematopoietic stem cells that are replicating in vivo. J Exp Med 1996; 183: 1797–1806
15. Bhatia M, Wang JC, Kapp U, Bonnet D, Dick JE. Purification of primitive human hematopoietic cells capable of repopulating immune-deficient mice. Proc Natl Acad Sci USA 1997; 94: 5320–5325

16. Moore KA, Ema H, Lemischka IR. *In vitro* maintenance of highly purified, transplantable hematopoietic stem cells. Blood 1997; 89: 4337–4347

17. Park HS, Goodlad RA, Wright NA. Crypt fission in the small intestine and colon. A mechanism for the emergence of G6PD locus-mutated crypts after treatment with mutagens. Am J Pathol 1995; 147: 1416–1427

18. Kirkland SC. Clonal origin of columnar, mucous, and endocrine cell lineages in human colorectal epithelium. Cancer 1988; 61: 1359–1363

19. Wright NA. Epithelial stem cell repertoire in the gut: clues to the origin of cell lineages, proliferative units and cancer. Int J Exp Pathol 2000; 81: 117–143

20. Brittan M, Wright NA. Gastrointestinal stem cells. J Pathol 2002; 197: 492–509

21. Watt FM. Epidermal stem cells: markers, patterning and the control of stem cell fate. Philos Trans Roy Soc London B Biol Sci 1998; 353: 831–837

22. Oshima H, Rochat A, Kedzia C, Kobayashi K, Barrandon Y. Morphogenesis and renewal of hair follicles from adult multipotent stem cells. Cell 2001; 104: 233–245

23. Ferraris C, Chevalier G, Favier B, Jahoda CA, Dhouailly D. Adult corneal epithelium basal cells possess the capacity to activate epidermal, pilosebaceous and sweat gland genetic programs in response to embryonic dermal stimuli. Development 2000; 127: 5487–5495

24. Alison M, Sarraf C. Hepatic stem cells. J Hepatol 1998; 29: 676–682

25. Lowes KN, Brennan BA, Yeoh GC, Olynyk JK. Oval cell numbers in human chronic liver diseases are directly related to disease severity. Am J Pathol 1999; 154: 537–541

26. McKay R. Stem cells in the central nervous system. Science 1997; 276: 66–71

27. Palmer TD, Takahashi J, Gage FH. The adult rat hippocampus contains primordial neural stem cells. Mol Cell Neurosci 1997; 8: 389–404

28. Roy NS, Wang S, Jiang L, Kang J, Benraiss A, Harrison-Restelli C *et al. In vitro* neurogenesis by progenitor cells isolated from the adult human hippocampus. Nat Med 2000; 6: 271–277

29. Flax JD, Aurora S, Yang C, Simonin C, Wills AM, Billinghurst LL *et al.* Engraftable human neural stem cells respond to developmental cues, replace neurons, and express foreign genes. Nat Biotechnol 1998; 16: 1033–1039

30. Fridenshtein A. Stromal bone marrow cells and the hematopoietic microenvironment. Arkh Patol 1982; 44: 3–11

31. Nilsson SK, Dooner MS, Weier HU, Frenkel B, Lian JB, Stein GS *et al.* Cells capable of bone production engraft from whole bone marrow transplants in nonablated mice. J Exp Med 1999; 189: 729–734

32. Pittenger MF, Mackay AM, Beck SC, Jaiswal RK, Douglas R, Mosca JD *et al.* Multilineage potential of adult human mesenchymal stem cells. Science 1999; 284: 143–147.

33. Prockop DJ. Marrow stromal cells as stem cells for nonhematopoietic tissues. Science 1997; 276: 71–74

34. Horwitz EM, Prockop DJ, Fitzpatrick LA, Koo WW, Gordon PL, Neel M *et al.* Transplantability and therapeutic effects of bone marrow-derived mesenchymal cells in children with osteogenesis imperfecta. Nat Med 1999; 5: 309–313

35. Hou Z, Nguyen Q, Frenkel B, Nilsson S, Milne M, van Wijnen A *et al.* Osteoblast-specific gene expression after transplantation of marrow cells: implications for skeletal gene therapy. Proc Natl Acad Sci USA 1999; 96: 7294–7299

36. Phinney D, Kopen G, Righter W, Webster S, Tremain N, Prockop D. Donor variation in the growth properties and osteogenic potential of human marrow stromal cells. J Cell Biochem 1999; 75: 424–436

37. Azizi S, Stokes D, Augelli B, DiGirolamo C, Prockop D. Engraftment and migration of human bone marrow stromal cells implanted in the brains of albino rats – similarities to astrocyte grafts. Proc Natl Acad Sci USA 1998; 95: 3908–3913

38. Andrews RG, Singer JW, Bernstein ID. Precursors of colony-forming cells in humans can be distinguished from colony-forming cells by expression of the CD33 and CD34 antigens and light scatter properties. J Exp Med 1989; 169: 1721–1731

39. Krause DS, Fackler MJ, Civin CI, May WS. CD34: structure, biology, and clinical utility. Blood 1996; 87: 1–13

40. Chan JY, Watt SM. Adhesion receptors on haematopoietic progenitor cells. Br J Haematol 2001; 112: 541–557

41. Jankowska-Wieczorek A, Majka M, Ratajczak J, Ratajczak M. Autocrine/paracrine mechanisms in human hematopoiesis. Stem Cells 2001; 19: 99–107

42. Weissman I. Stem cells: units of development, units of regeneration, and units in evolution. Cell 2000; 100: 157–168

43. Whetton A, Graham G. Homing and mobilization in the stem cell niche. Trends Cell Biol 1999; 9: 233–238

44. Quesenberry P, Becker P. Stem cell homing: rolling, crawling, and nesting. Proc Natl Acad Sci USA 1998; 95: 15155–15157

45. Friedenstein A, Ivanov-Smolenski A, Chajlakjan R, Gorskaya U, Kuralesova A, Latzinik N et al. Origin of bone marrow stromal mechanocytes in radiochimeras and heterotopic transplants. Exp Hematol 1978; 6: 440–444

46. Clark B, Keating A. Biology of bone marrow stroma. Ann NY Acad Sci 1995; 770: 70–78

47. Ogawa M. Differentiation and proliferation of hematopoietic stem cells. Blood 1993; 81: 2844–2853

48. Metcalf D. Hematopoietic regulators: redundancy or subtlety? Blood 1993; 82: 3515–3523

49. Prosper F, Stroncek D, McCarthy JB, Verfaillie CM. Mobilization and homing of peripheral blood progenitors is related to reversible downregulation of alpha4 beta1 integrin expression and function. J Clin Invest 1998; 101: 2456–2467

50. Zanjani E, Flake A, Almeida-Porada G, Tran N, Papayannopoulou T. Homing of human cells in the fetal sheep model: modulation by antibodies activating or inhibiting very late activation antigen-4-dependent function. Blood 1999; 94: 2515–2522

51. Peled A, Petit I, Kollet O, Magid M, Ponomaryov T, Byk T et al. Dependence of human stem cell engraftment and repopulation of NOD/SCID mice on CXCR4. Science 1999; 283: 845–848

52. Nilsson SK, Johnston HM, Coverdale JA. Spatial localization of transplanted hemopoietic stem cells: inferences for the localization of stem cell niches. Blood 2001; 97: 2293–2299

53. Krause D, Theise N, Collector M, Henegariu O, Hwang S, Gardner R et al. Multi-organ, multi-lineage engraftment by a single bone marrow-derived stem cell. Cell 2001; 105: 369–377

54. Alison MR, Poulsom R, Jeffery R, Dhillon AP, Quaglia A, Jacob J et al. Hepatocytes from non-hepatic adult stem cells. Nature 2000; 406: 257

55. Theise N, Nimmakalayu M, Gardner R, Illei P, Morgan G, Teperman L et al. Liver from bone marrow in humans. Hepatology 2000; 32: 11–16

56. Wagers AJ, Sherwood RI, Christensen JL, Weissman IL. Little evidence for developmental plasticity of adult hematopoietic stem cells. Science 2002; 297: 2256–2259

57. Yusa K, Tsuruo T. Reversal mechanism of multidrug resistance by verapamil: direct binding of verapamil to P-glycoprotein on specific sites and transport of verapamil outward across the plasma membrane of K562/ADM cells. Cancer Res 1989; 49: 5002–5006

58. Miller CL, Eaves CJ. Expansion in vitro of adult murine hematopoietic stem cells with transplantable lympho-myeloid reconstituting ability. Proc Natl Acad Sci USA 1997; 94: 13648–13653

59. Goodell MA, Rosenzweig M, Kim H, Marks DF, DeMaria M, Paradis G et al. Dye efflux studies suggest that hematopoietic stem cells expressing low or undetectable levels of CD34 antigen exist in multiple species. Nat Med 1997; 3: 1337–1345

60. Hall F, Han B, Kundu R, Yee A, Nimni M, Gordon E. Phenotypic differentiation of tgf-beta1-responsive pluripotent premesenchymal prehematopoietic progenitor (p4 stem) cells from murine bone marrow. J Hematoth Stem Cell Res 2001; 10: 261–271

61. Bunting KD. ABC transporters as phenotypic markers and functional regulators of stem cells. Stem Cells 2002; 20: 11–20

62. Beltrami AP, Urbanek K, Kajstura J, Yan SM, Finato N, Bussani R et al. Evidence that human cardiac myocytes divide after myocardial infarction. N Engl J Med 2001; 344: 1750–1757

63. Asahara T, Murohara T, Sullivan A, Silver M, van der Zee R, Li T et al. Isolation of putative progenitor endothelial cells for angiogenesis. Science 1997; 275: 964–967

64. Shi Q, Rafii S, Wu MH, Wijelath ES, Yu C, Ishida A et al. Evidence for circulating bone marrow-derived endothelial cells. Blood 1998; 92: 362–367

65. Takahashi T, Kalka C, Masuda H, Chen D, Silver M, Kearney M *et al*. Ischemia- and cytokine-induced mobilization of bone marrow-derived endothelial progenitor cells for neovascularization. Nat Med 1999; 5: 434–438

66. Asahara T, Masuda H, Takahashi T, Kalka C, Pastore C, Silver M *et al*. Bone marrow origin of endothelial progenitor cells responsible for postnatal vasculogenesis in physiological and pathological conditions. Circ Res 1999; 85: 221–228

67. Lin Y, Weisdorf D, Solovey A, Hebbel R. Origins of circulating endothelial cells and endothelial outgrowth from blood. J Clin Invest 2000; 105: 71–77

68. Kalka C, Masuda H, Takahashi T, Kalka-Moll W, Silver M, Kearney M *et al*. Transplantation of *ex vivo* expanded endothelial progenitor cells for therapeutic neovascularization. Proc Natl Acad Sci USA 2000; 97: 3422–3427

69. Williams G, Alvarez C. Host repopulation of the endothelium in allografts of kidneys and aorta. Surg Forum 1969; 20: 293–294

70. Sinclair R. Origin of endothelium in human renal allografts. Br Med J 1972; 4: 15–16

71. Lagaaij E, Cramer-Knijnenburg G, van Kemenade F, van Es L, Bruijn J, van Krieken J. Endothelial cell chimerism after renal transplantation and vascular rejection. Lancet 2001; 357: 33–37

72. Poulsom R, Forbes SJ, Hodivala-Dilke K, Ryan E, Wyles S, Navaratnarasah S *et al*. Bone marrow contributes to renal parenchymal turnover and regeneration. J Pathol 2001; 195: 229–235

73. Andersen CB, Ladefoged SD, Larsen S. Cellular inflammatory infiltrates and renal cell turnover in kidney allografts: a study using *in situ* hybridization and combined *in situ* hybridization and immunohistochemistry with a Y-chromosome-specific DNA probe and monoclonal antibodies. APMIS 1991; 99: 645–652

74. Williams G, Krajewski C, Dagher F, Ter Haar A, Roth J, Santos G. Host repopulation of endothelium. Transplant Proc 1971; III: 869–872

75. Gao Z-H, McAlister V, Williams G. Repopulation of liver endothelium by bone marrow-derived cells. Lancet 2001; 357: 932–933

76. Tomita S, Li R, Weisel R, Mickle D, Kim E, Sakai T *et al*. Autologous transplantation of bone marrow cells improves damaged heart function. Circulation 1999; 100: II247–II256

77. Kocher A, Schuster M, Szabolcs M, Takuma S, Burkhoff D, Wang J *et al*. Neovascularization of ischemic myocardium by human bone-marrow-derived angioblasts prevents cardiomyocyte apoptosis, reduces remodeling and improves cardiac function. Nat Med 2001; 7: 430–436

78. Gunsilius E, Duba H-C, Petzer A, Kähler C, Grünewald K, Stockhammer G *et al*. Evidence from a leukaemia model for maintenance of vascular endothelium by bone-marrow-derived endothelial cells. Lancet 2000; 355: 1688–1691

79. Klug MG, Soonpaa MH, Koh GY, Field LJ. Genetically selected cardiomyocytes from differentiating embronic stem cells form stable intracardiac grafts. J Clin Invest 1996; 98: 216–224

80. Makino S, Fukuda K, Miyoshi S, Konishi F, Kodama H, Pan J *et al*. Cardiomyocytes can be generated from marrow stromal cells *in vitro*. J Clin Invest 1999; 103: 697–705

81. Orlic D, Kajstura J, Chimenti S, Bodine DM, Leri A, Anversa P *et al*. Transplanted adult bone marrow cells repair myocardial infarcts in mice. Ann NY Acad Sci 2001; 938: 221–229; discussion 229–230

82. Orlic D, Kajstura J, Chimenti S, Jakoniuk I, Anderson S, Li B *et al*. Bone marrow cells regenerate infarcted myocardium. Nature 2001; 410: 701–704

83. Orlic D, Kajstura J, Chimenti S, Limana F, Jakoniuk I, Quaini F *et al*. Mobilized bone marrow cells repair the infarcted heart, improving function and survival. Proc Natl Acad Sci USA 2001; 98: 10344–10349

84. Jackson KA, Majka SM, Wang H, Pocius J, Hartley CJ, Majesky MW *et al*. Regeneration of ischemic cardiac muscle and vascular endothelium by adult stem cells. J Clin Invest 2001; 107: 1395–1402

85. Bittner R, Schofer C, Weipoltshammer K, Ivanova S, Streubel B, Hauser E *et al*. Recruitment of bone-marrow-derived cells by skeletal and cardiac muscle in adult dystrophic mdx mice. Anat Embryol 1999; 199: 391–396

86. Malouf N, Coleman W, Grisham J, Lininger R, Madden V, Sproul M *et al*. Adult-derived stem cells from the liver become myocytes in the heart *in vivo*. Am J Pathol 2001; 158: 1929–1935

87. Pereira R, O'Hara M, Laptev A, Halford K, Pollard M, Class R *et al*. Marrow stromal cells a source of progenitor cells for nonhematopoietic tissues in transgeneic mice with a phenotype of osteogenesis imperfecta. Proc Natl Acad Sci USA 1998; 95: 1142–1147

88. Quaini F, Urbanek K, Beltrami AP, Finato N, Beltrami CA, Nadal-Ginard B *et al*. Chimerism of the transplanted heart. N Engl J Med 2002; 346: 5–15

89. Strauer BE, Brehm M, Zeus T, Gattermann N, Hernandez A, Sorg RV *et al*. Intracoronary, human autologous stem cell transplantation for myocardial regeneration following myocardial infarction. Dtsch Med Wochenschr 2001; 126: 932–938

90. Boers JE, Ambergen AW, Thunnissen FB. Number and proliferation of clara cells in normal human airway epithelium. Am J Resp Crit Care Med 1999; 159: 1585–1591

91. Otto WR. Lung epithelial stem cells. J Pathol 2002; 197: 527–535

92. Janes S, Hunt T, Brittan M, Jeffery R, Forbes S, Hodivala-Dilke K *et al*. Lung repopulation by haematopoetic stem cells (HSC) after bone marrow transplant (BMT). Am J Resp Crit Care Med 2002; 165: A465

93. Kotton DN, Ma BY, Cardoso WV, Sanderson EA, Summer RS, Williams MC *et al*. Bone marrow-derived cells as progenitors of lung alveolar epithelium. Development 2001; 128: 5181–5188

94. Karam SM. Lineage commitment and maturation of epithelial cells in the gut. Front Biosci 1999; 4: D286–D298

95. Korbling M, Katz RL, Khanna A, Ruifrok AC, Rondon G, Albitar M *et al*. Hepatocytes and epithelial cells of donor origin in recipients of peripheral-blood stem cells. N Engl J Med 2002; 346: 738–746

96. Okamoto R, Yajima T, Yamazaki M, Kanai T, Mukai M, Okamoto S *et al*. Damaged epithelia regenerated by bone marrow derived cells in the human gastrointestinal tract. Nat Med 2002; 8: 1011–1017

97. Brittan M, Hunt T, Jeffery R, Poulsom R, Forbes SJ, Hodivala-Dilke K *et al*. Bone marrow derivation of pericryptal myofibroblasts in the mouse and human small intestine and colon. Gut 2002; 50: 752–757

98. Powell DW, Mifflin RC, Valentich JD, Crowe SE, Saada JI, West AB. Myofibroblasts. II. Intestinal subepithelial myofibroblasts. Am J Physiol 1999; 277: C183–C201

99. Powell DW, Mifflin RC, Valentich JD, Crowe SE, Saada JI, West AB. Myofibroblasts. I. Paracrine cells important in health and disease. Am J Physiol 1999; 277: C1–C9

100. Suzuki A, Zheng Yw YW, Kaneko S, Onodera M, Fukao K, Nakauchi H *et al*. Clonal identification and characterization of self-renewing pluripotent stem cells in the developing liver. J Cell Biol 2002; 156: 173–184

101. Clarke D, Johansson C, Wilbertz J, Veress B, Nilsson E, Karlström H *et al*. Generalized potential of adult neural stem cells. Science 2000; 288: 1660–1663

102. Alison MR, Poulsom R, Forbes SJ. Update on hepatic stem cells. Liver 2001; 21: 367–373

103. Paku S, Schnur J, Nagy P, Thorgeirsson SS. Origin and structural evolution of the early proliferating oval cells in rat liver. Am J Pathol 2001; 158: 1313–1323

104. Alison M. Liver stem cells: a two compartment system. Curr Opin Cell Biol 1998; 10: 710–715

105. Alison M, Golding M, Lalani el N, Sarraf C. Wound healing in the liver with particular reference to stem cells. Philos Trans Roy Soc London B Biol Sci 1998; 353: 877–894

106. Alison MR, Golding M, Sarraf CE. Liver stem cells: when the going gets tough they get going. Int J Exp Pathol 1997; 78: 365–381

107. Baumann U, Crosby HA, Ramani P, Kelly DA, Strain AJ. Expression of the stem cell factor receptor c-kit in normal and diseased pediatric liver: identification of a human hepatic progenitor cell? Hepatology 1999; 30: 112–117

108. Lemmer ER, Shepard EG, Blakolmer K, Kirsch RE, Robson SC. Isolation from human fetal liver of cells co-expressing CD34 haematopoietic stem cell and CAM 5.2 pancytokeratin markers. J Hepatol 1998; 29: 450–454

109. Omori N, Omori M, Evarts RP, Teramoto T, Miller MJ, Hoang TN *et al*. Partial cloning of rat CD34 cDNA and expression during stem cell-dependent liver regeneration in the adult rat. Hepatology 1997; 26: 720–727

110. Petersen BE, Goff JP, Greenberger JS, Michalopoulos GK. Hepatic oval cells express the hematopoietic stem cell marker Thy-1 in the rat. Hepatology 1998; 27: 433-445

111. Petersen B, Bowen W, Patrene K, Mars W, Sullivan A, Murase N *et al*. Bone marrow as a potential source of hepatic oval cells. Science 1999; 284: 1168–1170

112. Theise N, Badve S, Saxena R, Henegariu O, Sell S, Crawford J *et al.* Derivation of hepatocytes from bone marrow cells in mice after radiation-induced myeloablation. Hepatology 2000; 31: 234–240

113. Kleeberger W, Rothamel T, Glockner S, Flemming P, Lehmann U, Kreipe H. High frequency of epithelial chimerism in liver transplants demonstrated by microdissection and STR-analysis. Hepatology 2002; 35: 110–116

114. Petrenko O, Beavis A, Klaine M, Kittappa R, Godin I, Lemischka IR. The molecular characterization of the fetal stem cell marker AA4. Immunity 1999; 10: 691–700

115. Forbes SJ, Hodivala-Dilke KM, Jeffrey R *et al.* Hepatocytes derived from bone marrow stem cells demonstrate polyploidisation. J Hepatol 2001; 34: 20–21

116. Tada K, Roy-Chowdhury N, Prasad V, Kim BH, Manchikalapudi P, Fox IJ *et al.* Long-term amelioration of bilirubin glucuronidation defect in Gunn rats by transplanting genetically modified immortalized autologous hepatocytes. Cell Transplant 1998; 7: 607–616

117. Fox IJ, Chowdhury JR, Kaufman SS, Goertzen TC, Chowdhury NR, Warkentin PI *et al.* Treatment of the Crigler–Najjar syndrome type I with hepatocyte transplantation. N Engl J Med 1998; 338: 1422–1426

118. Strain AJ, Neuberger JM. A bioartificial liver – state of the art. Science 2002; 295: 1005–1009

119. Lumelsky N, Blondel O, Laeng P, Velasco I, Ravin R, McKay R. Differentiation of embryonic stem cells to insulin-secreting structures similar to pancreatic islets. Science 2001; 292: 1389–1394

120. Zulewski H, Abraham EJ, Gerlach MJ, Daniel PB, Moritz W, Muller B *et al.* Multipotential nestin-positive stem cells isolated from adult pancreatic islets differentiate *ex vivo* into pancreatic endocrine, exocrine, and hepatic phenotypes. Diabetes 2001; 50: 521–533

121. Guz Y, Nasir I, Teitelman G. Regeneration of pancreatic beta cells from intra-islet precursor cells in an experimental model of diabetes. Endocrinology 2001; 142: 4956–4968

122. Faris RA, Monfils BA, Dunsford HA, Hixson DC. Antigenic relationship between oval cells and a subpopulation of hepatic foci, nodules, and carcinomas induced by the 'resistant hepatocyte' model system. Cancer Res 1991; 51: 1308–1317

123. Bonner-Weir S. Beta-cell turnover: its assessment and implications. Diabetes 2001; 50: S20–S24

124. Bernard-Kargar C, Ktorza A. Endocrine pancreas plasticity under physiological and pathological conditions. Diabetes 2001; 50: S30-S35

125. Bonner-Weir S, Sharma A. Pancreatic stem cells. J Pathol 2002; 197: 519–526

126. Ramiya VK, Maraist M, Arfors KE, Schatz DA, Peck AB, Cornelius JG. Reversal of insulin-dependent diabetes using islets generated *in vitro* from pancreatic stem cells. Nat Med 2000; 6: 278–282

127. Strutz F, Müller G. Transdifferentiation comes of age. Nephrol Dial Transplant 2000; 15: 1729–1731

128. Ng Y, Fan J, Mu W, Nikolic-Paterson D, Yang W, Huang T *et al.* Glomerular epithelial–myofibroblast transdifferentiation in the evolution of glomerular crescent formation. Nephrol Dial Transplant 1999; 14: 2860–2872

129. Sun D, Fujigaki Y, Fujimoto T, Yonemura T, Hishida A. Possible involvement of myofibroblasts in cellular recovery of uranyl acetate-induced acute renal failure in rats. Am J Pathol 2000; 157: 1321–1335

130. Grimm PC, Nickerson P, Jeffery J, Savani RC, Gough J, McKenna RM *et al.* Neointimal and tubulointerstitial infiltration by recipient mesenchymal cells in chronic renal-allograft rejection. N Engl J Med 2001; 345: 93–97

131. Momma S, Johansson CB, Frisen J. Get to know your stem cells. Curr Opin Neurobiol 2000; 10: 45–49

132. Johansson CB, Momma S, Clarke DL, Risling M, Lendahl U, Frisen J *et al.* Identification of a neural stem cell in the adult mammalian central nervous system. Cell 1999; 96: 25–34

133. Lois C, Alvarez-Buylla A. Proliferating subventricular zone cells in the adult mammalian forebrain can differentiate into neurons and glia. Proc Natl Acad Sci USA 1993; 90: 2074–2077

134. Bayer SA, Yackel JW, Puri PS. Neurons in the rat dentate gyrus granular layer substantially increase during juvenile and adult life. Science 1982; 216: 890–892

135. Kaplan MS, Hinds JW. Neurogenesis in the adult rat: electron microscopic analysis of light radioautographs. Science 1977; 197: 1092–1094

136. Palmer T, Schwartz P, Taupin P, Kaspar B, Stein S, Gage F. Progenitor cells from human brain after death. Nature 2001; 411: 42–43

137. Bjornson C, Rietze R, Reynolds B, Magli M, Vescovi A. Turning brain into blood: a hematopoietic fate adopted by neural stem cells *in vivo*. Science 1999; 283: 534–537

138. Morshead CM, Benveniste P, Iscove NN, van Der Kooy D. Hematopoietic competence is a rare property of neural stem cells that may depend on genetic and epigenetic alterations. Nat Med 2002; 8: 268–273

139. Galli R, Borello U, Gritti A, Minasi M, Bjornson C, Coletta M *et al*. Skeletal myogenic potential of human and mouse neural stem cells. Nat Neurosci 2000; 3: 986–991

140. Mezey E, Chandross K, Harta G, Maki R, McKercher S. Turning blood into brain: cells bearing neuronal antigens generated *in vivo* from bone marrow. Science 2000; 290: 1779–1782

141. Eglitis MA, Mezey E. Hematopoietic cells differentiate into both microglia and macroglia in the brains of adult mice. Proc Natl Acad Sci USA 1997; 94: 4080–4085

142. Woodbury D, Schwartz E, Prockop D, Black I. Adult rat and human bone marrow stromal cells differentiate into neurons. J Neurosci Res 2000; 61: 364–370

143. Freed CR, Greene PE, Breeze RE, Tsai WY, DuMouchel W, Kao R *et al*. Transplantation of embryonic dopamine neurons for severe Parkinson's disease. N Engl J Med 2001; 344: 710–719

144. Carlen M, Cassidy RM, Brismar H, Smith GA, Enquist LW, Frisen J. Functional integration of adult-born neurons. Curr Biol 2002; 12: 606–608

145. Potten CS. Cell replacement in epidermis (keratopoiesis) via discrete units of proliferation. Int Rev Cytol 1981; 69: 271–318

146. Ghazizadeh S, Taichman LB. Multiple classes of stem cells in cutaneous epithelium: a lineage analysis of adult mouse skin. EMBO J 2001; 20: 1215–1222

147. Hunter JAA SJ, Dahl MV. In Clinical Dermatology. Oxford Blackwell Science, 1995; 831–837

148. Watt FM. Keratincyte integrins. In Leigh IM, Watt FM (Eds.) The Keratinocyte Handbook. Cambridge: Cambridge University Press, 1994; 153–163

149. Jones PH, Harper S, Watt FM, Eglitis MA, Mezey E. Stem cell patterning and fate in human epidermis. Cell 1995; 80: 83–93

150. Adams JC, Watt FM. Fibronectin inhibits the terminal differentiation of human keratinocytes. Nature 1989; 340: 307–309

151. Bickenbach JR. Identification and behavior of label-retaining cells in oral mucosa and skin. J Dent Res 1981; 60: 1611–1620

152. Reynolds AJ, Jahoda CA. Cultured dermal papilla cells induce follicle formation and hair growth by transdifferentiation of an adult epidermis. Development 1992; 115: 587–593

153. Liechty K, MacKenzie T, Shaaban A, Radu A, Moseley A-M, Deans R *et al*. Human mesenchymal stem cells engraft and demonstrate site-specific differentiation after *in utero* transplantation in sheep. Nat Med 2000; 6: 1282–1286

154. Toma JG, Akhavan M, Fernandes KJ, Barnabe-Heider F, Sadikot A, Kaplan DR *et al*. Isolation of multipotent adult stem cells from the dermis of mammalian skin. Nat Cell Biol 2001; 3: 778–784

155. Schultz E. Satellite cell behavior during skeletal muscle growth and regeneration. Med Sci Sports Exer 1989; 21: S181–S186

156. Lipton BH, Schultz E. Developmental fate of skeletal muscle satellite cells. Science 1979; 205: 1292–1294

157. Goldring K, Partridge T, Watt D. Muscle stem cells. J Pathol 2002; 197: 457–467

158. Ferrari G, Cusella-De Angelis G, Coletta M, Paolucci E, Stornaiuolo A, Cossu G *et al*. Muscle regeneration by bone marrow-derived myogenic progenitors. Science 1998; 279: 1528–1530

159. Gussoni E, Pavlath G, Lanctot A, Sharma K, Miller R, Steinman L *et al*. Normal dystrophin transcripts detected in Duchenne muscular dystrophy patients after myoblast transplantation. Nature 1992; 356: 435–438

160. Saito MD DJ, Lennon DP, Young RG, Caplan AI. Myogenic expression of mesenchymal stem cells within myotubes of mdx mice *in vivo* and *in vitro*. Tissue Eng 1995; 1: 327–343

161. Gussoni E, Soneoka Y, Strickland C, Buzney E, Khan M, Flint A *et al*. Dystrophin expression in the mdx mouse restored by stem cell transplantation. Nature 1999; 401: 390–394

162. Breton M, Li ZL, Paulin D, Harris JA, Rieger F, Pincon-Raymond M *et al*. Myotube driven myogenic recruitment of cells during *in vitro* myogenesis. Dev Dyn 1995; 202: 126–136

163. Wise CJ, Watt DJ, Jones GE. Conversion of dermal fibroblasts to a myogenic lineage is induced by a soluble factor derived from myoblasts. J Cell Biochem 1996; 61: 363–374

164. Gibson AJ, Karasinski J, Relvas J, Moss J, Sherratt TG, Strong PN *et al*. Dermal fibroblasts convert to a myogenic lineage in mdx mouse muscle. J Cell Sci 1995; 108: 207–214

165. Pye D, Watt DJ. Dermal fibroblasts participate in the formation of new muscle fibres when implanted into regenerating normal mouse muscle. J Anat 2001; 198: 163–173

166. Zuk PA, Zhu M, Mizuno H, Huang J, Futrell JW, Katz AJ *et al*. Multilineage cells from human adipose tissue: implications for cell-based therapies. Tissue Eng 2001; 7: 211–228

167. Lee J, Qu-Petersen Z, Cao B, Kimura S, Jankowski R, Cummins J *et al*. Clonal isolation of muscle-derived cells capable of enhancing muscle regeneration and bone healing. J Cell Biol 2000; 150: 1085–1099

168. Prockop D, Azizi S, Colter D, DiGirolamo C, Kopen G, Phinney D. Biotechnology of extracellular matrix. Biochem Soc Trans 2000; 28: 341–345

169. Mackay A, Beck S, Murphy J, Barry F, Chichester C, Pittenger M. Chondrogenic differentiation of cultured human mesenchymal stem cells from marrow. Tissue Eng 1998; 4: 415–428

170. Nakagawa S, Toritsuka Y, Wakitani S, Denno K, Tomita T, Owaki H *et al*. Bone marrow stromal cells contribute to synovial cell proliferation in rats with collagen induced arthritis. J Rheumatol 1996; 23: 2098–2103

171. Wang X, Montini E, Al-Dhalimy M, Lagasse E, Finegold M, Grompe M. Kinetics of liver repopulation after bone marrow transplantation. Am J Pathol 2002; 161: 565–574

172. Ying QL, Nichols J, Evans EP, Smith AG. Changing potency by spontaneous fusion. Nature 2002; 416: 545–548

173. Terada N, Hamazaki T, Oka M, Hoki M, Mastalerz DM, Nakano Y *et al*. Bone marrow cells adopt the phenotype of other cells by spontaneous cell fusion. Nature 2002; 416: 542–545

174. Srivatsa B, Srivatsa S, Johnson KL, Samura O, Lee SL, Bianchi DW. Microchimerism of presumed fetal origin in thyroid specimens from women: a case–control study. Lancet 2001; 358: 2034–2038

175. Jiang Y, Jahagirdar BN, Reinhardt RL, Schwartz RE, Keene CD, Ortiz-Gonzalez XR *et al*. Pluripotency of mesenchymal stem cells derived from adult marrow. Nature 2002; 418: 41–49

176. Campbell JH, Efendy JL, Han C, Girjes AA, Campbell GR. Haemopoietic origin of myofibroblasts formed in the peritoneal cavity in response to a foreign body. J Vasc Res 2000; 37: 364–371

177. Garcia SB, Novelli M, Wright NA. The clonal origin and clonal evolution of epithelial tumours. Int J Exp Pathol 2000; 81: 89–116

178. Garcia SB, Park HS, Novelli M, Wright NA. Field cancerization, clonality, and epithelial stem cells: the spread of mutated clones in epithelial sheets. J Pathol 1999; 187: 61–81

179. Tsao JL, Zhang J, Salovaara R, Li ZH, Jarvinen HJ, Mecklin JP *et al*. Tracing cell fates in human colorectal tumors from somatic microsatellite mutations: evidence of adenomas with stem cell architecture. Am J Pathol 1998; 153: 1189–1200

180. Steel G. Growth Kinetics of Tumours. Oxford: Clarendon Press, 1977

181. Fearon ER, Vogelstein B. A genetic model for colorectal tumorigenesis. Cell 1990; 61: 759–767

182. Woodford-Richens K, Williamson J, Bevan S, Young J, Leggett B, Frayling I *et al*. Allelic loss at SMAD4 in polyps from juvenile polyposis patients and use of fluorescence *in situ* hybridization to demonstrate clonal origin of the epithelium. Cancer Res 2000; 60: 2477–2482

183. Pereira R, Halford K, O'Hara M, Leeper D, Sokolov B, Pollard M *et al.* Cultured adherent cells from marrow can serve as long-lasting precusor cells for bone, cartilage, and lung in irradiated mice. Proc Natl Acad Sci USA 1995; 92: 4857–4861

184. Anderson D, Gage F, Weissman I. Can stem cells cross the lineage barrier? Nat Med 2001; 7: 393–395

185. Taniguchi H, Suzuki A, Zheng Y, Kondo R, Takada Y, Fukunaga K *et al.* Usefulness of flow-cytometric cell sorting for enrichment of hepatic stem and progenitor cells in the liver. Transplant Proc 2000; 32: 249–251

186. Mitaka T. Hepatic stem cells: from bone marrow cells to hepatocytes. Biochem Biophys Res Commun 2001; 281: 1–5

187. Forbes S, Vig P, Poulsom R, Thomas H, Alison M. Hepatic stem cells. J Pathol 2002; 197: 510–518

188. Holden C, Vogel G. Stem cells. Plasticity: time for a reappraisal? Science 2002; 296: 2126–2129

189. Janes SM, Lowell S, Hutter C. Epidermal stem cells. J Pathol 2002; 197: 479–491

190. Forbes SJ, Vig P, Poulsom R, Wright NA, Alison MR. Adult stem cell plasticity: new pathways of tissue regeneration become visible. Clin Sci (Lond) 2002; 103: 355–369

Index

Progress in Pathology

Volume 6

DATE DUE

1 5 DEC 2008		
	0 3 NOV 2012	

GAYLORD

PRINTED IN U.S.A.

West Sussex Health Libraries
COPY NUMBER   2061061